Penicillin

Penicillin

Triumph and Tragedy

Robert Bud

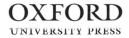

OXFORD
UNIVERSITY PRESS

OXFORD

UNIVERSITY PRESS

Great Clarendon Street, Oxford OX2 6DP

Oxford University Press is a department of the University of Oxford.
It furthers the University's objective of excellence in research, scholarship,
and education by publishing worldwide in

Oxford New York

Auckland Cape Town Dar es Salaam Hong Kong Karachi
Kuala Lumpur Madrid Melbourne Mexico City Nairobi
New Delhi Shanghai Taipei Toronto

With offices in

Argentina Austria Brazil Chile Czech Republic France Greece
Guatemala Hungary Italy Japan Poland Portugal Singapore
South Korea Switzerland Thailand Turkey Ukraine Vietnam

Oxford is a registered trade mark of Oxford University Press
in the UK and in certain other countries

Published in the United States
by Oxford University Press Inc., New York

© Board of Trustees of the Science Museum 2007

The moral rights of the author have been asserted
Database right Oxford University Press (maker)

First published 2007

British Library Cataloguing in Publication Data

Data available

Library of Congress Cataloging in Publication Data

Data available

Typeset by Laserwords Private Limited, Chennai, India
Printed in Great Britain
on acid-free paper by
Biddles Ltd, King's Lynn, Norfolk

ISBN 978–0–19–925406–4

10 9 8 7 6 5 4

To my Parents

Contents

Illustrations

Introduction: Penicillin—Chemical and Brand

A child is screaming with the pain of earache. The entire family is anxious. At last a doctor brings relief by prescribing penicillin. Even if the patient has not yet recovered, hope is now at hand. People, rather than bacteria, are in control and the parents can relax.

Such scenes have been familiar across the world for more than half a century. Ever since its introduction during the Second World War, penicillin has been among the most reassuring and most widely used of drugs. It was the prototype, and has remained the most familiar member, of the family of antibiotics—medicines for combating bacteria and other undesirable microbes, and themselves extracted from living organisms. Promising a break with humanity's enduring fear of infectious disease and enabling dramatic increases in life expectancy, its discovery has been widely regarded as the single most beneficial outcome of modern science.

The original discovery of penicillin has also been among the best-known events in the history of medicine. The achievements of Alexander Fleming, who in 1929 first reported the effects of a product of the penicillin mould on bacteria, and of scientists at the University of Oxford who pioneered the drug's isolation and use during the early 1940s—including Howard Florey, Ernst Chain, and Norman Heatley— have been frequently celebrated. In 1999, a study of more than 30,000 users of the news museum, the 'Newseum' in Washington DC, found that Fleming's discovery was the sixth most important story of the century and the highest-rated event not to have directly involved an American.[1] Three years later, Fleming was the only twentieth-century scientist to reach the 'top 20' in a British poll of top Britons of the past thousand years.

By the beginning of the twenty-first century, however, we have become used to prophecies of incurable plagues, which clash with the simple celebration of past successes. MRSA bacteria, resistant to attack from almost all medicines, infest many hospitals, and other bacteria are also fighting back. Government inquiries explain the evolution of such resistant strains by suggesting that patients consume antibiotics inappropriately, using the wrong amounts—often on the wrong germs. These reports blame the irresponsible use of a treasured resource, leading to threats to society as a whole.

Taking a historical perspective on penicillin means, therefore, encompassing not just the great triumphs of the discovery but also the subsequent discomfort with how this drug and the other antibiotics have been used. In this account, we will examine the two together. Such an approach demands not just a reflection on the development of a material product. So great is the drug's public presence that it transcends any divide between society and technology. In its combination of reassurance and medical benefit, penicillin could be compared to a marketing 'brand'.[2] Indeed, it could be said to be one of the globe's most powerful brands. Penicillin is so closely associated with 'strong medicine', scientific triumph, social improvement, and reliability that the very writing of a prescription gives hope to the patient and a sense of power to the doctor.

Not of course just a brand, penicillin is also a family of chemicals with a distinctive chemical structure and characteristic action on certain classes of bacteria. Many such chemicals are produced 'naturally' in tiny quantities from the microscopic fronds of the brush-like moulds in the penicillium family, while further members have been derived from those natural products. Generally, the penicillins prevent susceptible disease-causing bacteria from assembling walls on new cells as they reproduce. Without rigid walls to retain the chemical 'soup' within, the bacteria inflate and burst like balloons.

We can therefore think of the single entity 'penicillin' as both a brand and a family of chemicals. Over a period of more than half a century, the history of penicillin can be seen to have followed from the remarkable interaction of one quality with the other. In the course of that time, both the brand and the chemical have themselves changed. The balance of the benefits promised by the brand to the individual and to the community has shifted: towards the individual, and away from the community. The chemical has changed too: the single drug has been developed in ingenious ways to increase productivity and reduce cost, to widen its range of activity and to deepen its effectiveness against bacteria.

The drug's use has brought its qualities into a relationship that can be praised as mutually supportive or, alternatively, condemned as deeply dysfunctional. At first, the interaction between the brand and the chemical seemed a triumph. When the drug was introduced after the Second World War, small doses cured almost instantly such diseases as pneumonia, rheumatic fever, and syphilis, which had been greatly feared and often fatal. Penicillin brought not just hope to sufferers but also status to the institutions and nations that had promoted it. Medicine itself was transformed. Sir Macfarlane Burnet, Australian Nobel Prize-winning physician, described this divide in his *Natural History of Infectious Disease*, which went through three editions between 1950 and 1962. 'One can', he proclaimed, 'think of the middle of the twentieth century as the end of one of the most important social revolutions in history—the virtual elimination of infectious disease as a significant factor in social life.'[3]

Until the early 1960s, the history of penicillin in particular, and of antibiotics in general, might have been compared to a theatrical comedy—difficult problems were encountered but ultimately they were resolved. There were genuine triumphs: the great achievement of introducing a new drug quickly and safely, and also, at the day-to-day level, the cures of patients suffering from daunting infections. From the early 1960s, however, an alternative darker story was formulated by an increasing number of people dismayed by the misuse of valued medicines; rather than a comedy, this better resembled a tragedy.

A word with many connotations, tragedy can mean merely a story with a terrible ending. It can also signify the predictable, but inexorable, progression to a crisis and even a catastrophe, representing, in the words of the philosopher Hayden White, 'resignation of men to the conditions under which they must labor in the world'.[4] Penicillin has proved a triumph both for its discoverers and for millions of beneficiaries. At the same time, with its potentially disastrous outcome, its ineluctable progression to that end, and our inevitable submission to the essential constraints of the world, the story of penicillin can also be read as a tragic drama. In this tragedy, all of us who have ever taken penicillin or any other antibiotic have been actors.

1

Illness, Drugs, and Wonder Drugs before Penicillin

Even before penicillin was isolated at the beginning of the Second World War, conditions had been prepared for post-war optimism over the new medicine. A dynamic medical culture that flourished in the inter-war years was already building expectations for rapid change. Strong traditions of preventing disease through hygiene and morality were complemented by rising hopes for treatments promoted by a pharmaceutical industry sophisticated in both marketing and research, and even for instant cures. Lay people, medicine, and the media in America and Europe were celebrating the arrival of new 'wonder drugs'. At the same time, the misery widely experienced even in the richest of societies instilled, in many, a determination that the post-war future would be different.

Physical suffering from acute infection was still a widespread feature of Western societies in the 1930s. After retiring, a London social worker born in 1930 complained to an interviewer that: 'the past has sort of a romantic glow and people forget the dirt and the illness, the diphtheria, and the polio and the poverty and lack of hot water...it's all twaddle, they forget the children who died in infancy, and the women who died in childbirth and the men who were crippled and the lack of employment.'[1] Not just the poor were vulnerable to infection. America's finest doctors were helpless when, in 1924, the 16-year-old son of US President Calvin Coolidge contracted septicaemia from an infection of a blister on his toe—caused by a chafing tennis shoe. Within a few days the boy was dead. In the autumn of 1943, three-quarters of British civilians suffered a mild or serious malady.[2] Most of these conditions were mild—colds and influenza were the most common—but others were chronic, such as bronchitis and rheumatism, and a few were life threatening.

Such infectious and potentially fatal diseases as pneumonia and rheumatic fever, which particularly struck children, were especially feared. The trauma inflicted by an episode of rheumatic fever on an entire family has been described by American surgeon and writer Sherwin Nuland, in his account of his own teenage brother's illness in 1942. In Nuland's poor but not unusual American family, an elder brother had earlier died of bronchial pneumonia at the age of 3 and at the same age Sherwin himself had only just survived diphtheria. His mother had recently died. Such was the fear that the younger boy's rheumatic fever engendered that his father contemplated suicide as he coped with the fear of another loss in his family. The grandmother coped with her worries by plying the invalid with fattening foods. After six weeks in bed, the boy recovered, but he had lost forever his teenage athleticism.

By past standards, however, prevention was nonetheless proving startlingly effective against the horrifying experience of disease. Across the Western world, deaths from infectious diseases declined dramatically between 1900 and 1940, and infant life expectancy had greatly increased. Year on year up to 1937, deaths from infectious diseases in the USA fell by 2.8 per cent per annum. By 1940, pneumonia and influenza were responsible for only one quarter of the deaths they had been causing there forty years earlier. Deaths from tuberculosis had fallen slightly faster. Typhoid and dysentery, once major causes of death, were now responsible for killing only 2 people in every 100,000.[3]

The success of the preventive measures that sustained these major health improvements would be a constant presence in both the prehistory and the history of penicillin. Since the late nineteenth century such earlier public-health measures as efficient sewage disposal and clean water supplies had been widely supplemented by encouragements to citizens to stay healthy through 'hygiene'.[4] Whether qualified as 'personal' or 'social' hygiene, this involved not just a variety of exacting precautions, but also the more general taking of a personal responsibility for one's own welfare. Approved medical practices were linked therefore with moral responsibility for staying healthy and with the implication of moral failure in the case of illness.

Following medically recommended codes of behaviour could both enhance social standing and reduce the chances of falling victim to bacteria-induced illness. Texts on cleanliness and on child-rearing emphasized that morality, discipline, and hygiene were linked, and stressed the exclusion of both moral and physical filth. In 1915, the US National

Association for the Study and Prevention of Tuberculosis had formed the 'Health Crusade'. It enrolled children into an Order to which they pledged that they would follow health rules such as opening windows and brushing their teeth. Success was rewarded not just by health but also by elevation up a ladder of crusading ranks.[5] The Boy Scouts in Britain awarded a 'healthy man' badge to the well behaved. The inter-war years also saw the rise of such organizations in the USA as the optimistically entitled Health and Happiness League, whose members' pledges ranged from not using public drinking fountains to the destruction of every accessible housefly.

While taking responsibility for one's own welfare before the Second World War could be an effective measure, it was also a stressful obligation. A leading British doctor complained in 1931 that his patients were so obsessed with health that they were making themselves ill.[6] Failure to stay healthy was often punished not just with illness, but also with blame. 'Good' behaviour seemed to be key both to preventing disease in the individual and to the protection of society in general. Correspondingly, failure to prevent disease was, to some people, itself a sign of moral failing. Others were willing to grant that illness was not itself blameworthy, but felt, nonetheless, that it could be caused by blameworthy acts of carelessness.[7] In later life, a lady recalled: 'when she was younger she had travelled home from the seaside in a wet bathing suit, and this had caused her to catch a chill which had later developed into pneumonia. Catching pneumonia had therefore been her fault.'[8]

All infection could cause guilt, because it implied a lack of care in the face of germs. Syphilis, however, lies especially close to the centre of the penicillin story. It had long been linked, across Western cultures, to rules of appropriate sexual behaviour. The many levels of guilt that could be exquisitely experienced by an entire family are explored in Henrik Ibsen's 1881 play *Ghosts*. A victim moans, 'My whole life ruined—irreparably ruined—and all through my own thoughtlessness... If only it *had* been something I'd inherited—something I wasn't to blame for.'[9] He discovers that in fact he had inherited syphilis from his father. But his mother can then join in the feelings of guilt: 'Your poor father could never find any outlet for this overpowering joy of living that was in him. And I didn't bring any sunshine into his life either.'

Syphilis was particularly mysterious because the disease develops through four, often widely separate, phases. The symptoms of the first two are relatively mild, though in the second stage there is a rash inhabited by infectious bacteria, followed by a latent period without symptoms. The third stage, affecting about 30 per cent of sufferers, can appear years later. It leads to hideous wastage of the bones, and damage to the eyes and to the nervous system. The fourth stage of late syphilis ends in madness and death. Syphilis is generally spread by sexual contact, but could also enter through open wounds. The seats of public toilets were widely feared as the source of infection, even for the chaste. The babies of infected mothers could also inherit it—doctors with a black sense of humour described it as a disease 'from womb to tomb' or 'sperm to worm'.[10]

The repugnance and condemnation evoked by syphilis even in the mid-twentieth century were captured by a 1942 British opinion study of attitudes to sexually transmitted diseases, conducted by the Mass Observation group.[11] About one-fifth of the 150 respondents emphasized moral or social attitudes. One man, asked about his feelings on venereal disease, answered: 'I should also associate it with a certain feeling of degradation and disgust. I have a similar objection to boils and pimples—whether this is aesthetic or the relic of some nursery snobbery I don't know.' A retired vegetarian clerk opined, 'Horrible. Result of lust and lack of self-control. Sometimes innocent people suffer from the disease.' And a widowed mother and spiritualist was quoted: 'I am old fashioned enough to think that it should be a question of morals; failing that, people who contract it should be segregated and medically or surgically dealt with so that they can't be a Plague again.'

The respondents to Mass Observation enquiries displayed great uncertainty as to what caused venereal disease, its symptoms, and cures. Apparently many were not clear whether gonorrhoea and syphilis were separate conditions. Could they be contracted from drink, or through a handshake? Could only women catch syphilis? It seemed a 55-year-old man thought so.[12] As for cures, one respondent in the Mass Observation study reported the particularly counter-productive belief that sex with a virgin would cure such afflictions. Another was not sure that venereal diseases could be cured, but then felt that perhaps this fatalism was propaganda: 'It is quite possible that the venereal boggy [sic] is a substitute for the old eternal hell—it kind of keeps people good.'[13]

Building up one's health demanded the commitment of everyone, not just those immediately at risk of illness. Thus, the scout movement had been invented by Baden Powell in the wake of the Boer War at the beginning of the twentieth century because he was appalled by the physical condition of army recruits. The 'fossils' of official anxieties over the fitness of citizens can also be seen in the stark, unheated, open-air swimming pools built between the wars still to be found across Europe and North America. Their funding testifies to the belief that virtue, health, and happiness could jointly be improved through personal endeavour.[14] With increasing talk of war in Europe during the 1930s, enthusiasm for national fitness grew. In February 1933, Britain's *Morning Post* newspaper reported riots between communists and Nazis in Berlin, and the same issue described a new system of physical training which should 'sweep the country as a cleansing flame' to wipe away the tiredness and listlessness that had followed the trauma of the previous world war.[15] After Britain's dismal performance in the 1936 Olympics, the British government and the media took an interest in fitness.[16] In just the two months October and November 1936, *The Times* newspaper carried six editorials on the topic. Britain's emphasis on moral and educational incentives rather than on legal compulsion would make clear its distinction from the fascist countries.

Nonetheless, public figures and doctors complained repeatedly that people were being tempted to fall back on medicines rather than aspire to good behaviour. When Sir Leo Amery welcomed his guest speaker, the government Health Minister, to the annual meeting of the British Social Hygiene Council in June 1936, he complained, 'At present they are not taught to live healthily but only where to get physic if diseased.'[17]

Complementing the model of prevention, a new pharmaceutical model of treatment was growing, driven by consumers, industry, and science. The chaos of an economically and politically disrupted world was reflected in attitudes to medicine, as the author of an empirical study of New York City concluded in 1939: 'The families make numerous, varied and uncoordinated choices among physicians, clinics, hospitals, proprietary medicine, home remedies and other resources in time of illness.'[18] Even in a country where respect for medical science was high, there was therefore an established culture of treating medicines as consumer goods chosen by, or for, sick people and not principally as the intellectual property of doctors. Particularly for the financially stretched in the 1930s, taking medicine was often an alternative to consulting a doctor, a tradition that would prove important in the post-war era when penicillin, too, came to be the target of consumer ambition.

Patients of the 1930s were therefore well used to shopping for medicines in line with their own predilections and aspirations. With the exception of limited ranges of poisons, they could also generally purchase what they wished and could afford. Consumers could turn to the scientifically formulated and respected home remedies such as Milk of Magnesia (magnesium hydroxide) or aspirin (acetyl-salicylic acid), but also to so-called 'patent' medicines whose composition was kept secret, and, further, to a vast range of alternative therapies. Local traditions of what medicines 'worked' were deeply entrenched, and were respected even by doctors. In some areas it was normal to send a patient away with a bottle of liquid—brown if it was a cough mixture because most of them were based on morphine solutions. Tonics, however, were red, possibly to cover the green or yellow colour of iron salts, and most were bitter.[19] A reminiscence of a lady in the north of England shows the predominance of traditional remedies supplemented by the purchase of commercial products. 'I can remember two things used for colds: one was Dad's sock, thickened with camphorated oil, put round the neck, and I had to go to bed with that. When I think about what that safety pin could have done if it came open! The second was your vest thickened with camphorated oil. We always smelt of camphorated oil, no matter what time of the year it was.'[20]

Against the endurance of old medicines, the market in western Europe and America offered a wealth of new treatments. Although their success was rarely tested, and often controversial, many were nonetheless both economically important and part of health regimens in which millions of people believed. Marketing, public relations, and science made the difference between great wealth and commercial death for manufacturers in the newly energized modern pharmaceutical industry (see Ill. 1). In general, branding was more important than the purely pharmacological properties of products. On the other hand, in contrast to the model of disease control by discipline-driven prevention, the industry was seeking to have its products seen as both potent and scientific. Thus, even before the Second World War, the pharmaceutical industry was characterized by the twin qualities of marketing and science.

The scale of American consumption was indicated by a 1933 committee report on the costs of medical care. It estimated that the American public spent over $700 million a year on medicines.[21] One-third of this total was spent on doctors' prescriptions, and two-thirds on home remedies such as aspirin and patent medicines. In Britain, although expenditures per head were about half those in the USA, the distribution was similar.[22]

The drug industry grew with the advertising opportunities provided by the new media industries of the twentieth century: mass-market newspapers and the radio. In Britain during the 1930s pharmaceutical advertising constituted about a quarter of all advertising on all goods. The Beecham company, the country's leading purveyor of proprietary medicines, had an advertising budget of £1 million in 1939.[23] Radio

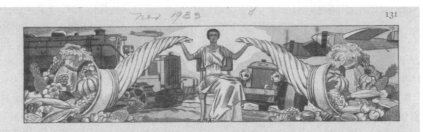

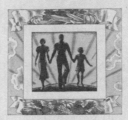

1. Celebration of science as the source of a cornucopia of benefits in a 1934 advertisement from the Squibb pharmaceutical company.

Bristol-Myers Squibb/Medicine and Madison Avenue On-Line Project—Ad #MM0211, John W. Hartman Center for Sales, Advertising & Marketing History, Rare Book, Manuscript, and Special Collections Library, Duke University, Durham, North Carolina.

offered special opportunities. In the USA during the mid-1930s, one-third of all commercially sponsored radio continuity announcements were related to medicines.[24] The British could also receive English-language commercial radio—beamed from Luxembourg and Normandy.[25] Thus in 1939 they could benefit from the Carter Liver Pills Troubadour whose programme on Radio Luxembourg 1293 metres was to be heard on Sunday, Monday, and Tuesday mornings and afternoons on Wednesday, Thursday, and Friday. Only on Saturdays was this happy poet of the laxative silent.[26]

Even the growth of science-based products during the inter-war period was coloured by marketing. A 1935 article published in the *Annals of Medical History* described the endless attempts to find a treatment for the sexually transmitted disease gonorrhoea. It was less dangerous, but much more prevalent, than syphilis.[27] The paper showed that statistically, every male in Berlin could expect to catch gonorrhoea once in his life, and poor seamen in towns such as Hamburg might suffer twice. Complications could turn a painful but temporary inconvenience into sterility and even blindness. As for cures for this disease, antiseptics—principally silver nitrate—had been used for a century, but they were unreliable and painful. Treatments went in and out of fashion. 'Some clever chemist synthesizes a new organic silver salt. His medical associate uses it on men afflicted with gonorrhoea. He is impressed favourably and says so. Others concur and the new compound is a success until another chemist brings out something else.'

A few new preparations did, however, have considerable and unprecedented power to protect, treat, and even cure. A new culture of drug development also underpinned the pre-war growth of the ethical pharmaceutical industry, whose achievements would be critical to the production and distribution of penicillin. The new disciplines of microbiology and bacteriology had yielded vaccines and sera which used the chemicals produced by the animal body to provide a defence against infections. Since the end of the nineteenth century, vaccinations against tuberculosis and diphtheria, for instance, had been developed, though they were not yet widely trusted. Antitoxin prepared from horses could protect against tetanus, and in the 1930s a serum prepared from rabbits could be used to treat pneumonia. Since the mid-1920s, injections of insulin prepared from pigs could mitigate the effects of diabetes. Complementing these 'biologicals', there were also a few physiologically powerful chemicals such as neosalvarsan, used to cure syphilis.

The vitamins were perhaps the most immediately important drug development of the inter-war years, to the public and the pharmaceutical industry. They offered hope to people uncertain of how to maintain their health, and, taken by an undernourished population, they averted the bow-legs of rickets and other deficiency conditions familiar in poverty-ridden industrial areas. In their reputation for efficacy—and also in their role in building the pharmaceutical industry—vitamins were the predecessors of penicillin. Even when taken in the form of old and trusted remedies and imbibed generously in the long-established tradition of tonics, vitamins won the support of leaders of modern physiology and became the focus of attention of major modern companies. They thus crossed the lines between folk medicines, proprietary medicines, and the officially sanctioned products of medical science.

The very category of 'vitamins' was still new. The Polish chemist Casimir Funk had only coined the word in 1912, after he had identified the amine whose absence in polished rice caused the disease beriberi. Within a few years, Edward Mellanby in London and McCollum in Madison, Wisconsin, showed that two factors, 'A' and 'B', could explain the therapeutic value of cod-liver oil to rats. Factor 'A' in turn was soon shown to comprise two vitamins given the names 'A' and 'D'. A veritable alphabet soup had been cooked.[28]

The old nostrum cod-liver oil proved to be a rich source of the newly named vitamins A and D. Several generations of children will share the memories of this elderly lady who remembered, 'We used to come home from school, and after our dinner, stand in line and take a spoonful of cod liver oil. If you were sick you had to take another one.'[29] This tonic had been intermittently popular with doctors in the nineteenth century, even if by the end of the century it was increasingly seen as old-fashioned and derided as foul-tasting. However, the use of steam to extract the fresh oil at sea rather than waiting for the rancid livers to be offloaded after a long fishing expedition did improve the quality somewhat, and a variety of other methods were used to make the oil less 'fishy'. Such commercial innovations made the product more palatable, and the support of Edward Mellanby made it once again scientifically acceptable.

Mellanby himself believed not only that a shortage of vitamins A and D was responsible for specific diseases of rickets, blindness, and general malaise, but also that vitamins could cure infectious disease.[30] The evidence for efficacy of vitamins in fighting infection may have been poor, the results were inconclusive, and most doctors remained unconvinced, but the British public, above all, continued to believe in the oil's great powers. Through the 1930s cod-liver oil was the topic of an average of six articles and letters a year in *The Times*. By 1937 Britain was exporting more than half a million kilograms of the oil per annum.[31] It was the mainstay not just of the fishing cooperative Seven Seas, but also of a drug company like Wellcome, much better known for its more modern medicines. As war threatened, administrators feared shortage if trawlers were requisitioned as minesweepers. An emergency meeting of civil servants decided that most adults probably did not need it, but children did, and they should get priority. From the outbreak of the Second World War, cod-liver oil was made available free of charge to British children. As many as 5,340,000 bottles were given out in 1948 and the arrangement continued until 1971.[32]

During the Second World War, when the deprivations of the wartime diet made people more health-conscious, a British survey, conducted by Mass Observation, concluded: 'The greatest increase in medicines is of the vitamin variety, two people in five of those who are taking more medicines mentioned that they are taking vitamins in some sort of chemical form.'[33] This belief was not just a British characteristic. The US historian Rima Apple quotes a company vice-president who administered capsules in work breaks in early 1941. 'Despite a mild influenza epidemic during the early weeks of the experiment, he found work attendance was 50% better than the same period the year before.'[34]

The vitamin business provided the infrastructure of the post-war pharmaceutical industry, which combined science with marketing. Many of the companies that became important in the post-war world were major purveyors of proprietary medicines in the 1930s. Even those which had previously focused on marketing raw materials to the pharmacist now took advantage of the vitamin craze. Ethical pharmaceutical companies such as Merck developed research and production facilities to meet market expectations. They were also introduced to the high-pressure marketing world by the vitamin business, based as it was on science but addressing the self-medicating needs of the general public.

Among the most innovative of the major pharmaceutical concerns was the Abbott company. Having avoided the low-margin cod-liver oil, it sought other even more nutritious fish products, and alighted on a Norwegian report on the benefits of halibut-liver oil which was tasteless and even richer in vitamins than cod-liver oil. From top to bottom, the company believed in the virtues of their products. At meetings of the board, directors passed around the capsules in which the oil was sold.[35] Sales representatives known as detail men visited doctors to sing their products' praises.

The marketing of vitamins was energetic, but it was also backed up by many scientific innovations, as vitamins came to be produced either synthetically or by using microorganisms. The best known development was Vitamin D production pioneered at the University of Wisconsin in the 1920s, by irradiating fatty foods such as milk. Research on such other vitamins as B and C lay at the forefront of chemistry.[36]

Although vitamins were more powerful as preventives than as cures, they provided a base for industry's hopes of new drugs as well as sustaining its profits. Late in the 1930s, this precedent would be built upon, as the sulphonamide drugs began to provide rapid relief for hitherto incurable infections. These new products went, however, much further than prevention, for they seemed to offer a new kind of redemption from illness by curing wide swathes of symptoms caused by common bacteria. They provoked exciting new aspirations for a future medicine, but these were based on very long-established hopes, and the terms through which they were interpreted were drawn from early modern Europe.

The terms 'wonder drug', 'miracle drug', and 'magic bullet', which later became key qualities of the penicillin 'brand', were widely used in the 1930s to interpret the significance of radically new materials. It was a strategy developed first in Germany, a country which was at the heart of the scientific world early in the twentieth century. German chemists were the world's leaders and, on both sides of the Atlantic, scientists and doctors looked to Germany for inspiration and education.

At the beginning of the twentieth century, the metaphor of the 'magic bullet' had been summoned up from the alchemical tradition of early modern Europe by Paul Ehrlich, professor of bacteriology of the University of Frankfurt, to communicate the significance of a new means of treating disease. He believed that scientists could provide a range of powerful drugs, so targeted that a single injection would deliver enough poison into the bacterial population for the body's defences to complete the cure. Athough in many ways a modern cosmopolitan, Ehrlich evoked German folklore as he explained the principle by which his drugs killed germs, using the term 'magic bullets' and creating one of most memorable metaphors of drug history. A recently published volume of the great Grimms' German dictionary had previously attributed this expression to the appendix of a biography of Faust originally published in 1674, but reprinted as recently as 1880. This described the use of magic bullets by the Lapps to convey poison to their targets, with exactly the same German word, *Zauberkugel*—magic bullet—as Ehrlich deployed.[37]

Ehrlich built on his philosophy of chemotherapy to develop his own powerful chemical cure for syphilis, Salvarsan, in 1909. This represented a profound advance on the earlier treatments based on bismuth, arsenic, and mercury, and it is the achievement for which Ehrlich is now remembered. Nonetheless, treatment with Salvarsan was not the one-shot cure he had anticipated in his vision of chemotherapy. It took two years and could cause toxic reactions and, occasionally, death. Careful management was needed—this alone would have made it difficult to control, and such problems were compounded by the stigma associated with sexual misconduct, which was scarcely mentionable. So Ehrlich's vision of chemotherapy was therefore only partially realized even by Salvarsan, but it did provide a philosophical basis for the use of the term 'magic bullet' and the sense that the new era of medicine was quite different from the recent era of palliatives and prevention.

The twentieth-century enthusiasm for interpreting the development of modern medicines in terms of early modern ambitions for miraculous transformations in health could also be seen in the veritable cult of Theophrastus Bombastus von Hohenheim or, as he styled himself, Paracelsus. This founder of chemistry, who was born in 1493, had seen himself as a 'wonder doctor', not only developing such practical drugs as mercury to combat the newly encountered disease of syphilis, but also believing in seeking the 'arcana' that would cure every ill. In Nazi Germany, he had a status comparable to that of Isaac Newton in England, Galileo in Italy, or Benjamin Franklin in the USA. Almost 100 historical books and fifty dissertations about him were published between 1933 and 1945 and the well-known director Georg Wilhelm Pabst marked the 450th anniversary of his birth with a still-celebrated movie.[38] This enthusiasm went beyond the borders of Germany: the history of alchemy and the faith in the single cure for all diseases attracted widespread interest in Britain and America too.[39]

Pabst's movie built on an already well-established genre of plays and books exploring the dreams wedding science with medicine and drawn to the fascination of wonder drugs. For example, in 1919, just a few months after the end of the First World War, theatregoers in Hamburg, Germany, were applauding a comedy with the title *Das Wundermittel (The Wonder Drug)*.[40] Denouncing the confidence tricks of modern medicine and of modern art—medical quackery and artistic theory—it dealt with the profound attraction of novelties which could not be comprehended but which were known to be powerful. The author was one of Germany's then-favourite playwrights, Ludwig Fulda, a mature author with an international reputation.[41]

Like Ehrlich's coinage, the plot of Fulda's play linked modernity to deeply entrenched hopes of a general cure for disease. The audiences to *The Wonder Drug* were treated to the story of two friends, one interested in making money from modern art and the other from science. Fritz, the chemist, at first claims that his discovery 'Mirakulin' is a wonder drug and cures all illnesses. When he attempts to retract what he had only meant to be an elaborate hoax, he finds it is too late: society has taken to the medicine and will not give it up. A duchess begs him not to disillusion her, rather losing her pearls and jewels than abandoning her faith in Mirakulin.[42] A friend reprimands Fritz: 'Your medicine may disappear: You will not root out Mirakulin; It has been eternal and will be eternal, just from time to time its name changes.'

When Fulda's *Wundermittel* was still new, the American writer Sinclair Lewis asked his friend, the science writer Paul De Kruif, 'Why shouldn't we collaborate on a book? About doctors? About what was alleged to be medical science? What would be funnier? What would be more sensational? What could be more timely?'[43] The outcome, the 1925 novel *Arrowsmith,* was perhaps the best known of all books about wonder drugs. It explored the tension between the ambition to do good science, to rescue humanity, and to build a personal career. The story follows a hero who finds a wonderful medicine, but in using it in the Caribbean to protect a population against plague, he is torn between rigorous scientific testing and saving lives. His own wife dies from the infection and he compromises his data. Although the story was fictional, the therapy described by Lewis, the bacteria-destroying 'phage' virus, was real and indeed has continued to attract attention as a potential cure for bacterial infection into the twenty-first century.

In these works, the fantasy of a wonder drug was expressed with some sense that it related to what might indeed exist, but also with a certain sceptical irony. They were also composed and consumed against a background of enthusiastic promotion, in which the line between 'real' and fantasy was often far from clear. In the United States, one of the classic works of early consumerism, *100,000,000 Guinea Pigs*, published in 1933 by two leading activists, Frederick Schlink and Arthur Kallet, condemned the large number of unregulated quack medicines foisted on the public.[44] Some of these offered relief from minor complaints; others of the quack medicines, however, would offer benefits eerily reflected in the penicillin story itself.

Among the most vivid of the advertised claims for a cure-all was for an antiseptic entitled Yadil, which became popular in Britain during the influenza pandemic of 1918. The parallel of the claims made for this quack medicine with the later realities of penicillin reflects the building of a brand before the reality of the chemical that would fulfil its promise. Yadil was first promoted just to the medical profession, but the owners became more ambitious. The manifesto produced in 1922 had a title as long as its claims were great: *The Yadil Book: The Careful Study of this Book and the Use of Yadil Everywhere for Every Disorder will Save Hundreds of Thousands of Lives Every Year.*[45] The next year's claims were no smaller though the title was slightly shorter, *Tuberculosis: The Problem Solved: Yadil Antiseptic Cures & Prevents the White Scourge.* Intense advertising took the message everywhere in Britain, except to readers of the *Daily Mail* newspaper, which refused to sell space to its promoters. That paper published a 1924 denunciation of the fraud by the distinguished chemist William Pope.[46] Instead of the proclaimed contents 'tri-methenal allylic carbide', which he scorned as nonsense, it was, effectively, a pleasantly scented solution of the formaldehyde used to preserve dead animals.

The phrases 'magic bullet' and 'wonder drug' therefore captured a category that had been developed through literature, through quackery, and through medical research. Fantastical as their promise might often appear, in the late 1930s they seemed to be transformed from dream to reality by the emergence of the sulphonamide drugs. These medicines, the first successful antibacterials, transformed not just the prospects for curing a particular individual's infection, but also attitudes to the prospects of medicine in general. Their example provided twin stimuli to the penicillin story—it encouraged the development of another successful chemical, and it provided the precedent for the integration of the cultural category of 'wonder drug' with a real pharmaceutical.

News of the first successful chemical attack on bacteria announced by the German chemist Carl Domagk in 1935 came as a revelation to the pharmaceutical industry and to physicians. At the world's largest chemical company, IG Farben, in Germany, Domagk had been experimenting for years with dyes which might kill microbes. The first positive results were obtained in December 1932, but the company did not publish for more than two years, possibly to assure its patent position. The product, named Prontosil, was a hitherto unknown red dye. French chemists, however, found that the colouring component could be easily eliminated to leave an equally effective colourless drug. In this process, Prontosil the patented dye became sulphanilamide, a long-known and therefore freely accessible chemical.

In 1936 the medical magazine *The Lancet* announced the startlingly positive results of Leonard Colebrook, the British doctor who had tested sulphanilamide on women suffering childbirth fever. *The Lancet's* editorial counselled caution and reminded readers that prevention should be the priority over cure.[47] Many others felt, however, that the sulphonamide drugs had near-miraculous potential. The distinguished American physician Perrin Long, excited by Colebrook's results, used sulphanilamide to cure the sinus affliction of President Roosevelt's son. He and his medicine were widely acclaimed. The contrast with the tragic death of Coolidge's son just a dozen years earlier was particularly telling.

The successful cure of the President's son had an immediate and compelling impact on the image of the new drug in the United States. At the American Medical Association meeting in June 1937, attendance at the session on sulphanilamide was overflowing. *Time* magazine reported that 'doctors believe they have a phenomenal all-round specific against many bacterial diseases'.[48] According to *Time*, Dr Henry Helmholtz of the Mayo Clinic summarized the opinion to the AMA Convention thus: 'We have only scratched the surface of the potentialities of sulfanilamide, the results to date have been so startling as to be fantastic.' At the same meeting, the AMA heard news that gonorrhoea, then affecting 2 million Americans, could be cured in four days for only 49 cents. The *New York Times* announced the probable victory over the streptococci in general and put it down to modern industrial research.[49]

More specifically this transformation in the prospect of modern medicine was widely interpreted as the outcome of the Ehrlich programme. *Newsweek*, in its report of December 1936, rendered the story as the outcome of persistence rewarded: 'On the heels of Ehrlich's brilliant work, hundreds of chemotherapists started raking shelves of chemicals, looking for similar killers. Setback followed setback...'[50] Similarly, sulphonamide drugs were introduced in the official popular magazine of the American Medical Association, *Hygeia*, in a 1937 article entitled 'Magic Bullets'. The text combined this allusion to Ehrlich with an excruciating paean to Paracelsus.[51] The same linkage was spelled out in *Behind the Sulfa Drugs* by the German-trained psychiatrist Iago Galdston, although Galdston had to admit that in fact the interference with a bacterium's metabolism by which the sulphonamide drugs worked (only articulated in 1940) was actually quite different from that of Ehrlich's Salvarsan.[52] Rather than poisoning bacteria, sulphonamides starved them.

A year after the seminal meeting at the American Medical Association, further news, even more reassuring than the announcement of sulphanilamide itself, was announced from England. At the May and Baker factory in Dagenham, east of London, chemists developed a sulphonamide drug, sulphapyridine, which seemed to cure pneumonia and meningitis, diseases which were still taking a very high toll. In the UK 31,000 people died of pneumonia in 1936.[53] Not all would be cured even with the new medicine (since some cases were, for instance, caused by viruses, which it did not affect), but a drug that seemed to promise cure to seven out of ten of these people really was of tremendous significance. Echoing Ehrlich, who had named his drug 606, because it was the 606th chemical he had screened, May and Baker called their drug M&B 693.

The success of M&B 693 widely popularized the descriptions 'wonder drug' and 'miracle drug'. The terms expressed, for instance, the unbounded enthusiasm awoken early in September 1938 by the miraculous cure of a little girl suffering from meningitis, in a story of magic through science that would shortly be frequently retold in the era of penicillin.[54] Betty Walters, a 7-year-old child from England's industrial Black Country, was admitted desperately ill to the Wolverhampton Royal Infirmary suffering with meningitis. She came from a family which was a victim of technological innovation. Her father, a carter, followed a trade rapidly becoming obsolete, and he had been made an invalid during the First World War. Because he had only worked for seven years in the previous twenty, the family of two adults and five surviving children lived on means-tested benefits. The new product rescued these victims of the modern world. Betty was treated with M&B 693 and recovered within twelve hours. The relief of her mother was reported by the local press:

If only this miracle drug had been invented earlier, perhaps my poor little Billy and my poor little Audrey, both of whom died of meningitis, would have been with me now . . . I thought that little Betty was going to be the third of my children to be stricken down in the same way. We were told we had little to hope for. Consequently, I was amazed to hear first that Betty might live, then that she would live, and finally that she would be completely cured.

Perhaps the reporter for the local newspaper had put words in the interviewee's mouth, but her relief was clearly real. The story of M&B 693 was given heightened significance by the drama of the times. News of patients such as Betty Walters was simultaneous with preparation for war. On 30 September, Chamberlain flew back from Munich with a piece of paper signed by Herr Hitler and promising 'peace for our time'. On 2 October the *Sunday Graphic* newspaper published a true-life story entitled 'A surgeon's case-book' by a London surgeon, James Harpole, which ended with the heart-warming story of a child brought back from the brink of death by M&B 693. 'Suddenly the blue eyes opened, the little face lit up, and a small piping voice said: "Nice man".' Hearing the sound of newsboys calling beneath, he told how the nurse opened the window 'and the voices now came distinctly—International crisis—hope of peace. A sudden relief came on us. "Everything is going to be all right now". I said with conviction.'[55]

Even if Chamberlain's hopes for peace were misplaced, the victory of the sulphonamides did spell real hope and a change in attitudes to disease. The new science provided the vindication of the old Paracelsian dream of a medical revolution. The will to revolt against the limitations of the past was so strong that the terms 'wonder drug' or 'miracle drug' were taken seriously and not, more ironically, to refer to their perhaps more natural American connotations of quack medicine. In January 1939, the *Star Weekly* published in Toronto, under the headline 'Fighting Death with "693"', reported that 'Medical men are tirelessly testing a miracle drug bordering on witch cures of the Middle Ages, that promises to wipe out pneumonia.'[56] 'Witch cure' was of course a reference to alchemists and above all to Paracelsus.

The sense that the sulphonamides were heralding a new age of medicines was incorporated into laws across the developed world. Drugs recognized by medical science were differentiated from more general stuff which people took for their health—despite the onset of the Second World War in 1939 and on both sides of the front, Ironically, though, it was not the novel curative efficacy of the sulphonamides that led to the first regulatory distinctions between modern prescription medicines, quack medicine, and household remedies. Instead it was their abuse through old-fashioned stupidity. The use of the sweet-tasting, but poisonous, solvent di-ethylene glycol to dissolve sulphanilamide by a small Tennessee company caused the deaths of a hundred people. After years of fruitless wrangling about the control of drugs, this disaster led to the passing of the US Food, Drug and Cosmetic Act in 1938 with hardly any debate. Even the advertising industry's own magazine argued that it was obvious that 'sin and sulfanilamide' needed to be controlled.[57] The new law regulated for the first time in the USA both the medicines available only through prescription and drugs whose contents were carefully enough spelled out for the customers to make a judgement for themselves.[58] Similarly, in France a 1938 law distinguished between remedies and scientific medicines, and regulations were strengthened three years later, on the other side of defeat, by the Vichy government.

In Britain, new legislation controlling the advertising of drugs was passed also in the autumn of 1941, again despite the otherwise pressing concerns of war. As in the USA and France, the new British law responded to the urgent need to distinguish between modern medicine, quack medicine, and household remedies. Advertising of products that claimed to cure such diseases as cancer and TB was banned absolutely, and advertisements for any medicine without a specified composition were also banned. Science, not popular culture, was given the legislative keys to health. When a proponent pleaded for exemption from the new drug regulations for herbalists, and described what good people they were, the intervention was dismissed by the formidable parliamentarian Edith Summerskill, who asked, 'Can the honourable member say whether, in addition to their charm and social standing, they have any scientific qualifications?'[59]

Development took place so fast that, even as war was declared, a new generation of wonder drugs was announced. The French-born scientist René Dubos, then working at New York's famous Rockefeller Institute, had been stirred by the success of Prontosil and sought to go one better. In the late 1920s he had systematically searched soils looking for an enzyme which could destroy the sugar-based coating of the pneumococcus bacterium responsible for pneumonia and in the 1930s widened his search to killers of other bacteria. Introducing bacteria into samples of soil, he sought an ingredient of the dirt that would kill the microbes he had added. In July 1939 he announced the discovery of an organism in the soil which indeed did assault the dreaded microbes staphylococci and salmonellae. He called the toxic chemical that was being exuded by his organism 'tyrothricin'. That year the Third International Congress on Microbiology was held in New York City's Waldorf-Astoria Hotel, and on 8 September Dubos stood on the podium with a bottle containing 500 grams of his bacterium killer and announced that he had enough medicine here to protect 5 trillion mice.[60]

Over a period of two years, the Rockefeller Institute and drug companies put considerable effort towards developing tyrothricin. Dubos himself quickly identified and chemically isolated two products, known as gramicidin and tyrocidine. These chemicals proved to be too toxic to be used internally, but they could be used topically (tyrothricin is an ingredient of a popular brand of throat lozenges) and they did offer the prospect of further improvement.

By the end of the 1930s, therefore, scientific medicines effectively regulated by governments seemed to offer a radically new future to medicine.

21

To an audience at the opening of a new hospital in Birmingham, England, vitamin pioneer and now medical administrator Edward Mellanby in July 1938 prophesied that within fifty years a hospital would no longer be needed to treat infections. 'It may, of course', he proclaimed, 'be full of motor accidents (laughter); or it may be full of very old people whiling away their last years of life in peace and happiness.'[61]

Expectations were well developed, industry had grown, developments had been rapid, and improvements were tangible, but no existing drug could fulfil the expectations that had been aroused. The limitations of the first wave of 'wonder drugs' were becoming quickly apparent. Sulphonamide drugs proved problematic: many patients suffered bad reactions, wounds that had become infected could not be treated, and bacteria quickly developed high levels of resistance. Dubos's antibiotics were toxic.

This was the moment at which penicillin arrived in the public arena. Expectations for the new drug would be coloured deeply by reaction to pre-war conceptions of disease, by hopes for wonder drugs, and the taste of sulphonamides. The brand was coloured, too, by the particular experience of penicillin's creation, which proved to be among the most famous episodes in the history of science.

2

Penicillin from Organized Science

Penicillin had not yet been isolated in September 1939, when war was declared, but by D-Day in June 1944, less than five years later, it was being made in large factories to meet the needs of invasion and of deserving civilians. The effort had not just produced chemicals and knowledge, it had also displayed the power of a new process of scientific development with great promise for the post-war years.

Penicillin was a biological product whose manufacture would require the integration of a variety of scientific and engineering disciplines. On a scale unprecedented in bioscience, collaborating teams of researchers were deployed to meet the challenge. Expertise in bacteria had to be linked to experience with moulds, chemistry, and the engineering of sterile systems for the support of living creatures. Beyond the drug itself, novel technologies for the mass production of natural substances through fermentation were generated through its development. Overwhelming the scepticism of chemists, these technologies transformed the products, and the scale, of the pharmaceutical industry. By 1960 they had been given the collective title of biotechnology.

This network of innovations also bred personal and national pride, resentments, jealousies, and stories which would themselves be an important component of the penicillin brand. Such feelings were strong, and difficult to articulate, in part because the development moved precipitously between a small scale involving a few talented scientists and a large international project with impersonal corporate achievements. In addition, this transformation was associated with a shifting geography, as the centre moved from the United Kingdom to the United States. Yet, even across that divide, the challenges of bringing together diverse specialisms would characterize every stage of the development.

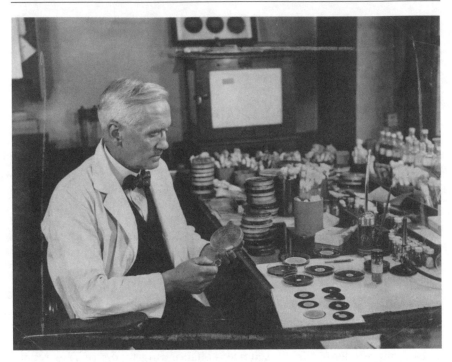

2. Alexander Fleming shown at work in his laboratory in 1943. This iconic image by the well-known photographer James Jarche celebrated as contemporary an achievement 15 years previously. The picture was published in the *Daily Herald* newspaper.
NMPFT/Science & Society Picture Library.

The multidisciplinary challenge of penicillin would be significant from the very beginning of the story. While it may have been discovered through the accidental experience of a single man, the response of scientists from a variety of backgrounds was critical to the development of the drug—and the community's early limitations would underscore the meaning of later developments in scientific organization.

The discoverer, Alexander Fleming, was a respected bacteriologist at the Pathological Institute at St Mary's Hospital Medical School, a striving and productive centre (see Ill. 2). His colleague Leonard Colebrook would be among the most influential of pioneers of the use of sulphonamide drugs, while the school's dean, Sir Charles Wilson (later honoured as Lord Moran), had the ambition to achieve a standing for his institution comparable to Johns Hopkins Medical School. This would require facilities that he estimated in the mid-1920s would cost £100,000, then equivalent to half a million US dollars.[1] Prophetically, Wilson appealed in May 1929 to Lord Beaverbrook, owner of Britain's biggest-selling newspaper, the *Daily Express*. 'Salvarsan', he wrote, 'was discovered on the continent, not as a happy accident, but as the result of years of systematic investigation. Similar advances cannot be made in England until money is found for whole time workers in this subject.'[2] Within two weeks he had been given £63,000. St Mary's was, for its time, a commercially savvy institute competing to be as famous as the world's best.

Early in the 1920s, Fleming had been excited briefly by the properties of a germ-killing compound he had found in human tears, which he named lysozyme. This proved to be of no direct medical benefit, since its victims were exclusively harmless organisms. However, lysozyme proved to be a chemically interesting enzyme and, through his experiments, Fleming developed a range of techniques for investigating the effect of a chemical on bacteria that would stand him in good stead for the future.

Fleming's experience of lysozyme would be critical to exploiting the accident in September 1928. Returning from a month's holiday, he found a heap of dirty dishes needing to be washed out. He discarded them, but, on reflection, recovered the dish with a small growth of dark green felty mould surrounded by a sterile ring separating it from the 'staph' bacteria. Reasoning that perhaps the mould was exuding a substance similar to lysozyme, Fleming studied the effects of the filtered broth of nutrient on which the mould had grown, using techniques he himself had developed for the earlier investigation (see Ill. 3). Showing that it killed, or prevented

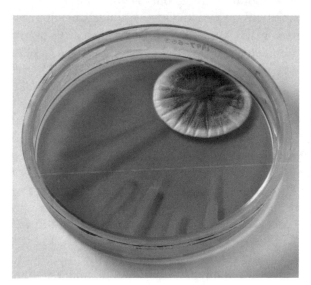

3. Replica of an early experiment by Fleming showing the effect of penicillin produced by mould on the growth of bacteria. This plate was produced for use in the 1944 ICI-sponsored film on penicillin in which Fleming himself appeared. Science Museum inventory number 1997–663.

Science Museum/Science & Society Picture Library.

25

4. Sample of penicillium mould given by Alexander Fleming to his friend Douglas Macleod about 1935, after a conversation about the superiority of penicillin over the newly discovered Prontosil. This sample may be seen to have marked the transformation of penicillin to potential medicine. The mounting dates from the 1960s. Science Museum inventory number 1997–731.

Science Museum/Science & Society Picture Library.

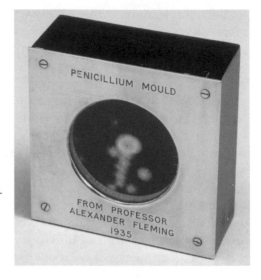

the growth of, some bacteria but not others, Fleming published a report of his observations in the *British Journal of Experimental Pathology*.[3]

Fleming failed to separate whatever mysterious chemical within the liquid was affecting the bacteria, so he gave the name 'penicillin' to the mould juice as a whole. Whereas there had long been folk traditions of the therapeutic benefits of moulds, and whatever good fortune had attended his first observation, it was Fleming who inserted penicillin into the life of science. As a contemporary pointed out, 'Fleming put penicillin on the map.'[4] He published his results in an easily available journal article and then distributed widely the culture that produced his active substance. Samples were sent across Europe and the United States. When, later, renewed attention was paid to the mould, samples were found in the stores of laboratories in Oxford, Columbia, Paris, Baarn (the Netherlands), and Copenhagen.

With a London location and distinguished colleagues, Fleming attracted interest to his work, but its further development suffered from a fractured scientific community. Two research students at St Mary's were interested in the therapeutic potential of the drug, but they were medically, not chemically, trained, and in any case could only give Fleming a few months' assistance before moving on.[5] Across the city, in the London School of Hygiene and Tropical Medicine a leading biochemist, Harold Raistrick, tried to extract the elusive principle from its broth. Whatever he did seemed to destroy the delicate chemical structure. On the other hand, Raistrick did find how to grow it reliably. Furthermore, he sent a sample to his American friend Charles Thom, who clarified its botanical name, *Penicillium notatum*, a fungus first identified as early as 1911 by the Danish biologist P. Westling. While Raistrick's links with Fleming on the one hand and Thom on the other were critical to the advances he made, he was strictly limited in the range of skills on which he could draw. Raistrick complained that he could not raise the interest of bacteriologists in the curious mould juice.[6] Conversely, Fleming would later claim that he could not get chemists interested in the problem of separation. Even he was bemused by these fractures within the scientific community of his time.[7]

The fragmentation of science in London was reflected elsewhere, and much of the interest in penicillin that emerged during the 1930s can be compared to bubbles that grew briefly and then burst suddenly. The precedents of sulphonamide and, later, Dubos's tyrothricin were, however, elevating what had been a curiosity into a challenge. At a 1935 London lecture Fleming learned of Domagk's discovery of the properties of Prontosil, and he is reported to have said to his friend MacLeod, 'I've got something much better than Prontosil, but no one'll listen to me.'[8] (See Ill.4) Fleming may have been frustrated in the short term, but already there were widening horizons for a potential medicine.

Beyond medicine, the context of penicillin was changed by a 1930s transformation in the organization of science. The challenge of the drug had defeated a community in London divided between chemists and bacteriologists. Now, however, biological scientists in leading universities were increasingly consulting with companies and collaborating with industry. Interdisciplinary teams were being established.[9] The experiences of the work on vitamins, insulin, and plant steroids were providing precedents for the successful collaboration of academic and industrial researchers.

The new organization of science won purchase even at Oxford. Despite its conservative reputation, as Britain slowly recovered from the depths of the Depression during the 1930s, the university aspired to be modern. In 1934 it allocated a large science area within its campus.[10] At the physics department, the German-educated Frederick Lindemann was establishing a world-class low-temperature laboratory, recruiting Jewish refugees expelled by the Nazi government from previously distinguished German universities. The chemistry departments had close relations with the newly formed chemical combine Imperial Chemical Industries (I.C.I). The professor of organic chemistry, Robert Robinson, was closely associated with the company and personally obtained nine patents during the 1930s.[11]

A multidisciplinary research school which, including research students, numbered two dozen active researchers was being built up by the new professor of pathology, Howard Florey. The William Dunn School he oversaw, had been opened in 1926 at the heart of the new science area and next to the organic chemistry department in the Dyson-Perrins Laboratory. With an interest in addressing the underlying causes of illness, Florey established strengths in clinical pathology, experimental pathology, and bacteriology, but focused upon projects that crossed the divides between these specialities. The enzyme discovered by Alexander Fleming, lysozyme, and lymphocytes were early subjects of attack. Grants were tiny and money was short, obtained in bits and pieces by, in Florey's words, 'shaking a hat in all possible directions'.[12]

Rather than mere poverty, such shortages indicated the victory of ambition over prudence. Indeed, the technologies and skills the team could deploy, the number of people on whom it could draw internally, the support it could muster internationally, and the results it achieved highlight its standing among the elite of world science in terms of both quality and scale. With a tenacity that would be the key to the success of penicillin, Florey ensured that the disconnection between disciplinary concerns, which had been such a feature of the penicillin story early in the 1930s, would not be repeated.

The achievements of Florey's team were still associated with particular individuals and a focus on basic science. Ernst Boris Chain, a German refugee biochemist just finishing a second doctorate in Cambridge, was recruited by Florey in 1937.[13] It was he who first grasped the chemical challenge of separating penicillin and, over more than twenty years, his life would be intertwined with the drug. His interest grew out of a concern with such enzymes as lysozyme in which the laboratory was already interested. Scanning the literature, Chain came across reports of penicillin. Finding a sample of Fleming's mould in a nearby laboratory, and believing its product to be another enzyme, Chain addressed the problems of separating the active principle. This would be an interesting scientific challenge, and Florey agreed the mould was worthy of further study. Certainly Chain was ambitious, but he was not looking for a medicine. His goal was, instead, to achieve a separation that had defeated all others.

The priority of Chain's problem was, however, not immediately obvious at a time of international crisis. Even though the Medical Research Council did agree to fund Chain's salary, the laboratory's ambitions ran far ahead of its resources. Despite the beginning of war, the solution was to turn to the Rockefeller Foundation of New York, the world's richest funder of scientific research.[14] On 20 November 1939, Chain and Florey submitted a grant proposal for three years of support to look at proteins which might attack bacteria. Among several topics included in the proposal was a study of penicillin.

Whereas the style of research funded by grant application may have resembled modern practice, the reality of the 1930s was still very different from that of the more anonymous world to come. The application was received at the Foundation's European office in France on 30 November: the very same day the desk officer sent a telegram to the Foundation's New York-based head of science, Warren Weaver, recommending that a grant be awarded.[15] Within hours, Weaver had responded to his telegram, 'the application of Florey appeals to me, but I seriously question whether a three-year grant is justified under present circumstances. Could this not be handled on a year to year basis?'[16] A few days had to elapse as transatlantic airmail letters communicated a more measured correspondence. Florey was then given an informal assurance that funding would be renewed, so long as the situation did not change radically for the worse.[17] Weaver's support would be critical at several stages in this process. He had, for many years, been determined to bring a hard scientific basis to the often-descriptive biological disciplines. During the 1930s he supported studies of genetics and of the processes that explain the nature of life.[18] Thus, when Chain assumed penicillin was a protein and decided it might therefore be worth studying, he was linking it not only to his own previous studies of snake venom and lysozyme, but also to the big questions of contemporary science. He was dealing with the chemicals of life at the centre of Warren Weaver's interests.

The separation of penicillin had defeated others. The Oxford team succeeded by using the novel technique of freeze-drying which was being explored in Cambridge to produce dried blood plasma in preparation for war. Successfully separating a biologically active dry powder, even though it proved later to be just 1 per cent pure penicillin, was a very considerable achievement. The penicillin, described at the time as 'as unstable as an opera singer', had made up just one part in a million of the original broth.[19]

A single experiment can be seen as translating penicillin from a narrowly scientific challenge into the medical realm. In March 1940, Chain tested much of his entire supply, 40 mg, scarcely more than one-thousandth part of an ounce, on two mice.[20] The mice showed no immune response, no swelling or illness. Chain interpreted this to mean that penicillin was not a protein. As a scientist, he was profoundly disappointed, for, while there may have been other evidence, this experiment proved to him that, instead of being a member of the scientifically important family of proteins, penicillin was a small and probably scientifically boring molecule.[21] But if the problem was less interesting, the product was more valuable. Chain, for one, changed gear from a scientific to a medical project at that point. He had shown penicillin could be isolated, and the product, complete with impurities, was, seemingly, non-toxic.

Although Florey was irritated that the experiment had been conducted in his absence, it increased his interest too. He was assisted by the variety of expertise in Oxford, which was critical to the quick success of the team. The night before Chain's experiment on the mice, Norman Heatley, a biochemist who had been marooned in Oxford by the war instead of taking up a post-doctoral fellowship in Denmark, suggested that they could create a much more concentrated solution by passing the penicillin from its original watery broth into the organic solvent ether, which does not mix with water, and then back into an alkaline solution in water. Each time, impurities would be left behind.[22] The contrast between the charming Heatley and the irascible Chain would become legendary, and indeed their relationship was so bad that Heatley refused to work for Chain and reported directly to Florey.[23] The apparatus Heatley built no longer exists, but forty-five years later he made a replica for London's Science Museum (Ill. 5).[24]

By combining the techniques of Heatley and Chain, extraction was improved. The urgency was also increasing. In May 1940, France fell to the German invasion. At Oxford University, penicillin was tested on eight sick mice. The untreated mice died, while the four treated mice survived. Florey and Chain reflected on a miracle.[25]

From this moment onward, Florey focused his laboratory's work on penicillin. Progressively, he established parallel projects on the chemistry and biochemistry of penicillin, production, bacteriology, large-scale extraction, pharmacology and biology, and clinical testing. His managerial skills were tested by the strong personalities within the team and his own ambiguous relationships with some of its members. Florey's own wife was responsible for the clinical trials. She had to work closely with Margaret Jennings, whom she knew to be conducting an affair with her husband, yet the two women maintained a professional relationship. Ethel Florey's

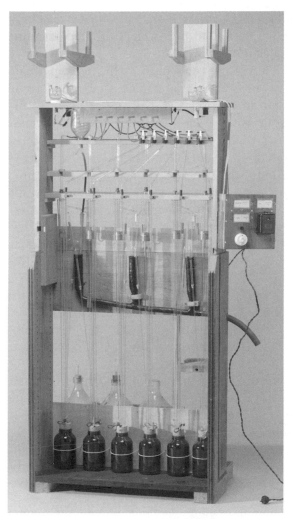

5. Replica of his original apparatus for the separation of penicillin from the juice exuded by mould, built by Norman Heatley himself in 1986. Less well known than the bedpan fermenters, the design of this separation device was critical to early laboratory manufacture. In the collections of the Science Museum, inventory number 1986–1116.

Science Museum/Science & Society Picture Library.

secretary Muriel Burge later recalled having to convey draft academic papers between wife and mistress: Ethel's numerous reports were checked by Margaret Jennings on behalf of Howard Florey.[26]

Since the penicillin needed for a single patient had to be extracted from hundreds of litres of fermentation liquid, the Oxford team needed to find efficient means of growing the penicillium mould. Heatley found that the mould which formed on the surface of the nutrients would continue to produce penicillin if the saturated broth beneath it was removed and new nutrient added. Shallow flat dishes that allowed the broth to be poured

31

without damaging the surface mould were therefore sought.[27] Stacks of pots made to Heatley's design by a friend of Florey in the Staffordshire potteries were arrayed in the Dunn institute (Ill. 6).

Nonetheless, Florey was continually challenged by the need to obtain sufficient penicillin to carry out a substantial clinical study. This would require industrial interest, but in wartime speculative investment would be hard to win. How better to win attention than through a therapeutic triumph? Within six months, therefore, the Oxford team went from an experiment on eight mice to human experimentation. First, the safety of the drug was proved by administering a dose to a woman dying from cancer. Early in 1941, with a further small quantity available, Florey and his colleagues administered a small dose to Albert Alexander, a policeman. A simple prick from a rose thorn had caused an infection which had already cost him his eye, and his entire body was badly infected. At first, the penicillin injection really seemed to improve Alexander's condition. A miraculous recovery appeared to be in the offing, but supplies were running low. At first they were supplemented by recycling the half of the penicillin that was excreted into the patient's urine rather than absorbed by the body. Each morning, one of the team collected it from the hospital and carried it back to the laboratory by bicycle, on what was referred to as the 'P-Patrol'.[28]

Depending on its own resources, the laboratory was forced to a small-scale and ad hoc approach. This was captured in the laboratory notes made at the time by Edward Abraham, a member of the Oxford team. On 18 February 1941, Abraham reported: 3.7 litres of the patient's urine had been combined with one-third volume of the organic solvents chloroform and ether. Then extracted into ether and then re-extracted into dilute sodium hydroxide solution. 550 ml of water solution were now re-extracted with

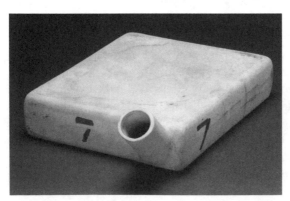

6. Bedpan-like fermenter for growing penicillium mould developed by Norman Heatley and used in Oxford 1941–3. Now in the collections of the Science Museum, inventory number 1976–628.
Science Museum/Science & Society Picture Library.

ether. This was once again mixed with ether. Once again extracted with sodium hydroxide solution, finally freeze dried. The output reported from this labour was just more than half a gram of impure penicillin.[29] The effort was heroic but inadequate. Such methods had stretched supplies, but not sufficiently. The patient relapsed and died. The doctors treated five more victims of infection, with mixed results. While four made impressive recoveries, one other died.[30]

Cottage in scale, the results obtained in Oxford were sufficiently reassuring to capture the further support of the Rockefeller Foundation, which would be critical to their subsequent development. In the spring of 1941 Warren Weaver visited England. Florey shared with him the team's results and his sense of frustration caused by his inability to get penicillin made by British companies. Weaver and he discussed the possibility of bringing Florey and Heatley to the USA to find and instruct 'some American mold or yeast raiser who would undertake a large-scale production of this material for a test, say, 10,000 gallons for the first run'.[31] Weaver was impressed: his internal Rockefeller report suggested that 'It is probable that this new chemotherapeutic agent will outrank the sulfa drugs in combating a long series of infectious diseases.'[32] This enthusiastic commitment to the potential of penicillin was made at a time when experimental and clinical data were still very limited. It testified to the persuasiveness of his Oxford host but also to the attraction of the model of the 'wonder drug' and the compelling precedent of the sulphonamide drugs.

The commitment made for Florey to cross the Atlantic was substantial, even by the standards of the Rockefeller Foundation. The $6,000 grant Weaver arranged made up a sixth of the funds still available for science that year.[33] Of course, money would not be enough: space on one of the increasingly scarce flights would be required. Priority on the London–Lisbon plane was obtained by the intervention of Mellanby of the Medical Research Council, while US Surgeon General Thomas Parran offered his services to get priority for the two scientists on the Lisbon–New York plane.[34] Science was still a small, elite business. They left on 27 June 1941. Chain knew nothing of the visit until he saw the suitcases of his departing colleagues in the laboratory at Oxford and, of course, was apoplectic with rage that he was to be excluded.[35]

Florey and Heatley descended upon an American scientific community that had been primed to recognize the importance of their mission. Just two months earlier, a Columbia University team concluded that penicillin would be an outstanding drug. A month after Weaver's internal memorandum to his Rockefeller colleagues, they issued a prophecy in terms very similar to Weaver's, suggesting that penicillin might 'prove as useful or even more useful than the sulfonamides'.[36]

The British visitors were conducted rapidly from one contact to another through the famously tight-knit Washington community. Introduced by his old friend John Fulton, professor at Yale, Florey met the chairman of the National Research Council, who then passed him on to America's leading expert on moulds, Charles Thom, who had originally classified Fleming's penicillium. Thom, who had no connection with the newly formed National Institutes of Health, worked instead at the far larger Department of Agriculture. This brought the problem of producing penicillin into the purview of one of the world's largest research enterprises. Within a week of Florey's arrival in the USA, Thom had introduced him in turn to an agriculture department scientist, Percy Wells, then deputizing for a boss who was motoring out of town.[37] As Thom introduced the two Englishmen to Wells, it was obvious to him what should be done. Instead of directing the visitors to the leading academic centre of fermentation science at the University of Wisconsin in Madison, he directed them instead to former colleagues who had just been redeployed to the newly established 'Northern Regional Research Laboratory' amid the cornfields of Peoria, Illinois.[38] A year later, Wells commented that all he had then in mind was that Peoria take the British results and upscale them.[39]

It would be tempting to contrast the poor British with a luxuriously appointed US department. However, it was technical skill, not commercial scale, that distinguished the Peoria laboratory. The small group in Illinois had been evicted from a government site known as 'The Color Laboratory' outside Washington, DC, where the new Pentagon was to be built. Congress had voted the money in 1938, but would not allow it to be spent till the scientists were in place, which meant that the new laboratory had only opened in late 1940.[40]

Small and new though it still was, the Peoria laboratory brought expertise in the cultivation of mould to the penicillin enterprise and specifically, too, an engineering perspective, which complemented the microbiological expertise of the British. The overall mission of the new laboratory was to make useful chemicals from otherwise surplus agricultural waste, then known as 'chemurgy'.[41] Biological materials made from farmers' produce might, for instance, prove useful as the raw materials for the acids used as flavourings and preservatives in the newly popular non-alcoholic carbonated drinks such as lemonade and colas. Citric acid (still used in many carbonated drinks), lactic acid, which was more favoured in unrefrigerated

European drinks (and used in sparkling glucose drinks) and gluconic acid (from penicillium mould) could each be produced from microbes using techniques of fermentation. Even while still based in Washington, the USDA team had become interested in the possibility of developing these techniques. The moulds such as penicillium resembled plants—indeed, it was the botanists who were the experts on them—and the layer of mould was often referred to by them as a 'moss'. Thus, while the extractive techniques practised by the Oxford scientists might be compared to cookery, the USDA team were expert gardeners.

The team that had moved to Peoria already had experience in growing moulds in deep fermenters, rather than merely on the surface of nutrients as the British had done. This was a technology pioneered early in the 1930s in Delft, now in German-occupied Netherlands, and the Peoria expertise was still rare in the United States and unknown in Britain.[42] In principle attractive, the technology raised difficult problems later characterized as 'the three As' of deep fermentation: Asepsis, Aeration, and Agitation.[43] While still based in Washington, a distinguished Color Laboratory team of Percy Wells, David Lynch, Henry Herrick, and Orville May (three of whom were soon made directors of their own laboratories) partially filled a rotating drum lying on its side, so that it constantly mixed oxygen with its mouldy soup as it turned.[44] This was not just science—the team may have been small but it did things on a large scale. A pilot vessel completed in 1936 held almost a tonne of soup, with a capacity of 2,000 litres.[45] Its interior was equipped with buckets and obstructions, which would ensure proper mixing. To prevent the growth of unwanted organisms, only sterile air was admitted and the drum was made of high-purity aluminium. Other non-rusting metals such as copper would have stunted the growth of mould. This created new engineering problems: since aluminium is soft, weight-bearing components had to be made of bronze.

The new technology proved significantly more effective than the current state-of-the-art techniques for growing penicillium to make gluconic acid using shallow aluminium pans. Using the traditional approach, a factory could make in eleven days half the yield theoretically possible. With the rotary drum, the team could improve the yield impressively: to more than four-fifths of theoretical limit in much less time, just two days. The increasing speed did not just mean more efficiency. It also meant there was less time for a wild spore of some alien species to float into the fermentation and ruin all the work. Ironically, the team also made another improvement. They abandoned the use of the penicillium, because it was

35

difficult to work with and did not reproduce fast enough, and replaced it with a different micro-organism.

The USDA scientists had also made a far-reaching discovery in the feeding of the penicillium. The substantial quantity, and significant cost, of nutrients used by the large fermenter was an attraction to the agricultural supplier of raw materials. It was, however, a problem for the impoverished chemical laboratory. In seeking to make sorbose, a sweetener, in 1937, Andrew Moyer of the USDA laboratory had stumbled upon a discovery that would be key to the development of penicillin manufacture.[46] One important nutrient supplying nitrogen to the mould cost $30 for each experiment. With restricted budgets, this seemed a lot, and people looked around for a replacement. Someone found a gallon bottle covered in dust labelled 'corn steep water concentrate', which had come from the Staley Manufacturing Company in Illinois. The people there had been looking for a use for this by-product. Now it was tested, found to work beautifully, and instead of costing $30 per experiment, it would cost only 60 cents. After that they tested cornsteep liquor in all their experiments.

Cornsteep liquor would prove the key to cheap penicillin. Florey himself stayed in Peoria just long enough to make arrangements and then moved on to visit other centres. Heatley, however, stayed to communicate his hard-won expertise and shared a bench with Andrew Moyer, the gruff, rather Anglophobic pioneer of cornsteep liquor. Heatley went away for a few days and, on his return, instead of the penicillium producing two units per millilitre, it was making four or five times as much. Moyer was secretive about what he had done at first. In response to Heatley's query of how he had achieved his spectacular yields, he replied merely, 'adjuvants'.[47] Later Heatley would learn that Moyer had replaced the artificial medium the Oxford team had used with the cornsteep liquour that had already proved so useful in other fermentations. He had also added the milk sugar lactose. Now a millilitre gave 100 units of activity.[48] Moyer's attempt later to patent his developments would create bad feeling with his allies for years to come.[49]

The following year the Peoria laboratory would make a second breakthrough, finding a new, much more productive strain of penicillium mould. The US army had sent samples from its bases all over the world, but the best, ironically, was found growing locally on a melon in the Peoria market.[50] This was particularly important, because the new strain was better adapted to being grown in the deep fermenter than Fleming's original. If penicillin could be made from penicillium grown not just on the surface of a dish but submerged in the body of a vat, the productivity could be substantially increased, as the production of the organic acids had already demonstrated. Even if the yield were to be no better than in bottles, a single tank of 45,000 litres would give the same amount of penicillin as 60,000 to 70,000 two-litre bottles.[51] Two years later Wells would congratulate Moyer on the achievements made since that visit in July 1941: 'The story of how you found the organism discontented with the set-up and your improvement of its lot was what I would have expected; nevertheless the accomplishment is outstanding. Your long years of experience in making the "bugs" jump through the hoop were just what was needed.'[52]

Florey, as what would be called a 'product champion' and, in his words, a 'carpet-bagman', was still needed to enthuse his American hosts. Travelling on his Rockefeller grant, after leaving Peoria, Florey sought out companies that would take his discovery seriously. He succeeded in persuading one of the most respected corporations, Merck, to accept Norman Heatley's help to get production going.[53] Their output thereby increased greatly.[54] Squibb, which had initially examined the opportunity to develop penicillin in 1936, was once again interested. Pfizer also saw prospects in this area. Nonetheless, while these organizations were not large, and heavy pressure was put on them to take an interest in penicillin, at first they were hesitant about working together for fear of falling foul of powerful legislation against any apparent industrial conspiracy.

When Florey returned to the United Kingdom, neither did a flood of American penicillin follow him, nor was he pursued by great press interest at home. Instead he found, as he complained to his American host John Fulton, that in his absence 'a certain number of people with not enough to do have been dipping their oars here and made the situation much more complicated than it need ever have been'.[55] In retrospect, the development of penicillin from small-scale laboratory phenomenon to major industry took place very rapidly. At the time, however, take-up seemed, to the participants, to be slow. There was a war on. Provisions were short. For the British government, there were many other priorities—radar, the early years of the atomic bomb, the bombing of Germany, and fighting in North Africa.

Until the summer of 1942, a few perceptive and well-meaning scientists making important conceptual and practical developments dominated the story of penicillin. Work on it was part of the private life of science as it had long been conducted. On both sides of the Atlantic, interdisciplinary teams had formed and were drawing on unique expertise and leadership. The budgets were, however, still small, and the public was largely ignorant of the new medicine. With its few characters, the story rather resembled an intimate play on a small stage.

That autumn, penicillin became public property and part of the history of wartime culture, resembling a Hollywood movie with an enormous cast, a major marketing campaign, and impressive budgets. Now it involved governments, big business, and the great instruments of wartime propaganda. This irreversible transition would define the penicillin brand as no longer under the control of either scientists or physicians.

Such a transition might seem to reflect merely the natural move of the penicillin story from a research phase to development and manufacturing. That, however, would be too simplistic. The injection of funds, people, companies' and government interest meant a transformation in the ways of doing science. The process of development in which the scientists found themselves was radically new. From the familiar interchange within small hierarchical elites, the scientific process itself was transformed into a very much larger, more complex system encompassing industry and the public. Over a thousand chemists were involved in one aspect of the work alone. Teams of scientists from many institutions, dependent on collaboration rather than deference, worked together, transgressing deeply entrenched divides between professors and students, between academic and industrial research, and between science and technology. At about the same time, the idea of an atomic weapon was also moving from the brains of individual physicists to the vast organization that would be required for the realization of a working weapon.

The effort to modify penicillium mould genetically by means of radiation illustrates the new style of work. Although this programme is little known, its importance to the production of penicillin proved to be great. The capacity of radiation to change the genes of living things had been explored since the 1920s, principally as a means of studying genetics, but at the newly formed National Institutes of Health outside Washington, the German-born Alexander Hollaender became interested in mutating moulds to make them better producers of organic acids.[56] Whilst that project was not successful, when penicillin became known Hollaender was naturally attracted to the possibility of improving productivity by modifying moulds.

In the autumn of 1942, forming a consortium with the group at Peoria and the leading US genetics laboratory at Cold Spring Harbor on Long Island near New York, Hollaender tried to raise support for experiments on penicillium. He wrote to Demerec, director of Cold Spring Harbor, of the contribution he felt genetics could make to this urgent war work.

'*Much more* has to be done to bring this organism to a level where it will be commercial to produce it profitably. It *won't* be an easy job.'[57]

At first Hollaender and Demerec found it hard to get support. They sought to supply the Merck corporation with possibly high-yielding mutants. This avenue was frustrated when Merck showed little interest in the work.[58] Their higher-status competitor on the west coast, the Californian geneticist George Beadle at the University of Stanford, did get funding to make and test mutants, but his results were unimpressive.[59] So it was not until May 1944 that funding was approved for Demerec and his colleagues.[60]

The Cold Spring Harbor team would arrange the irradiation of the mould, send promising samples to the University of Minnesota for investigation, and from there a few of the most promising moulds would be sent on to the University of Wisconsin in Madison, which had pilot plant facilities for deep fermentation.

Even today Madison is the world's dairy capital, and the campus of the university still boasts a massive silo at its centre. It had already attracted talented scientists, but even they sought to address the practical interests of the university's constituency. In the 1920s, it was Wisconsin staff who had discovered that by irradiating milk they could radically enhance its vitamin D content. Despite initial reservations, and the traditions of medicine, the university had patented the discovery, setting up the Wisconsin Alumni Research Fund (WARF) as a vehicle. This provided a new funding stream for its staff. In keeping with this practical bent, its department of microbiology was particularly distinguished, including the famously unambitious Marvin Johnson, an expert on fermentation who had studied in Europe during the early 1930s.[61]

Several groups at the university came to be interested in the penicillin production problem. Johnson had acquired pilot-scale 450-litre fermenters from the Commercial Solvents company, which gave the university a valuable asset at a time when other groups were working either with much smaller laboratory-scale equipment or with fermenters holding thousands of litres. In addition, the botany department came to be involved, bringing an expertise in the genetics of moulds. A Ph.D. student who would later become a leader in the area recalled:

This team approach was nearly unique in the history of research at Wisconsin. It had successfully flourished between Professors Peterson (Biochemistry) and Fred (Bacteriology) beginning in 1916, so the pattern had existed for nearly 25 years. But, in 1943–4 the numbers of persons involved was much larger . . . 7 faculty and nearly 20 students and staff. This necessitated frequent group meetings (sometimes at less than weekly intervals), preparation of reports and of course clear definitions of responsibilities (to minimise overlapping efforts). As might be expected with so many diverse personalities involved and committed to the program, rather vigorous discussions were frequently held and an element of competition was evident.[62]

Within a month, the inter-institutional team of the Universities of Minnesota and Wisconsin and Cold Spring Harbor had created and grown an outstanding organism exuding 500 units per millilitre by irradiating Peoria's finest with X-rays. Two Wisconsin botanists, funded by the WARF, went further and set out to breed what they called an 'albino' mould: that is without any of the yellow discoloration which caused pain when the drug was injected.[63] The project would take a decade but, almost immediately, it was attended by startling success. A burst of ultraviolet rays further altered the Cold Spring Harbor mutant's genes, so that the penicillium, known as Q-176, produced over 1,000 units of penicillin in every millilitre of broth. This was a huge increase compared with the first Oxford results of 2 units per millilitre. There was a slight chemical difference from the most therapeutically efficacious penicillin structure, but this problem was solved by control of the fermentation. The resulting mould spores, ten times as productive as their natural ancestors, were sent freely worldwide to over 150 laboratories.[64]

Organization was, of course, not historically associated with the creative urge. Artists and geniuses had usually been seen as individually inspired. That the blending of the individualistic model of academic science and the group-oriented industrial styles created tensions was not merely an administrative convenience: it challenged the allocation of credit, the fundamental currency of scientific life. Even the trivial tensions it caused are instructive. In a letter to his friend John Fulton at Yale, Florey described a bizarre new world that was unfolding in England during 1943, as in Burma the British were desperately trying to save India and in Italy the Allies were approaching Rome. In Oxford, Florey reported conflict too:

There is a frightful scramble going on amongst the chemists which gives me a slight pain in the neck. I am getting very worried about getting too much credit for what is going on and if you get a chance to emphasise how much is due to Chain in particular and all the other people here. I am frightfully worried about this whole publicity and credit business as I'm afraid it is only going to lead to inevitable trouble.[65]

Certanly Florey was right to worry about Chain. When the Oxford team produced a post-war two-volume account of their work, Chain complained on numerous counts.[66] He made a major issue out of the credit allocated to each of the seven authors.

The scientists involved in this scramble might seem narrow minded or even stupid, worrying about trivia at a time of total war. Their squabbles can, however, also be interpreted as interesting disorientation caused by immersion in a seemingly bizarre system. In other words, the arguments about credit tell us what a new scientific world was now being explored by veterans trained in an older environment. In the development of penicillin, men who might have been the most worldly wise demonstrated a disorientation and lack of balance. The phrase 'moral economy', used to describe the aspects of society dependent on relationships, has proved useful to historians of science.[67] This phrase, coined originally to describe how early nineteenth-century radicals expressed outrage in careful measure, described their sense of propriety and transgression. Since much of science too is based on non-financial exchange whose currency is taught through professional formation, the squabbles about credit can be interpreted in terms of an encounter with a new moral economy of science.[68]

The model for the new pattern of scientific work was to be found in industrial research. There, large teams had been responsible for such breakthroughs as the tungsten lightbulb and nylon. In general, the group, not the individual, was given credit, a style very different from past science. In the 1950s it would be denounced as signifying the triumph of 'The Organization Man'.[69] On the other hand, its successes meant that, while it had once been the preserve of the chemical and electrical industries, it was becoming more widespread.

With the power of big business behind it, in the United States industrial research was just then becoming the major employer of scientists in general. Between the 1920s and the 1950s, the standing of industrial research, compared to universities, shifted from a dwarf to a giant, and it was in wartime that the reversal of roles became evident.[70] A survey conducted by the American Chemical Society of its members in 1941 showed that in 1926 approaching a quarter had been teaching in university, but only one-sixth had been employed in industrial research. Over the succeeding fifteen years, progressively more had come to work in industry and fewer in teaching so that, by 1941, the 1926 ratios had been exactly reversed: one-quarter worked in industrial research and one-sixth in academe. Britain and the rest of the world were behind, but on the same trajectory. If in retrospect we can see that the 1930s had already experienced the growth of a new moral economy that linked science and industry, the cultural assimilation of such shifts had been a slow process, which had accelerated rapidly under the pressure of wartime development, and particularly that of penicillin.

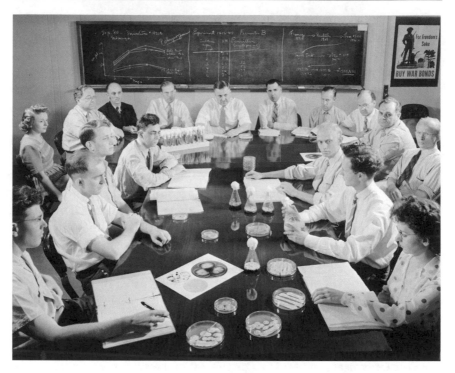

7. The team at the Northern Regional Research Laboratory discussing penicillin. This scale of collaborative work was characteristic of industry but new to academic and even government science.

Fritz Goro/Time-Life/Getty Images.

The significance of the industrial model could be seen most clearly in the fermentation group at the Peoria laboratory, which expanded considerably during the war from its small beginnings. A wartime photograph shows a group of fifteen people around a table (see Ill.7). The team had become so large that even those closely connected with it were not aware of the contributions made by each participant. When, some years later, Chester Keefer, who had been responsible for distributing penicillin during the war, sent the draft of a historical article to the laboratory for checking, he received a critical response. The laboratory suggested that names of the key people be omitted completely, rather than accepting a very partial list.[71] Heatley himself was similarly chastised when he sent the draft of an article for a two-volume summary of penicillin being prepared by the British. His adviser at the Northern Regional Research Laboratory commented on the text submitted: 'I may say that throughout our studies there was a great deal of team work, and it is often very difficult to say just who was responsible for one phase of the development and who was responsible for another.... I would suggest that possibly the best solution is to leave out any references to names of persons and to refer to the work as developments at the Northern Regional Research Laboratory.'[72]

Thus not only did research conducted by industry itself become more important in the penicillin story—its culture also pervaded the teamwork, whether it was conducted in government laboratories, academe, or industry. The boundaries of science itself became blurred: the public in the USA and Britain were not only patients but also—through the press, public opinion, and anxious politicians—actors in the development itself. This new, complex system was difficult to comprehend: to many scientists, businessmen, and government administrators it seemed that they were trapped in iron webs of bureaucracy and beset by busybodies.

The transition from small to large scale was made possible by privately organized collaboration between companies and through the intervention of the US government into the scientific process. When Florey toured the USA in 1941, among his most important achievements had been to meet and convert his friend A. N. Richards, head of the US government's Committee on Medical Research of the OSRD (Office of Scientific Research and Development), and through him his boss, OSRD supremo Vannevar Bush. From a first meeting with companies in October 1941, the Committee on Medical Research would become the central point in the USA through which all data flowed. From 1944, as production increased, the War Production Board became the centre of a large network sharing expertise across twenty-five companies.

In Britain, official sponsorship of collaboration was less well organized. Late in 1942, through Fleming's Scottish connections, a minister responsible for the provision of war supplies became interested in the penicillin problem. Knowing Fleming through the Ayrshire Society, he convened a meeting of experts in industry and academe to see what could be done to resolve problems of supply.[73] Production of penicillin through fermentation was taken out of the hands of the MRC and given to the much more powerful Ministry of Supply, which had the backing of Prime Minister Churchill himself.[74]

Richards, the head of the US Committee on Medical Research, was himself a physiologist and pharmacologist. He believed that the best prospect for cheap penicillin lay with chemical synthesis, but the wealth of the United States and its distance from the war meant that its industry could afford to follow three paths to penicillin. Richards supported three parallel approaches: penicillin manufacture for immediate use, development of new methods of fermentation, and a major attempt at synthesis. It was he who met with the companies and persuaded them to engage with the challenges of the new medicine. While individual companies followed their own paths, their joint achievement was to give US industry a central role in the future of antibiotics.

The first fermentation projects were urgent and craft based. Perhaps surprisingly, the first company to make progress was the Chester County Mushroom Laboratories in West Chester, Pennsylvania, a suburb of Philadelphia. Although its business was the growing of mushrooms as food, the technical director, Raymond Rettew, had made a hobby out of studying the chemical substances produced by the fungi. Now he was interested in seeing whether his business could contribute to the war effort.[75] By the middle of 1943, Chester County Mushroom Laboratories were processing 42,000 surface cultures a day. thereby producing the majority of the world's penicillin. Other companies quickly followed, several applying the traditional method of fermenting vinegar and, still in 1943, growing penicillium on bran.[76]

The outlook for deep fermentation had, however, been transformed from distant prospect to an imminent practice in mid-1943. Although, as late as July, Coghill, head of fermentation in Peoria, told the British that submerged culture was only a long-term prospect, in August the Pfizer Corporation opened a 2,000-gallon pilot plant.[77]

Pfizer was a small New York chemical company, specializing in making citric acid, but even before the war it had already acquired unique industrial experience with deep fermentation, producing fumaric acid in this way. In December 1941 the Merck and Squibb corporations had signed an agreement to formally lead the American effort, and Pfizer joined them in September 1942. The vice-president of Pfizer, John Smith, whose own daughter had died of an infection before the advent of penicillin, decided eventually to bet his company on the submerged fermentation process. The board backed him, and the company unilaterally put all its resources into developing the new process. Within four months of the opening of its 2,000-gallon fermenter, half the company's production was coming from that one tank.

The company then decided to build a full-scale plant immediately. Even in the United States, resources were short in wartime. Needing to convert a Brooklyn ice factory, Pfizer had problems obtaining even an elevator to move materials. A faulty vacuum on the freeze-dryer held up production. The fermenters that were installed were difficult to sterilize.

Smith, who 'followed every tank, every potency and everything on a day to day basis', used to invite staff to join him for lunch on what was informally known as the 'ulcer table', because of the level of worry.[78] Through such worrying and concern for detail, the company achieved success beyond anybody else's expectation. The following February, Pfizer opened the first commercial submerged fermentation plant. Containing fourteen main production tanks, each of 34,000-litre capacity, the plant was described by Florey as 'a miracle of construction and organisation'.[79] A visitor from another company put the success down to a century of experience in fermentation and an obsession with cleanliness.[80]

In 1944, Pfizer produced half America's penicillin. So it was at first dominant, but it was not alone. During the course of the war, over twenty US companies were involved in penicillin manufacture. With government permission and exemption from anti-trust legislation, they shared technology with each other and with academic institutions. In the industrial concerns seeking to make the drug by means of large-scale fermentation, scientists and engineers overcame novel challenges that have often been overlooked.[81] Never before had they had to handle biological processes of such sensitivity on an industrial scale. Contamination in water supplies, a leaking refrigerator, or strains mutating under the genetic pressure of ultraviolet lights used to sterilize air could create crises whose effects were easy to see but whose causes were hard to diagnose. An entirely new system for enhancing and mass-producing potent moulds, and extracting active chemicals, had to be devised. This aggregation of skills would be the subject of a journal established in 1957 and first entitled *Journal of Microbiological and Biochemical Engineering*, which in 1960 was condensed to *Biotechnology and Bioengineering*.[82] Penicillin technology thus became biotechnology.

Whereas, before the war, US companies in the pharmaceutical industry were far behind their German competitors, there was no doubt, in the early post-war years, that US companies dominated the world market. The development of the new drug had required an impressive growth of research. The laboratories at Merck, for instance, grew from thirty-five employees in 1933 to 500 in 1945.[83] It was not only traditional drug companies that had improved their standing. Pfizer, which had not even been involved in pharmaceuticals before the war, became a major world player by the early 1950s, largely on the back of penicillin.

The US production of more than 4 tonnes of pure drug in 1945 was about 300 times greater than just two years earlier.[84] The companies received hefty amounts of government support for the plants they built—more than $7 million during the war—which were purchased back at half the price thereafter.[85] However, industry invested much more of its own money too—and made a major commitment, even if much of their money might otherwise have been taken by the government as excess profits tax. In all, the fourteen wartime penicillin plants cost about $30 million.

For US industry the penicillin story was a triumph, but the manufacturers in the country of Fleming, Florey, and Chain have had a bad reputation. It was Florey's low opinion of the capacity of British industry that had encouraged him to go to America. Yet, had it not been for the even more impressive work of the Americans, the British performance might have seemed remarkable. They overcame their lack of experience with the cultivation of moulds without the assistance of such a centre as Peoria. To compensate for individual weakness, the companies tried to work closely together, and established their own hierarchy of collaborative organizations, the Therapeutic Research Corporation, which brought manufacturers together and ran a meeting, the 'Penicillin Producers' Conference', every six weeks or so. This involved not just major companies, but also academic advisers and researchers working on penicillin, including Alexander Fleming, Harold Raistrick from the London School of Hygiene, and Ian Heilbron and A. H. Cook from Imperial College London.[86]

British firms confronted conditions different from those which proved so fruitful in the USA. In a summary published immediately after the war, two participants contrasted the British with the American experience:

[In the United States the problems of plant design] were also solved thanks to the energy and skill of American engineers. In Great Britain energy and skill had to be expressed in the effective use of plant that was in part 'ersatz' and largely improvised and of labour that was largely 'directed' and almost entirely unskilled.[87]

The immediate needs imposed by conflict determined the perspective of industry in Britain. We can follow the experience of four key companies: Boots, I.C.I, Kemball Bishop, and Glaxo.[88] They were not much smaller than their American counterparts: indeed, Boots and ICI were both larger companies, although neither was well established in the new scientific drugs business. Above all, they lacked experience in deep fermentation. Luck also played a role.

The Boots story is an instructive lesson in the role of bad luck. It shows the uncertainty that surrounded the identity and prospects of the new drug during the early 1940s. The company was Britain's foremost chain of chemists; it also had substantial research and production arm facilities in Nottingham, including a complex, with some of Britain's foremost modernist buildings.[89]

The head of bacteriology, C. E. Coulthard, had met Alexander Fleming in the 1920s and seems to have kept up a close relationship with him. Some time in the early 1930s, Fleming gave a sample of his mould to Coulthard in the hope that 'we' might 'be able to get our chemists working on it'.[90] Working with scientists in other organizations, Coulthard explored another much more plentiful germ killer produced by the mould when it was fed the sugar glucose.[91] This material was at first thought to be possibly a penicillin and was called 'Penicillin A', but its properties and behaviour were quite different from those of penicillin and the team renamed it 'Notatin'.[92] Scientists in the US came upon the same product which later proved to be of considerable scientific interest, even if it was not penicillin.[93]

So the first company to make penicillin industrially was Britain's largest chemical company, Imperial Chemical Industries (I.C.I.). This was a large company on a global scale with dozens of times the number of employees such a company as Merck. Deciding to overcome its total lack of experience in fermentation and the cultivation of microbes, it built a small production line on the site of its Manchester dyeworks at the end of 1941, which came to produce about thirty doses a week, and in early 1943 senior staff toured the USA.[94] They were impressed by the Chester County Mushroom works, and came back to design production facilities with a projected investment of £300,000.

Immediately after I.C.I. had started taking an interest in penicillin, in the middle of 1942, a company much more experienced in fermentation offered its help to Florey. The Pfizer associate Kemball Bishop was an old-established London company specializing in making citric acid by fermentation on large trays, a process that it had learned from Pfizer. Unlike the American company, it did not achieve deep fermentation, but it overcame the problems of infection to apply its tray technology to penicillin production.[95] Every week it could supply 400 litres of the soup containing in all about one-third of a gram of penicillin to Oxford, where the drug was extracted.[96] This albeit limited output kept Oxford going during the hard year of 1942.

So short were supplies from British industry that the Royal Navy established its own small production unit in 1942. Its production of 200 million units a week (roughly appropriate for 200 patients) was comparable with the output of industrial companies until the middle of 1943. Based at the Royal Naval Medical School in Clevedon, it was a significant training centre as well as a production unit. Rather than the bedpans used in Oxford, the navy used gin bottles, of which it had a large supply.[97]

In 1943, the British manufacturers increased their interest and planned to begin mass production. Most of them planned facilities that were essentially expanded versions of Florey's academic pilot plant. They were much slower than the American companies to go for deep fermentation—partly because materials essential to maintain sterility, such as stainless steel, were in short supply, and partly because they lacked the American expertise in fermentation.[98] It was a misfortune that, at the crucial moment in the decision making of the key companies in July 1943, Americans advised a meeting of the 'Penicillin conference' that submerged culture still had to be considered a long-term prospect.[99] Moreover, the advice of the distinguished chemist Sir Robert Robinson, Oxford professor and a grand panjandrum, was also immensely influential. He was quite confident that penicillin would be synthesized in a chemical plant and that therefore a deep fermentation plant would be a costly irrelevance.[100] Rather than investing in this clearly risky long-term technology, the British companies focused on maximizing manufacture by the most reliable means available: surface culture.

The chemical engineer Frederick Warner did design a deep fermentation plant. But it would require a considerable amount of scarce stainless steel, and the Ministry of Supply rejected the request on the advice of Sir Robert. Although the British did finally decide to build submerged fermenter plants in the middle of 1944, these did not start producing penicillin until the end of 1945—eighteen months later.[101] This lag of eighteen months was in fact not dissimilar to the experience of several US manufacturers.

When, by contrast, Boots built a large Oxford-type plant, with a million milk bottles, it was producing within six months of the first soil being cut. So, whether or not a submerged fermentation plant would have been commercially advantageous to the British, there would have been little prospect of it being useful in war. A Boots company brochure compared its surface fermentation plant to a 'Bailey Bridge'—serviceable but temporary. Its demands did, however, lead to a national shortage of milk bottles.[102] Similarly pragmatic, Kemball Bishop maintained their early surface culture technology, just increasing the scale of production, which went up from 50 trays in 1942 to 200 trays in 1944 and then 600 trays a year later.[103]

The most important of the British manufacturers during the war was the Glaxo company. Formerly a producer of dried milk, during the 1930s its interests had moved via nutrition to vitamins and thence to the fermentation production of vitamin B. Without a long scientific background but deploying an outward-looking approach, Glaxo obtained from the Americans information and the idea of using cornsteep liquor as well as the improved Peoria strain. Starting with a small plant in 1942, Glaxo scaled up quickly, so that in 1943 its production was roughly equivalent to a kilo and a half of pure penicillin, about a third as much as Pfizer.[104]

While Pfizer moved to submerged culture, the British fought gamely on to improve surface methods. A new Glaxo plant used 300,000 flasks—a far cry from the few hundred at Oxford.[105] Early in 1944 the impact of the new facilities was beginning to show. In May Britain's production was over 2,000 million units, the equivalent to about a kilogram of pure product, say the same size as a domestic bag of sugar or flour. This was almost seven times the production rate at the beginning of the year. Glaxo supplied the raw drug to Burroughs Wellcome, who packaged it for bulk distribution, and to individual scientists for research. Alexander Fleming himself was asked to test samples.[106] A Glaxo plant opened at Stratford in East London in 1945 produced at the rate of over 30 kilograms a year of pure penicillin.[107] This was twenty times more than the plant of two years earlier, but not much compared to the USA's production measured in tonnes or thousands of kilograms.

In 1943, British production had been comparable to the American, but the next year it would be less than 2.5 per cent of the American.[108] The British were able to meet just one-twentieth of their own requirements, importing the rest from the USA. Companies in the country where penicillin had been discovered had fallen behind. In response, Glaxo bought rights from Merck and Squibb to build a plant in Durham's Barnard Castle. With its cathedral-like fermenter hall, the new factory, opened in 1946, was the equal of an American plant. A writer in the company newsletter joked, 'I almost begin to feel sorry for the Yanks.'[109]

Struggling to make up for lost ground, the British government went into partnership with the US Commercial Solvents Corporation, the second-largest producer in the USA. In Speke near Liverpool they spent £1.3 million to build the world's largest penicillin factory.[110] This was then transferred to the UK's alcohol company Distillers which had limited experience of chemical manufacture through fermentation though none in pharmaceutical manufacture.[111] At the end of the war, therefore, two large submerged fermentation plants were under construction in Britain, with others due to follow. All the surface plants had closed by the end of 1946; total British production was approaching a third of the American, and per head of population it had once again reached parity.[112] The lag that seemed so significant at the time was therefore short-lived.

Shortages caused by the war had certainly been important to the slower pace of British development. Perhaps, as importantly, the country had lacked fermentation experience and know-how. While it was a centre of expertise in bacteriology, at the beginning of the Second World War it was a backwater in the development of modern fermentation technologies. There were no relevant skills to bring together. Thirdly, the microbiologists had to compete with chemists who were powerful both in academe, and, through the great chemical combine I.C.I. in industry.

To most chemists, the future of penicillin manufacture was a synthesis from simpler chemicals without the need for the messy intervention of a mould. In both the UK and the USA, the best long-term prospect seemed to be this procedure, which had worked for a hundred years. Brewing might be suitable for making an impure food like beer, but in 1942 the model of manufacture was chemical synthesis. Through much of the war it seemed, both in the USA and in the UK, that penicillin would be synthetically manufactured in the long run and therefore that a major effort should be made to find the chemical route. The synthesis enterprise used the work of more than a thousand chemists working in 'four British and five American universities, five British and ten American pharmaceutical and chemical firms, one British and four American government agencies, and two British and two American research foundations'.[113] Private companies invested over three million dollars of their own money in the attempt—Merck alone spent $800,000.

The fermentation route was bedevilled by patent disputes, and it seemed to penicillin policy makers both in the USA and in the UK that it would be important to prevent a similar problem recurring in what seemed, in the longer term, the more important area of chemical synthesis. Thus, introducing the issue of a patent pool in December 1944, the Secretary of the MRC, Edward Mellanby, said it was certain that biological methods of production would be replaced.[114] A formal international treaty specifying the conditions for the exchange of information, licensing rights, and the allocation of patenting rights on synthesis between the various parties was negotiated between the United States of America and Her Britannic Majesty's government. Alfred Elder, who was appointed coordinator of the US penicillin programme in 1943, later recalled, 'I was ridiculed by some of my closest scientific friends for allowing myself to become associated with what obviously was to be a flop—namely, the commercial production of penicillin by a fermentation process.'[115] In the event, penicillin proved very hard to synthesize, and even when a full synthesis was developed in the late 1950s, it was not commercially competitive with the fermentation-derived product. Nonetheless, many of the results derived through this programme fed back into the broader project and would make an important contribution to it. The science and the technology of the penicillin projects would be closely interconnected.

Thus the synthesis project gave high priority to the problem of under-standing penicillin's structure. The solution would prove valuable to refining the fermentation process too, but this challenge alone proved practically, institutionally, and above all intellectually challenging, ulti-mately requiring the most modern of technologies. Practically, it was made more difficult by the shortage of pure material to analyse. Not until early 1943 was it possible to obtain penicillin pure enough to work out what kind of elements it contained. In their early analyses, the chemists missed a sulphur atom, which of course misled them in determining the structure. Institutionally, the problem was worsened when Robert Robin-son committed himself to a chemical structure that did not admit to a sulphur atom. Such was his status that it was hard to challenge his belief. Crystals were essential for testing this, and not until late 1943, at just the time the problems of submerged fermentation were being overcome, was a penicillin salt finally crystallized—at roughly the same time by Squibb in the USA and at Oxford. At this point it transpired that the British and Americans were working with two slightly different compounds. The use of cornsteep liquor to grow the penicillium mould had actually changed the product—for the good. Penicillin was in fact a family of products, not a single compound, and already four penicillins could be identified. The British penicillin was known as Penicillin F (probably for Florey) and the American as Penicillin G.[116] Such analytical success gave the chemists hope that synthesis was now within their grasp. Nonetheless, it still took two years to prove Robert Robinson wrong.

The structure was finally established through the X-ray crystallography of Dorothy Hodgkin at the University of Oxford, already a well-respected X-ray crystallographer and future Nobel Prize winner (see Ill.8).[117] In her attack on penicillin, Hodgkin interpreted the very large amounts of data by using the calculating power of modern electromagnetic punch-card machines otherwise used to plan convoys. Her funders at the Medical Research Council were so shocked by the size of her bill for computation, greater than everything else, that they wrote saying they were confident there had been an error.[118] Hodgkin's reply assured them there was no error and pointed out that in fact the calculations had been done with remarkable economy. Meanwhile, at nearby Bletchley Park the new digital computer, COLOSSUS, was being used to decode German signals, in Philadelphia the ENIAC computer was being used for atomic bomb calculations, and in Germany Konrad Zuse's S1 computer had been used for aircraft design. Computation was becoming a new scientific discipline.

The increasing chemical understanding of the drug enabled refinement of the growing media. At first, developing the mix of nutrients had been an ad hoc, not to say arcane, art. It had, for instance, been discovered emprically that adding hair cuttings to the nutrients improved the penicillin yield.[119] When the sulphur content of penicillin was confirmed, this need was both explained and superseded, as better means of adding sulphur were used. Equally, phenylacetic acid was added, as it was understood that a branch using this chemical was characteristic of Penicillin G.[120] Other improvements related not to the production of raw penicillin but to its compounding into a medicine. Because it was an acid, it could be combined with an alkali to make what is called a salt. A variety of salts were tried in the early days: sodium and potassium were the most common. Chemists at Eli Lilly, the pharmaceutical company

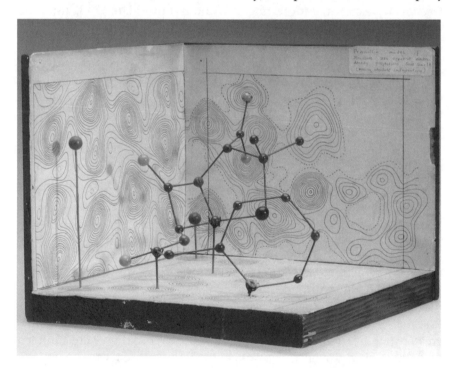

8. Model of the penicillin molecule devised by Professor Dorothy Hodgkin in 1945. Now in the collection of the Science Museum, inventory number 1996–206.
Science Museum/Science & Society Picture Library.

based in Indianapolis in America's Mid-West, became especially adept at modifying the chemical groups attached to the central core by changing the nutrients supplied during fermentation.[121] Soon the penicillins were distinguished not just by letters, but by understanding of the differences between the chemical groups that made them up. So penicillin G came to be known as benzyl penicillin.

Mass production by fermentation made possible the widespread distribution of penicillin to the military and to the public. In the first half of 1943, the USA produced less than one billion units of penicillin. In the second half of the same year, more than 20 billion were produced. The next year, when submerged fermentation plants started coming in, production was 1,663 billion units—an eightyfold increase on the previous year. The US government purchased penicillin at an agreed price, roughly equivalent to $9,000 an ounce (28g) in mid-1943—weight for weight about 250 times the price of gold.[122] Within a year, the cost fell by a factor of ten and kept falling. A dose that might have cost $20 in 1943 would be only 6.5 cents by the end of the war.[123]

The collapse in the price had been made possible by the organized collaboration among scientists whose fabled power would colour the opinion of penicillin in the future. Such processes were not unique to this drug, but the pencillin initiative was so much larger than any other in the medical sphere that it became iconic. This experience, and the experience of the medical impact of penicillin, would be translated into popular expectations by the mass media and shaped by expectations for what was quickly called a wonder drug. The brand, as well as the chemical, was refined in wartime, and it is to that we now turn.

3

Creating the Brand in the Era of Propaganda

The new drug's effects were so dramatic that they had a powerful impact on all who heard of or saw them. Such infections as pneumonia, rheumatic fever, gas gangrene, syphilis, and gonorrhoea, as well as sore throats, earaches, and boils, often yielded remarkably quickly. A 1946 report for pharmacists produced by Britain's Pharmaceutical Society reported that 'susceptible diseases... generally respond to a few massive doses'.[1] The Society then went on to observe that patients were demanding that 'no person should be allowed to die without having been given penicillin'.[2] This gruesome, latter-day version of the last rites expressed a belief in the brand that went beyond any mundane interpretation of its medical significance. The drama of penicillin's story itself fostered medical interest and patients' optimism. These were important in the 'selling' of the drug to the medical profession, to industry, and to the authorities during the war. The drug's medical influence, the perceived triumph of the new model of collaborative bioscience, and propaganda were intimately interconnected.

Inappropriate as it may, initially, seem to compare the early accounts of penicillin's development to propaganda, in the wake of the war, and against the legacy of the Depression, the penicillin story was used to serve widespread reform and exemplify 'modernization'. Accounts of the use and history of the drug appeared in newspapers and magazines, a major documentary was made, books were commissioned, and the story was retold in Parliament and Congress. Such interpretations of history to construct policy and culture did not detract from an appreciation of the medical potential; instead, they continually re-emphasized the qualities of the penicillin brand.

Penicillin became available to patients at a time when publics across the world yearned for good news. It was not just the war itself that was wearying. In many countries, rationing lasted till well after the Second World War. Even in Canada it outlasted the war by two years, and other less well-endowed countries suffered longer. The very word 'austerity' long evoked the legacy of the post-war years. Against the shortage of many luxuries, penicillin was a symbol of the wider range of effective medicines then becoming available. More than that, as the historian David Adams has pointed out, it symbolized the prospect of a new, more luxurious life that would be born through the suffering of war.[3]

Public perception was intimately connected with stories of how the drug could be used and its benefits. Time and again early accounts of the medical effect were linked to predictions of the future. Thus, in the USA, a dramatic demonstration of the power of penicillin was provided after it was used for the first time on large numbers of civilians in November 1942, in the aftermath of America's worst fire, at the Cocoanut Grove night club.[4] This Boston dance hall was packed with more than a thousand people, many of them servicemen with their sweethearts. By the next morning 492 people had died, and the fearfully burned survivors were in danger of long-term infection as well as suffering. Although the scarce supply of surface-fermented penicillin had been reserved for clinical trials, stocks were released and many patients were saved. The press was ecstatic. *Time* magazine reported that 'the wonder drug of 1943 may prove to be penicillin'.[5]

Florey himself used the prospective rhetorical power of a healing miracle to stir industrial interest in 1941, when he conducted his very first clinical trial on Police Constable Alexander. Although he achieved neither a medical nor a public relations breakthrough on that occasion, the principle of seeking the two together was established.

The earliest systematic experiments on servicemen were conducted in 1942 under the supervision of Ethel, Howard Florey's wife, on airmen recovering from burns in a few hospitals across Britain.[6] This was a time when bomber crews were returning with terrible burns. Other experiments were conducted at the Glasgow Royal Infirmary and the General Military Hospital near Oxford. During 1942, Ethel Florey also conducted studies of the use of penicillin on patients with infections of the eye and also of the inner ear's mastoid bone. Together with the dramatic study of Fleming and the American work, penicillin's general utility was now being proven. However, could the army be convinced?

In July 1942 the first samples of penicillin were sent to the front in North Africa. These were tiny quantities, which the local medical officer,

Major Pulvertaft, tried to supplement by growing the mould himself and using the juice directly on patients. That autumn, after the battle of Alamein, more supplies arrived from I.C.I. Florey himself visited North Africa early in 1943 to try out the effects of his drug. Ironically, his arrival coincided with a lull in fighting and there were no casualties with fresh wounds on whom to demonstrate his medicine. Treating the badly infected chronically ill soldiers he saw would not provide the dramatic demonstration to the army that he needed. However, in July 1943, Sicily was invaded, and wounded soldiers were returned to North Africa for treatment. Testing his medicine in novel conditions, Florey merely put penicillin powder into a wound and sewed it up. To the amazement of medical colleagues, infection was totally prevented. The dramatic findings of Florey in North Africa convinced the British army of the benefits of penicillin. On returning from his travels, Florey worked with the War Office to train 200 pathologists and 500 clinicians in the use of the new drug.[7]

Investigations of the drug's potential for the US military, were conducted separately—and at first more slowly. Up to February 1943, American physicians had studied just 143 patients. Then their work accelerated. About twenty physicians were working on the project, and the repute of their work spread. In April 1943 a report from the main centre of testing, the Bushnell Hospital in Utah, reported magnificent results.[8] The researchers confirmed the ability of penicillin to defeat infections caused by large classes of bacteria. Thus a soldier with multiple machine gun wounds in his leg had been protected from infection. Many soldiers with already horribly infected wounds, who would otherwise have died, could now be saved. Still the military were not particularly enthusiastic to find adequate resources. Champ Lyons, in charge of a second centre in Staten Island, New York, complained in June 1943 that the army was 'feeling its way' and that the red tape around the project 'was made of tempered steel'. He felt the drug should either be used or withdrawn. Urging the Surgeon General's office to make up its mind, he wrote that they need 'to fish or cut bait'.[9]

However, the results on wounds that Lyons reported and the success of the drug against gonorrhoea greatly impressed the US military.[10] From the end of the North Africa campaign in 1943, British and American soldiers began to get penicillin in significant quantities. By the time of the subsequent invasion of Sicily and then the fighting in Italy, there was enough for all the wounded. The doctors even successfully argued that it be given to German as well as Allied casualties.[11] In the words of two British surgeons, some of the medical teams were sceptical about the effects on the wounded of the 'quasi-scientific blunderbuss of modern prophylaxis and therapy'.[12] The effects on infection were, however, seen to be dramatic. The same surgeons noted the shifting state of wounds: in the first phase of the retreat from France, the average wound was 'an angry inflamed affair'. The North Africa campaign had seen the sulpha drug phase, in which the spreading of infection became much more rare but wounds remained 'the site of an active local infection'. With the subsequent widespread use of penicillin, infection was typically 'depressed to an almost negligible quantity'.[13]

Statistically it is difficult to separate the benefit of penicillin from the generally well-developed medical treatment of wounded and sick soldiers. The historian Mark Harrison has explored the sophisticated pattern of infection management by the British army.[14] Across the war its soldiers wounded in battle who managed to reach surgical care had a nine to one chance of survival.[15] Harrison points out that even at the time of the battle of Alamein, before penicillin was available, the British troops were much healthier than their German opponents.[16] At the battle itself one in five of the German troops were already sick. Even Rommel, their distinguished general, was suffering from hepatitis. Harrison points out the complex mix of reasons which included the long experience of the British in fighting in hot climates, and a generally more protective attitude to their men.[17] So, when, later, penicillin became available, its use was integrated into an already sophisticated medical culture.

Even an early post-war official study found difficulty in separating out the effect that penicillin had when it was introduced progressively more widely from 1943.[18] Although the collection of accurate and comparative clinical data had not been a high priority in battle conditions, a remarkably conscientious attempt was made to analyse the fate of casualties. A few of the statistics that could be compiled did seem to underpin the ecstatic response of military doctors to the new drug. Of soldiers who suffered arterial wounds about half suffered infective complications if they did not get penicillin but the infection rate was halved for those with penicillin. Similarly of soldiers with chest wounds, the death from infection fell almost two-thirds if penicillin treatment was used.[19] The impact of penicillin of course could really seem miraculous. By the time of the last year of the war only one wounded British soldier (below the rank of officer) in thirteen died from his wounds if he could reach medical assistance. A further two in thirteen were subsequently invalided out of the army. Ironically this number was twice as great as it had been in the

First World War, perhaps because, an official medical history surmised, the lives of more severely wounded men were now being saved.[20]

The benefits of penicillin in the treatment of the venereal diseases syphilis and gonorrhoea had a special meaning to patients, to doctors, to the image of these diseases in the wider society, and to the future of penicillin. These infections have always been a particular threat in wartime, and in the Second World War, with young men a long way from home, there was a constant danger of infection from prostitutes. Until penicillin, the treatment of syphilis in particular was slow and uncertain. Gonorrhoea was susceptible, in principle, to sulphonamides, but many strains of the disease had become resistant to them. Penicillin proved to heal marvellously quickly. Uncomplicated gonorrhoea could now be cured by a single day of treatment of penicillin, which was 98 per cent effective.[21] A sailor treated in 1944 remarked that now the disease was of less significance than a cold.[22] Even more excitement was raised by the discovery that syphilis would also yield instantly.

In June 1943, the director of the venereal disease research laboratory at New York's massive Staten Island Marine Hospital, John Mahoney, tested penicillin on four syphilis sufferers.[23] Within a week, all four were completely cured. When in October Mahoney presented his results to a conference of the American Public Health Association in New York, 'Everyone strained to hear what was said, and the impact was electrifying', in the words of one participant.[24]

Syphilis would be the single most important target of penicillin for the next few years, both in war and in peace. An irreverent note on the desk of Albert Elder, the project leader for the US production programme, read: 'The goal—to make penicillin so cheaply that it costs less to cure it than to get it!'[25] In the North Africa campaign, both US and British surgeons were told: if units of penicillin given to victims of gonorrhoea would get men back to the front faster than the same scarce medicine given to soldiers wounded in battle, then victims of the bordello had priority.[26]

Compared to the existing sulphonamides, penicillin had turned out to have several great advantages. The older medicine often caused side-effects ranging from nausea and sickness to rashes and inflammation, while, although some patients did react allergically to penicillin, most people could take therapeutic doses of the new drug without experiencing any side-effects.[27] Penicillin could also be used in a number of contexts in which sulphonamides were just ineffective. Wounds that were already infected, for instance, posed great challenges to such drugs, whose action was much weaker in the presence of pus and dirt. Nor did they have any effect on syphilis, which was speedily cured with penicillin. Finally, many bacteria, such as those which caused gonorrhoea, had rapidly developed resistance to the sulphonamides, and a new medicine was needed to treat cases that had recently become incurable.

The line between careful observation and ecstatic response was hard to keep. In February 1943 Mellanby, as Secretary of the Medical Research Council, sought to broaden tests of penicillin away from the Oxford team. He suggested to Florey that having now had the 'cream' of the investigation he should let others follow up.[28] So, despite Florey's concerns that he would have to compete for still scarce supplies, the Penicillin Clinical Trials Committee was established by the Council. Against this still cautious scientific approach, the desperate sick were turning to penicillin in unmanageable numbers. Although both British and American clinicians hoped to focus attention and scarce material on systematic trials, they were under enormous pressure from patients anxious for a last chance of life. The papers of Howard Florey are full of pleading from total strangers and from their physicians for a last-chance treatment with the wonder drug.[29]

In April 1943, for instance, the mother of quadruplets born in 1937 wrote in desperation. One of her children having successfully reached the age of 5 in healthy condition was now in a high fever. Infection had spread across his body and the sulphonamides being used to control some of the symptoms were making the child vomit, while failing to cure him. Florey marked the letter, 'none available'. Two weeks later he received a letter from a physican at the very Wolverhampton hospital at which M&B 693 had been so successfully used a few years earlier. Bacteria infecting a six-week-old child were producing uncontrollable boils across the infant's body. Florey wrote back, 'I am sorry we cannot do anything about it.'

In the USA, too, special requests were made to the controllers of this life-giving medicine. In March 1942, Anne Miller, a Connecticut patient with a worsening staphylococcal infection, shared a physician with a fellow patient at the New Haven hospital, John Fulton, Howard Florey's friend. When her temperature reached 107 °F, her physician turned to Fulton for help.[30] Although no American had yet been cured with penicillin, he got on the telephone and within a few days had obtained a small quantity. The drug was injected, the patient's temperature returned to normal, and she was to live a further fifty-seven years until her death in May 1999.

Celebrities could, naturally, be accorded special treatment: penicillin saved the life of actress and singer Marlene Dietrich, who contracted pneumonia in Bari, Italy, in 1943 while entertaining the troops.[31] Meanwhile, ordinary civilians could only get such treatment on an experimental basis through a few hospitals. The media reported numerous stories of children at death's door receiving a life-giving injection, often after the intervention of a newspaper or a benevolent industrialist.[32] The wonderful nature of penicillin, the relief of the children and the elderly, and the crusading ambitions of newspapers went together like a jigsaw puzzle.

Above all, there were calls to release supplies to treat those with heart disease caused by bacterial infection. News of the military experiments caused great excitement and raised expectations. News of penicillin's benefits resonated with pre-war expectation of a wonder drug. By June 1943, the Medical Research Council's liaison officer in Washington was reporting, 'Penicillin is surging upwards and is going to have a tremendous vogue here.'[33] Paul De Kruif, the science journalist, later recalled how the *Reader's Digest* had backed Jack Smith of Pfizer, who again in June 1943 had given a large quantity of penicillin to a child dying in a New York hospital from subacute bacterial endocarditis. The doctor, Leo Loewe, had suggested that enormous doses, equivalent to two months of the entire British production, would cure a patient, against the judgement of OSRD. Penicillin was still scarce and needed by the troops. Allocating such a large quantity to one sick child was not efficient, but it did move the audience of *Reader's Digest*. De Kruif described how his article had changed the medical mood:

But the *Digest* editors, trusting us, bet their chips on Leo and Jack Smith and published our story and in a few months Leo had cured so many incurable endocarditis victims that it would have caused a real stink if the OSRD hadn't eased penicillin for subacute bacterial endocarditis. So they released it.[34]

As supplies increased in 1944, penicillin moved from experimental treatment to icon. Within the USA, there was enough for civilians as well as military patients. On 1 May 1944, 1,000 US civilian hospitals were allocated penicillin. Just five weeks later, on D-Day, 6 June 1944, Allied troops landed well supplied on French beaches. The preparations for the US army invasion specified that penicillin was to be administered by powder in open wounds and parentarally (by means of a drip) as close to the battle front as possible.[35] The images of soldiers being treated on the beaches would become widely distributed testimonies to a wonder drug. Such a picture was, for instance, incorporated in the well-known advertisement for the manufacturer Schenley Laboratories published in *Life* magazine, under the heading 'Thanks to Penicillin He Will Come

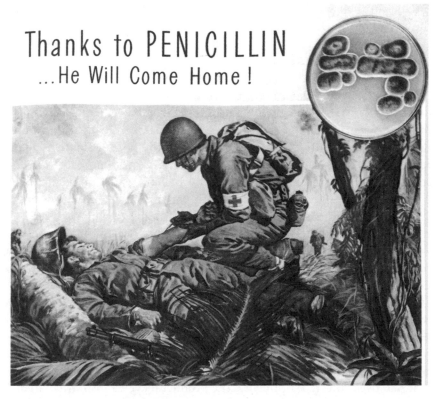

9. Classic illustration from a wartime penicillin advertisement for the products of Schenley Laboratories.

British Library P.P.6383 cke.

Home!' (Ill. 9). The use of the drug was therefore intimately interconnected with national propaganda and commercial marketing.

In August 1945 the drug became freely available through US pharmacies, in most states, to all who wanted to buy it. Britain was about a year behind its transatlantic ally in supplying penicillin to its people, and stories about Americans getting the drug caused bitter envy, while in the land of its discovery war victims were dying for the lack of it. Although the British government was still trying to reserve its scarce supplies for the military, from the middle of 1944 it succumbed to pressure and released a dribble to selected civilian patients.[36] With increasing production and imports from the USA, the pressure quickly eased there too, and in June 1946, less than a year after the war's end, any doctor was free to prescribe penicillin. The period of relative shortage was over, and pharmacies advertised the product in their windows as, one day, computer stores would announce the arrival of the latest operating system.

It is striking that the public image of early penicillin seems to have omitted the pain of the injection. Penicillin tended to be destroyed by the stomach's acids so, to eliminate substantial infections, the stomach needed to be bypassed, and that meant a drip into a vein or injections. At first injections had to be given eight times a day, and the impurity of the product meant that this could be very painful. Czechoslovak Armoured Brigade soldier Walter Ehrlich, associated with the British forces, later remembered his experience after he had been badly wounded in northern France and taken back to a hospital in Basingstoke, England.[37] He described a nurse going from patient to patient with her 'large syringe', injecting penicillin as she went, without bothering to change needles. 'I was told changing the needle was not necessary because penicillin prevents infections.' On the other hand, Ehrlich had received a serious injury; had penicillin not been available, his leg would have been amputated. Each injection could cause 'burning and smarting' that lasted up to half an hour. Jessie Carter, a young civilian, was treated at the very end of the war. She describes the feeling as if 'they'd injected boiling water. It was a very uncomfortable injection. Very uncomfortable.'[38]

Some improvements were, it is true, made quickly. Wartime penicillin was generally impure, and the body often reacted to the protein impurities that had been injected. Ironically, the product recycled from the patient's urine was often the purest available. Particularly after 1944, when the crystalline product became available, the problem of extraneous impurities was reduced. Release into the bloodstream was also slowed by adding impurities intentionally. One early solution was to suspend penicillin in a mixture of beeswax and peanut oil: this reduced the frequency of injections from eight times a day to three. However, while the beeswax reduced the frequency of injections, it increased the pain. An alternative solution proved to be more satisfactory. At the RAF hospital in Halton, Flight-Lieutenant Dennis Bodenham treated burned bomber crews.[39] He found that he could slow the metabolism of penicillin by adding the anaesthetic procaine, also known as Novocaine. The anaesthetic and the antibiotic, which he injected separately, were later chemically combined as the procaine salt of penicillin.

Although the injection was medically preferred, it is perhaps not surprising that some patients did seek out easier methods of taking the drug. For diseases of the mouth or throat, attractive lozenges and pastilles were soon available, although their effect was five times less than that when the medicine was injected or introduced directly into the body with a drip.[40] Other treatments for sore throats were also tried. At the US Naval Training Center in San Diego, physicians experimented with ice cream laced with penicillin.[41] So even before the more robust Penicillin V that could stand up to the rigours of the stomach became available in the mid-1950s, oral use had become common.

To the most enthusiastic visionaries, the promise of impregnated lipsticks linking red lips, sexual indiscretion, and syphilis, as well as lip sores, was irresistible. In his 1946 book *The Conquest of Disease*, the Russian-born British surgeon Alexis Milankovich (George Bankoff), told the public:

Soon young ladies will be able to buy their lipsticks impregnated with penicillin.... Penicillin will be like a guardian angel ready to halt any intruder that is unwelcome.... Penicillin given in sufficient doses to any would be dictator, or any evil genius trying to discover more potent rockets or liquid air bombs, will perhaps mellow their brain and subdue their evil desires.[42]

This promised performance in the theatre of unrealizable dreams would be but the forerunner of many more extravagant hopes as penicillin would be used to treat every infection and indeed many other complaints besides.

The story of penicillin's discovery was itself put to the service of propaganda. The early history which has come to be so well known was constructed at a time when all war stories were in some way national propaganda, but this one served particular institutional interests too. From mid-1942, just as the first airmen were being treated, but penicillin was still a very experimental drug, the benefits of therapy, the story of discovery, and prospects for the future came to be intimately connected. The Second World War was at its peak, and the fortunes of the Allies at their lowest. Although the United States had joined in the war and Britain was no longer alone, the Japanese were sweeping through the Pacific. In Europe, country after country had fallen to German invasion. The victories of Stalingrad in the Soviet Union and Alamein in North Africa would turn the tide, but they were still in the future. Good news was hard to come by. In July an employee in the optical company of Fleming's brother Robert suffered a brain infection. Fleming obtained some penicillin from Oxford and treated him successfully.

On 27 August an editorial in *The Times* newspaper in London announced: a wonder drug that would cure infection without side-effects had been developed by a British team.[43] Four days later, the public was told in a letter from St Mary's Hospital in London that the 'garland of honour' for the discovery was due to Alexander Fleming, who worked at the hospital.[44] A letter to *The Times* can be little more than the expression of a strong personal feeling, but this time it announced the beginning of a campaign. Journalists from London's *Evening Standard* newspaper were at the laboratory of Alexander Fleming looking for an interview even before *The Times* published its article.[45] Other journalists followed in rapid succession. Florey and Chain could not understand what had happened. An overwhelming press interest built up and focused upon the contribution of Fleming. Within a few days therefore Fleming had been made into a badly needed national hero and the discovery of penicillin a welcome triumph. His image appeared repeatedly in British magazines and in American ones too. Fleming's face dominated the front cover of a May 1944 issue of *Time* magazine, the very symbol of celebrity (see Ill. 10).[46] Inside he was described as a '20th century seer'.

The entry of penicillin into public life did not happen just through the activities of journalists. Grandees of British society also willed it. Their role lurks behind the activities of scientists, as the work of club chairmen and television executives frames the reputation of football clubs and their players. They propelled the fortunes of penicillin itself and its fabled discoverer Alexander Fleming into the realm of legend. St Mary's Hospital of course did not fail to prosper either. Even today a large plaque on the medical school's wall announces that Fleming discovered penicillin.

Seeking an explanation for the phenomenal transformation of penicillin, Florey and Chain saw the hand of Sir Charles Wilson.[47] He was no active scientist, but he was undeniably an interested and influential member of the establishment: the Dean of St Mary's, the physician to Prime Minister Winston Churchill, and from 1943, ennobled as Lord Moran. He may indeed have been instrumental in the 31 August letter to *The Times*. Certainly he ensured that St Mary's would be a beneficiary of the penicillin story and found opportunities to put down the influence of the Oxford team. So when Moran was asked to write a briefing note for Churchill on the reasons for the US lead in penicillin, he blamed Florey for giving British expertise away.[48]

A biographer of Alexander Fleming, Gwyn Macfarlane, has pointed to the importance of a second promoter of the St Mary's campaign, the long-time patient of Wilson, Lord Beaverbrook, owner of the *Evening Standard* and also of Britain's best-selling newspaper, the *Daily Express*.[49] Beaverbrook was an old friend of St Mary's. He had been a patron of the hospital since 1928, and may also have been specially interested in its asthma research (which was probably the accidental source of Fleming's

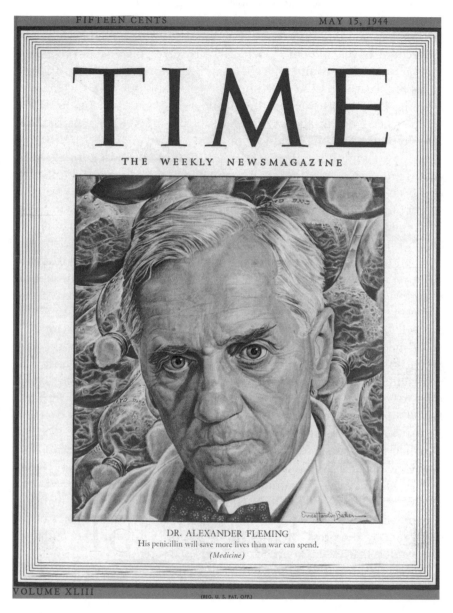

FIFTEEN CENTS   MAY 15, 1944

TIME
THE   WEEKLY   NEWSMAGAZINE

DR. ALEXANDER FLEMING
His penicillin will save more lives than war can spend.
(Medicine)

VOLUME XLIII   (REG. U. S. PAT. OFF.)

10. This cover shot of Alexander Fleming in *Time* in May 1944 confirmed his coronation as an American celebrity and created deep irritation amongst the Oxford team.

penicillium mould), for he was obsessed with his own asthma. Famous as the Minister of Aircraft Production responsible for transforming the prospects of building sufficient Spitfires and Hurricanes, he had resigned on account of his ailment.[50] Certainly his correspondence, even before the war, was full of complaints about his condition.[51] In 1955, at the end of his life, Beaverbrook recalled how he could not but help the cause of Fleming. On the other hand, he did not intervene often in the affairs of his papers and, in any case, it was not just Beaverbrook papers that jumped on the Fleming bandwagon.

As if two lords-a-leaping were not sufficient, a third jumped in as well. Lord McGowan, the chairman of Imperial Chemical Industries, had been a friend of Lord Beaverbrook since 1915. He had given his support to Beaverbrook's British Empire Campaign of the 1920s and they continued to be frequent correspondents. At the battle of Alamein in October 1942 McGowan's own son William was badly wounded. The I.C.I. pilot plant that had been gearing up sent penicillin immediately to Cairo and thereby saved William's life.[52] McGowan continued his support after the war, managing the financial side of the St Mary's Hospital Appeal and personally signing letters inviting support, sent together with a flyer headed 'Pay your debt to penicillin. Write a cheque to St Mary's now.'[53]

The medical research establishment, traditionally disdainful of the public's attitudes, was less self-conscious about the propaganda benefits of penicillin and more closely linked to the distinguished scientists at Oxford than to St Mary's. For instance, the President of the Royal Society was Robert Robinson, the Oxford chemist. Churchill's one-time adviser Sir Henry Tizard had retired to the mastership of Magdalen College, Oxford, of which Florey was a fellow. Tizard had to hear out Chain's complaints about the apparent conspiracy against the Oxford team seemingly being played out by Moran in London. Sir Edward Mellanby, Secretary of the Medical Research Council, despised the coverage received by Fleming as ephemeral.[54] When Florey complained about the relative neglect of his own team by the press, Mellanby assured him that it was the verdict of science that mattered. Chain, for one, was not convinced.

However, Oxford too acquired support from a more publicity-conscious nobleman. Lord Nuffield, head of Britain's largest car manufacturer, Morris Motors, itself based near the university, had a long-standing interest in medicine. Before the war he had offered to give an iron lung to every hospital in the British empire.[55] Nuffield had also fallen out with Beaverbrook who, while Minister of Aircraft Production, had dared to bully him.[56] Nuffield funded the Oxford team.

It would be a caricature of British society to portray its espousal of penicillin as the result of an antique aristocracy. In fact, Beaverbrook, McGowan, Moran, and Nuffield had all made their own way in life from humble beginnings. Their noble titles represented not inherited privilege, but the country's recognition of the formidable achievements they had each attained. Moreover, each was interested in public perception. They wanted to promote not just knowledge of penicillin among the elite, but also pride among the general public. Reckoning that pride could do work for the image of their organizations and of penicillin, they linked hopes for the new drug to national and institutional achievements.

The American pharmaceutical industry also saw the propaganda benefits of a penicillin story. The standing of an industry perennially attacked for the prices it charged would long benefit from its role in risky but triumphant development. The history as it became familiar in the USA was expressed in an industry-supported book published to coincide with the launch of penicillin on the public market in 1945.[57] Entitled *Yellow Magic*, its very title helped forge a link between long-held dreams and the new chemical. Alfred Newton Richards, the tsar of penicillin production, consulted on the manuscript, described it as the sort of writing he disliked. It contained reconstructed thoughts, and in places ran counter to the history that Richards knew.[58] The work of Fleming was covered in sixteen pages, Dubos got fourteen, and the Oxford team another fourteen. American industry warranted the remaining 120 pages. Richards's resentment remained private, and he too had become unimportant to the dissemination of the story. Here was another expert who had found he could no longer control penicillin-mania.

So well known did the penicillin story become that it could be used as a moral tale, with messages for new developments as challenges for a world after the conflict loomed. Lessons were, for instance, drawn in the United States by policy makers agonizing over the organization of post-war science. The shift of scientific leadership from Europe to the USA seemed to have been exemplified by the penicillin story, in which the first discoveries were made in pre-war Europe but the later ones in the USA. When, in 1947, America's National Institutes of Health called for more money, the director Rolla Dyer needed only to say: 'I do not myself feel justified in taking the responsibility for postponing anything in medical research. If Sir Alexander Fleming had delayed 1 year in starting his research on penicillin, you can add up for yourselves the number of lives that would have been lost.'[59] Of course the answer is none. But any small historical confusion over details did not obscure the point of his argument. He got his money.

The isolation of Alexander Fleming, both professionally and in time from the rest of the penicillin story, could puzzle admirers but it also provoked reflections on a new scientific world. While, for some, Fleming's discovery had been the great breakthrough and its sequel was mere development, for others Fleming was just the latest of a series of observers who had had a lucky break that he could not exploit and it was only later that penicillin was properly 'invented' through the power of organized science. His individual contribution would continually be contrasted with the teamwork that so often characterized the penicillin story. These competing models were reflected in polemical articles and historical books, documentary films and personal disputes.

Thus, the story of penicillin was used to introduce *Science, the Endless Frontier*. This key report on the future of American scientific research was written by Vannevar Bush, who had been head of the US government's wartime research programme. Urging that now research should be funded by government grants to the nation's best scientists, he began:

We all know how much the new drug, penicillin, has meant to our grievously wounded men on the grim battlefields of this war—the countless lives it has saved—the incalculable suffering which its use has prevented. Science and the great practical genius of this nation has made this achievement possible.[60]

In Britain the penicillin story was used to highlight the benefits of organized science to the country's reconstruction. The team approach had seemingly been exemplified by the Oxford work, which involved perhaps a dozen colleagues in 1941. Although within a few years that would seem small, this group continued to be recognized as a fundamentally different creative unit from the isolated Fleming. On the other hand the creative but isolated individual was a favoured hero of all scientific stories, and particularly at a time when the Cold War propaganda was highlighting the difference between the anonymous labourers under communism and democratic individualism.[61]

This tension between the individual model of invention and the team came to be subsumed within a broader political debate about the role of the individual in mass society. For Beaverbrook's *Daily Express*, the self-starting individualist was the kind of person who made Britain great; to the Harvard historian, I. B. Cohen, Fleming represented the free-thinking scientist.[62] To both he was the modern hero. If the success of penicillin did not follow quickly on the initial observation, that was because science had not been ready. On the other hand, for scientists and commentators on the political left, the future would belong to the working class, to the organization, or to the profession, rather than to the individualistic hero. Thus Cohen's book was criticized by the corporatist science journalist Waldemar Kaempffert for being insufficiently positive about the wartime achievement. At about the same time, organized cancer chemotherapy research was being promoted at New York's Sloan Kettering Institute on the model of penicillin.[63] With its close links to industry and collaborative nature, the teamwork of the Oxford discoverers seemed to exemplify modern technoscience. Thus *The Lancet* published an article in 1950 under the title 'Penicillin and Modern Research' contrasting the brilliant but old-fashioned style of Fleming and the modern organization of the Oxford team.[64]

A second conflict would be repeatedly reargued in the UK: had penicillin been given to the USA too cheaply? While, for the USA, victory in the Second World War meant widespread prosperity as well as military success, for the British, in the austere post-war years, symbols of their success were more scarce. At a time when dollars, prestige, and medicine were desperately wanted, the development of the wonder drug seemed to promise all three. The role of I.C.I. in particular meshed the story both with national politics and with USA–UK relations.

A sense that Britain had been robbed spread. Early in February 1944, Pfizer got their deep fermentation operating and suddenly were producing vastly more penicillin than the British. Just at that moment, a British patent-medicine manufacturer complained to his Member of Parliament about the rejection of a request to visit the USA to examine the application of mushroom technology to penicillin manufacture.[65] Of course, that approach was by now completely obsolete. The complaint, however, led to a question in the House of Commons about whether the British manufacturers were trying to prevent other firms entering the industry, and to a newspaper assault on industrial inertia and the abuse of monopoly.[66] The existing manufacturers responded immediately in the press, but the enquiry had attracted the attention of Prime Minister Winston Churchill, who detected the risk of political trouble. He consulted his scientific advisers, including Lindemann and Lord Moran. On Lindemann's reassuring note that an increase in production was planned, he replied, 'Good good. Press on report soon.'[67] Stories about attempts by American companies to trademark Fleming's word 'penicillin' were sent by local consuls in South America. The defence that this was just to protect the word against misuse by others was taken badly, and the attempts were defeated by a combination of efforts by the British government and I.C.I..[68]

This was a particularly difficult moment for the I.C.I. organization, whose size and importance made it the main target for press criticism. The Labour Party was already rumbling about nationalizing this peak of British industry. The same month as I.C.I. was criticized at home for letting British penicillin production fall behind that of the Americans, in the USA its close relations with the Du Pont Company were suddenly being investigated by the Department of Justice, threatening a post-war anti-trust suit.[69] I.C.I. did, however, defend their position with energetic public-relations campaigns. The company trumpeted the benefits of its standing by highlighting its technological contributions. When the company's ebullient chairman Lord McGowan gave a speech denouncing nationalization and evoking the company's success, including penicillin, copies of a newspaper were specially printed to include the speech in full and then distributed to many of the employees. The BBC also carried a report in its news bulletin.[70]

The key communication tool, however, in these pre-television times was the documentary movie. In March 1941, I.C.I. had decided to mount a major publicity campaign overseas to maintain its profile while it had few goods to sell. It had allocated to the project the large sum of £100,000. This had paid for the launch of a magazine about science for free distribution to influential people overseas, entitled *Endeavour*, and funding went on producing and distributing films. So it was in character and within existing strategy that, early in 1944, I.C.I. further responded to its wartime challenges by commissioning a film on the development and current manufacture of penicillin from Britain's major documentary producers the Realist Film Unit.[71]

In I.C.I.'s film, emotional and dramatic power was combined with a carefully fabricated sense of historical authenticity. The film spliced together the experience of a wounded soldier, miraculously rescued by the new drug, with a history of the development, including a re-enactment of Fleming making his discovery, shots of Florey, Chain, and Heatley apparently at work in their Oxford laboratory, and I.C.I. manufacturing the product. The script was carefully negotiated with Fleming and the Oxford team, yet the film as a whole still communicates a sense of journalistic integrity.[72] The documentary style was dramatically enhanced by the black and white photography of the cameraman, the later famous Austrian refugee photojournalist and social realist Wolfgang Suschitzky (see Ill. 11). At the same time, as Florey was told, the objective was self-consciously propagandistic—against the Americans.[73] The intended message was that it had been British scientists who had discovered penicillin and I.C.I. was

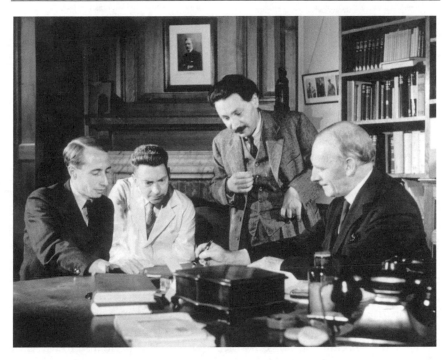

11. Iconic picture of penicillin researchers at Oxford taken by Wolfgang Suschitzky, the cameraman for the 1944 ICI-sponsored film about penicillin. The men shown are: Edward Abraham, Wilson Baker, Ernst Chain, and Robert Robinson.
Wolfgang Suschitzky/National Portrait Gallery.

making it. The film was widely shown and even reissued in 1947. Modern television documentaries about the time still frequently use clips from it.

The film expressed, but did not cure, British resentment about the behaviour of the Americans. Even after the penicillin shortage eased, many Britons resented the 'fact' that they had given the Americans a money-spinner, for the use of which 'we' now had to pay 'them' royalties.[74] Public resentment rumbled on and flared up in mid-1952, just when the Korean War was re-establishing Anglo-American friendships. Two leaders of wartime science, James Conant, President of Harvard, and Vannevar Bush, now President of MIT, received strongly worded letters communicating British feeling against the Americans for stealing penicillin, or at least taking advantage of British weakness.[75] Rather than merely dismissing the charge, Bush commissioned a formal report on the British allegations from John Connor, counsel for Merck and later the company president. Connor's report exonerated the American position. Connor concluded that in fact no licences for submerged fermentation had been paid for by the British pharmaceutical industry. Even if British firms had paid such US firms as Merck for know-how on the operation of penicillin plants, so far as he could see, 'people of good-will' could argue that America 'stole' penicillin from the British only by misunderstanding the issues.[76] Nonetheless, data from the British Glaxo company show that the funds transferred were significant: over ten years to 1956, Glaxo paid Merck £0.5 million for rights relating to penicillin and streptomycin, a significant sum at a time when its annual net profit was about £1.5 million.[77]

The anger over the 'theft' of penicillin resonated with other stories about the jet engine, television, radar, and atomic weapons, all technologies in which British engineers and scientists felt they had won a lead that had been lost, too cheaply, to the USA. The BBC had started the world's first high-definition public television service in 1938, only to see it suspended in wartime. Pride in radar, where the British had made the major advance of connecting receivers to create a network, was converted, in the public imagination, into the belief 'we' had invented radar. The earliest Allied work on the atomic bomb project had been begun in Britain, including the critical calculations on the amount of uranium that would one day be needed in a bomb. So the story of Britain 'giving' penicillin to the USA became a symbol of the passing of many of the trappings of power from the old empire to the new superpower.

In the 1940s era of reconstruction, Britain's apparent mistakes were as much a guide to future action as its successes. In 1945 the Labour Party came into power with a modernizing socialist agenda and a rejection not just of pre-war policies but of pre-war society. Moral tales were taken to heart from the story of penicillin at a time when being on the side of modernity was a political necessity. No sooner was the war over than moves were made to set up an organization that would promote patenting of government-originated ideas, particularly in the medical field. The memory of the failure to patent penicillin haunted the parliamentary debate over setting up the National Research Development Corporation. When it was finally launched in 1948 with the intention of taking patents for work carried out with government money, the Corporation was hailed by the *Daily Herald* newspaper, '£5 million to stop foreigners filching our ideas'.[78] In the new era, 'our ideas' symbolized by penicillin were becoming a key national asset.

As 1946 began, Lord Beaverbrook wrote an editorial in the *Daily Express*, which he owned, proclaiming, 'The British empire and its development is now and will be for evermore, the ark of the Covenant.'[79] Despite such protestations, the early post-war years saw the diminution of Britain's empire overseas and austerity at home. Instead of rule over a quarter of the world, the British people turned to their recent martial and technological accomplishments and the new welfare state as foci of national pride. The mood symbolized by the 1951 Festival of Britain could be described as 'defiant modernism'.[80] 'Nationalism, imperialism, obscurantism and insularity were crumbling; so was disease,' recalls the raconteur and historian Peter Vansittart.[81] When Fleming died in March 1955, his ashes were placed in the crypt of London's St Paul's Cathedral near the tombs of such military leaders as Lord Nelson and the Duke of Wellington. The *Daily Telegraph* newspaper commemorated the day with a photomontage showing nurses leaving the funeral, below a new radar installation for London's Heathrow airport (Ill. 12).[82] The story of penicillin had brought together accounts of the role of the scientist in the country's post-war future, of modernization in attitudes to patents, the functions of the state, industry, and academe, the needs of a new industry, the ambiguous role of

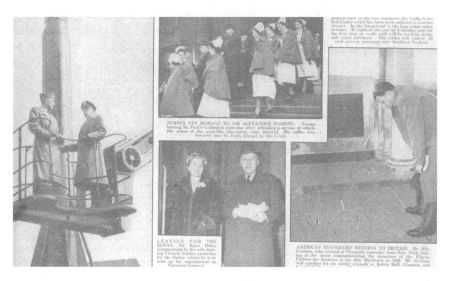

12. Defiant Modernism and penicillin. Nurses leaving the funeral service of Alexander Fleming (centre) were pictured by the *Daily Telegraph* below the new radar system at Heathrow airport and above a picture of the newly appointed Governor General of the Sudan setting off for his new realm. On the left and right are reminders of the importance of the American connection: Billy Graham is shown on the right inspecting the place from which the Pilgrim Fathers set off to the Americas in 1620. On the left an American general inspects a missile based in England, 19 March 1955.
©The Telegraph Group Ltd, 1955.

the United States, and the running of the proud new National Health Service. Together the pictures expressed the pride of a country reconstructing itself after war, and symbolically at their centre was the story of penicillin.

The largest British Commonwealth countries, Canada and Australia, each had their own connections with penicillin, in which each took special pride as they affirmed their own identities separate from that of the former mother country. Although material supplies were everywhere limited, as the war ended, penicillin was being made in Australia and Canada as well as in Britain. Florey, as an Australian, took special trouble to keep in contact with his home country. Indeed, Australia's Commonwealth Serum Laboratories were so good at producing penicillin that the country released the drug to its civilians even before the Americans did.[83] The Connaught Laboratories in Toronto, Canada, had developed insulin as a diabetes treatment, and they too developed penicillin production during the later part of the war. With their wish to have their global status recognized independently from the British, the expertise of the Canadians would have special importance.

Penicillin's image had been carefully wrought during the Second World War. To win the resources needed for its development, the drug's potential had been dramatically demonstrated and successes widely trumpeted. At a time when the world was about to be reconstructed, the achievement was exploited by institutions, companies, and hospitals and even research organizations and by nations struggling for their place in the post-war world. Their interests and ambitions framed the telling of its story which served their own self-understanding but also the interpretation of the drug. A strong brand associated with unprecedented power, science, and modern medicine emerged therefore out of the Second World War.

4

Making Penicillin across the World

During the decade following the end of the Second World War in 1945, people across the globe struggled to get access to penicillin. In the immediate wake of the conflict, many societies were in peril of mass epidemics. 'Defeat had reduced the peoples of Austria and Germany to a state of complete disorganisation, destitution and despair,' noted an eloquent British civil servant to his minister in September 1945.[1] At the very moment the atomic bomb was bringing new means of mass killing, mass protection was provided by penicillin. Syphilis might have proved the medical and social catastrophe for Europe that AIDS became in 1990s Africa, but thanks to penicillin, disaster was averted.

In controlling epidemics penicillin did not just raise the hopes of the individual but also promised benefits to entire nations. Its use was a practical step towards promoting public health, as well as a romantic weapon in the worldwide attempts to surmount the legacy of the past and the menaces of the future. In the USA there were sufficient penicillin supplies by 1945, and the UK had enough by 1946. In eastern Europe, Asia, and Africa, however, supplies continued to be inadequate. To increase supply and ensure they had control over a key national resource, across Europe and in China, Japan, and soon India, governments installed their own maufacturing plants. These measures led to worldwide availability of the drug and dissemination of the brand. Developments in Italy, Austria, and Japan during the early 1950s would also lead to the transformation of the chemical itself, with profound implications for penicillin worldwide.

Penicillin manufacture depended on new concepts and disciplines of biological technology, yet within a short time of the end of the war it was spread around the world. This surprising achievement was made possible by widespread wartime experiences with the manufacture and testing of small quantities of the drug. Despite a clampdown by the

Allies on details about what was seen to be a weapon, scientists in Axis countries had learned about the new wonder drug from the early publications of the Oxford team, which were not embargoed, and could draw upon long-stored samples of the mould that had been identified by Fleming.[2] Even if knowledge was often sketchy and any attempt to manufacture substantial supplies was frustrated, several teams, both approved by the Axis governments and in secret, made small quantities to test for themselves and to develop their own competence, preparing for the post-war world.

German soldiers encountered penicillin in prisoner of war camps and from captured Allied supplies. The astonishment of a German field-hospital physician at the effect of this *Wundermittel* is vividly expressed in a novelized story of an early German use of the drug, published less than a decade after the end of the war.[3] While the accuracy of some of its historical detail is unclear, the book evocatively describes in clinical terms the fate of a wounded German airman whose wounds are badly infected, who remains infected even after an ineffective leg amputation, and who seems destined for an early death. The tale describes how this typical, and—even with the best German drugs—unstoppable progression was reversed by regular injections of penicillin, provided by a captured British medical officer. Elsewhere, for lack of such a drug, many patients were succumbing to infection. A report appearing immediately after hostilities in Europe had ceased, in the military newsletter *Eighth Army News*, expressed shock at the often septic wounds of German soldiers in hospitals overrun by the British. The author, who was of course himself British, claimed that the better treatment of his side's wounded was the result both of penicillin and also of better attention to health and welfare of soldiers.[4]

Nonetheless, many teams across the wartime German Reich did themselves make the drug, albeit in small quantities. Across occupied Europe, scientists in such countries as the Netherlands and France were making and testing penicillin surreptitiously, and in Prague both official German and unofficial Czech researches were conducted simultaneously. The Japanese, with scraps of knowledge, were also making small amounts of penicillin as the war ended. The Chinese and the Russians, at first hardly better informed than their enemies, used the little they could glean from their Western allies and the scarce resources they could spare so that they could emulate the results reported in the West. If the facilities they had built were immediately superseded, their expertise was crucial to the subsequent building of a global industry. Several scientists who would be important in developing penicillin in the post-war years, and indeed would later be global leaders in biotechnology, were introduced to penicillin through those small-scale wartime experiments.[5]

Repression gave the impression of order and will, but behind this mask the Nazi regime also engendered corrupt links between the army, entrepreneurs, and senior party patrons, personal empires fighting turf wars, and private investment against the increasing probability of eventual defeat. Penicillin specifically was the object of ambivalence. On the one hand, it was a prestige medicine wanted by the army. On the other hand, German science had been the father of the sulphonamides and its industry was comfortable with their manufacture.

German scientists learned about penicillin from the *Lancet* articles published by Florey and his team in 1940 and 1941. These were transmitted by the neutral Swiss and Swedes with no difficulty.[6] Within Germany, however, bureaucratic muddle and contradictions compounded the technical difficulties of developing the drug. Although such well-known companies as Hoechst and Zeiss did experiment with its manufacture, there was no centrally organized programme.[7] The national research council established a network of academic groups, but this had only weak links to parallel small-scale industrial work. Instead, official patronage was the key to winning resources. Theodor Morell, Hitler's own doctor, had his own pharmaceutical interests. A recent comprehensive study of the German enterprise names five factories he acquired from Jewish owners. In one of these, in Olmütz (now Olomouc) in Czechoslovakia, penicillin was extracted, and then administered through Morell—on one occasion even to Hitler himself. After the attempt to assassinate Hitler in July 1944, Morell noted in his diary that he had treated a superficial arm wound with penicillin powder.[8] Whether this was German made or taken from an enemy soldier is unclear. However, a competing German physician whom Morell had once slighted proved it had little potency, and was possibly even toxic. Even at the beginning of 1945, German monthly production of penicillin, amounting to about 30 grams or 50 million units, was on a similar experimental scale to that of the British long before in 1942.

Leaking across a front and through neutral countries, information about penicillin was often fragmentary and vague. Had there not been a war, such centres as Prague, Delft, or Paris might have been the much more likely places for the development of penicillin technology than either Oxford or Peoria. For the moment, lacking detailed knowledge, all that scientists in occupied countries could know for sure was that cures for infection could be obtained from certain strains of mould. Fleming's work of the 1920s had been widely publicized, and there were samples of his mould in the great culture collection in the Netherlands and in Paris at the Pasteur Institute, which were both in German hands in 1940.

This approach could be seen clearly in German-occupied Czechoslovakia, where most of the Reich's penicillin was actually made. Before the war, this area had been a world centre in brewing and fermentation technology. American scientists, such as Wisconsin's Marvin Johnson, studied at the German university in Prague, where the citric-acid fermentation specialist Konrad Bernhauer taught.[9] His course became a textbook published in both 1936 and 1939 editions and translated into English.[10] The book was among the first texts to deal with submerged fermentation of air-dependent moulds.

During the war, the German university in Prague was flourishing, while the national technological institute was abolished.[11] In 1941 Bernhauer was given the rare resource of a 'four-year plan' research institute on enzymology. Its main focus would be the manufacture of alcohol and vinegar from carbohydrate, but penicillin was also on the agenda. Since Goering was behind the four-year plan, it has been suggested he himself must have been Bernhauer's backer.[12] With relatively lavish resources and strong pre-war tradition, the German university team explored the production of penicillin both through surface fermentation and also under submerged conditions. But as this work was becoming practical, Allied bombing of industrial areas became intense.[13]

Wartime news of the success of the Oxford team also inspired groups working in Prague without the knowledge of the Germans. When news of Alexander Fleming's work had reached Prague, a decade earlier, Czech scientists such as the young microbiologist Ivan Málek had taken an interest in antibiotic therapy.[14] With the German takeover in 1939, and closure of the bacteriology department in the Charles University, scientists such as he were in danger of being sidelined into routine epidemiological monitoring. However, to protect established men such as Málek, and students who might otherwise have been pressganged into forced labour, the Prague pharmaceutical company of Jiri Fragner recruited them to a newly created research laboratory.

Within the company, young employees attempted to emulate the Oxford team's work. Málek later recalled how, surveying samples of rabbit droppings, they found an extract that seemed to correlate with penicillin. It had the same yellow colour. What should Fragner do? In 1943 he consulted Málek, who advised that, after a German defeat, any process that the Czechs had developed would be rendered entirely uneconomic by the achievements of the victorious Allies. Nonetheless, by working on the product, they might develop some expertise. So Fragner approved continuing work. The team developed their own antibiotic, possibly a penicillin, which they called Mykoin BF510. For more than a year the work was conducted in secret from the occupying Germans lest they benefit from it.

Many of the same processes of separation as were being used in Britain and America were adopted by the isolated Fragner team. They managed to separate a drug using modern chromatographic techniques and even to test it, first on animals and then on people. The achievement was staggering, given the conditions of the time. At bottom, it testified to the professional standards and community that just a very few years before had linked Czech, British, and German scientists. After the war, the chemist on the team, Karel Wiesner, would move to Canada and become one of the world's leading natural products chemists.[15] The long-standing international ties of the team's members as well as their individual distinction also explained how, within a couple of years of the war's end, those scientists could be accumulating expertise in the technology so laboriously developed by the British and Americans.[16]

Scientists in occupied Netherlands and France also found ways of testing small quantities of the new drug. It was at the University of Delft in the west of the Netherlands that deep fermentation had first been explored early in the 1930s.[17] During the war, with the assistance of gin as a bribe, information about penicillin moved among Swiss journals, assistants in the university laboratory, and the gin manufacturing company NG&SF. From July 1944 to March 1945, the Dutch secretly experimented with a drug they called 'Bacinol'. It was used in desperation during that dreadful 'hunger winter' when the western province was cut off from food supplies by German troops and a rail boycott. Because of the wartime isolation of Delft, it was only later confirmed that the medication made in isolation and secrecy really was the same as the miracle drug of the British and the Americans about which the Dutch had heard.[18] The French, too, made penicillin underground during the war from pre-war cultures.[19] In France, the Netherlands, and Czechoslovakia, therefore, doctors and microbiologists had made great efforts and taken considerable risks to see for themselves the effects of this new drug and to prepare themselves for a time when they would be able to use it freely. Some of the largest penicillin plants in the world at the end of the twentieth century owed their origins to those teams.

The implications of penicillin for public health in Europe were substantial, but they were greater even in China. Although torn by war with

Japan, tensions between nationalists and communists, and held down by poverty, the country had rich and respected expertise, not just within its own tradition, but also developing expertise in Western science and medicine. Its scientists therefore took an interest in news of penicillin as they received it, and even produced their own, despite a desperate lack of resources. With the Japanese invading from the west, much of China's scientific activity had been moved to the far south-west, to Kunming in Yunnan province, close to the border with Vietnam.[20] It was visited in 1943 by the British scientific attaché Joseph Needham, who reported on his findings in the journal *Nature*.[21] His account both showed the urgent drive to modernize in nationalist China and also reported the development of penicillin.

Outside the town of Kunming, accessible by charcoal-burning bus, horse-drawn cart, jeep, or car, lay the National Epidemics Prevention Bureau. Its major responsibility in the early 1940s was the making of vaccines for typhoid and diphtheria, the traditional Chinese inoculant against smallpox, and sera for tetanus. Working conditions were primitive in the extreme and supplies from outside hard to obtain. Nonetheless, the head of the institute, the leading bacteriologist Dr Fei Fan Tang, ran a journal club to discuss developments about which they heard.[22] News of penicillin arrived in 1941 after the Oxford group had published in *Nature*. The Chinese scientists sought their own mould samples on clothes, boots, bean curd, meat broth, and shoe polish. Simple clinical experiments were carried out using the raw mould juice. When in 1944 Dr Tang was flown to India to join a public-health seminar, he returned with a further nine strains and some more information.

Finding conditions to grow the mould was difficult, due to Kunming's hot weather, but possible. Extraction was much harder. In Kunming, where even a refrigerator was rare, instead of the freeze-dryers used in Britain and America a simple freezing system was home built using an ice bath. And in September 1944 five bottles of penicillin were made. Two were sent abroad to Oxford and to Wisconsin for testing and to prove success, two were tested on patients, and one was kept for reference. The quantities made by the Chinese were tiny, enough perhaps for a dozen patients a month, but this did serve the purpose of building some expertise within the country.[23] This was supplemented by American supplies. From August 1944, several hundred ampoules a month were flown into Kunming.[24] For some months in 1944 the charity American Aid for China contemplated building a plant in the USA and developing means of adapting its technology to Chinese conditions but when they learned of the work at Kunming the project was terminated.[25] The Chinese had been able to make the first key steps in penicillin manufacture, drawing on their own expertise and skills (see Ill. 13).

Of course, having access to small quantities of the drug was very far from using it on a large scale. The Western Allies not only made penicillin but could also introduce it into a conflict which was only gradually reaching a crescendo. Scientists in the Soviet Union also experimented with its 'homegrown' product as early as 1942, but in the midst of an intensely fought war could not readily make use of it.

Shortly after the ending of the siege of Moscow, 200 patients were given penicillin produced from a culture originally scraped from the wall of a damp air-raid shelter.[26] The product proved effective, but, for the Soviets, a more easily made gramicidin, a variant of the first antibiotic that had been pioneered by René Dubos in the 1930s, was a more suitable solution to urgent needs. It was a much more stable chemical than penicillin, it addressed the worst difficulty of sulphonamides (their weak action on the staphylococci bacteria), and could be used on battle wounds. With the progress of war, more detailed information came from the West and in

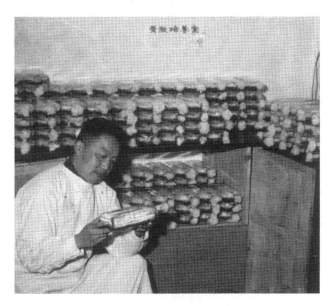

13. Penicillin research in Kunming, China, in 1943. This photograph was taken by Joseph Needham, then British scientific attaché, and published in his book *Science Outpost*.
By permission of the Syndics of Cambridge University Library.

1943 four British and American scientists visited in a formal capacity to bring information about Allied developments. Their visit was friendly but did not suffice to make penicillin widely available.[27]

Even in wartime, therefore, penicillin was widely known of, and desired across the globe. If beyond America, Britain, and the most developed parts of the British empire its use still touched very few people, as the war ended doctors feared that penicillin would now be widely needed to address the epidemics that, otherwise, were bound to follow. Diarrhoea, pneumonia, famine, and epidemics of every kind were experienced. The new drug helped the occupiers prevent the total collapse of the societies of their former enemies. Here, penicillin's role was not to help the isolated individual, as it later became, but to rescue entire societies.

As the war ended, British Prime Minister Clement Attlee feared a global famine. In the autumn of 1945 the harvest failed catastrophically cross Europe, North Africa, and East Asia.[28] European food production was 25 per cent below pre-war production, and rice production in the Far East was 15 per cent below normal.[29] The destruction of the world's transport infrastructure worsened the threat still further. Convinced by Attlee, President Harry Truman spoke on the radio to the American people, whom he starkly warned, 'Europe today is hungry.'[30] Just as peacetime hopes lifted, the weather declined. The winter of 1947 was the worst Europe had experienced in a generation.

With famine would come the threat of epidemic disease spreading among a weakened and starving population. The local infrastructure had broken down, and most supplies had to come from the occupying forces. In the autumn of 1945 a working party reported that the British had provided sufficient medical supplies to entirely support 75 million people for two months.[31] Even more onerous were the responsibilities of the USA, and it had supplied twice as much again. A grim poetic picture of the world at this time is given by the titles of the files assembled by British civil servants at the time. Carefully, they catalogued their papers under such titles as: 'Infectious Diseases: Pneumonia and Plague, outbreaks. 1943–1946'.

A British Health Minister was shocked to be told by a Dutch former resistance leader that Germans, for whom his government was responsible, would themselves experience concentration camp-like conditions and Berlin would become an 'Allied Buchenwald'.[32] He decided to check this judgement with his own generals, only to find that they agreed. In November 1945 the British 8 Corps was occupying north Germany. A specially printed brochure specifying beds, ambulances, and medical supplies ended in traditional stirring tones, 'The "Battle of the Winter" must be pushed on relentlessly and with determination as it is only by actual cooperation by all that it can be won.' Instead of just the name of the season, 'Winter' was now the enemy itself, and the casualties to be minimized were German.[33]

The greatest risks were judged by the British to be from 'typhus, dysentery, enteric fever, influenza, smallpox, venereal disease, poliomyelitis, malaria and possibly cerebro-spinal meningitis'.[34] Even three years later, in 1948, when the World Health Organization was founded, three priorities were still seen as so pressing that they could not wait for the formal bureaucracy to be established: influenza, infant mortality, and venereal diseases.[35] Since women infected with syphilis were at risk of bearing disabled children, the newly established UNICEF was also involved in protecting the health of the mothers.

Combining genuine altruism with straight self-interest, penicillin was made available particularly for the assault on syphilis. As during the war, both British and American forces were threatened by venereal disease. The British administration of north-west Germany under the formal title 'Control Commission Germany' was nicknamed 'Charlie Chaplin's Grenadiers' or 'Complete Chaos Guaranteed'.[36] Twelve million US troops, mostly sexually frustrated young men, were overseas in 1945.[37] For them VD was said to stand for 'Veronika Dankeschoen'. Rape was widespread. Many women also depended on what later would be called 'hunger-prostitution' for survival.[38]

Even before the war had ended, control over venereal disease had broken down in Germany. Bureaucratic regulations had become impenetrably complex as subdepartments of the Reich stopped communicating. Doctors responded by avoiding a practice which might well not be reimbursed. By August 1945 the venereal disease rate in the north Rhine region of Germany was running at ten times the rate of 1939.[39] Penicillin, when it was available, was effective at curing gonorrhoea, but demand far outstripped supply. A competitive spirit animated the wording of a press release issued by the British administration in the north Rhine region in 1946. 'With a high regional VD figure of 190 case of syphilis and 400 cases of gonorrhea, notified weekly, penicillin clinic centres may well compete on equal terms shortly with food queues.'[40] Early in 1948 it was reported to the Ministry of Health that one-sixth of Britain's entire penicillin production was being directed to Germany.[41]

This was the grey and battered world that Graham Greene described in his script for the movie *The Third Man* (see Ill. 14). He wrote of the villainous Harry Lime, who organizes a black market in stolen penicillin that

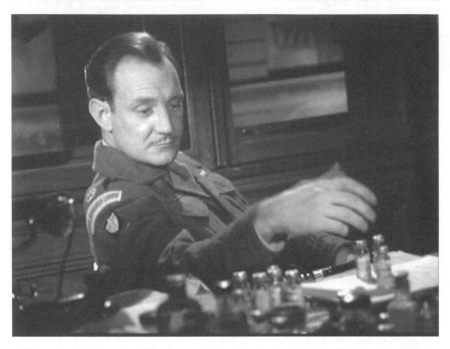

14. Sometimes claimed to be the best British film ever made, *The Third Man* was about a crook selling fake penicillin in post Second World War Vienna. Here fake penicillin is being exposed by Trevor Howard.
Canal + Image UK.

is diluted with sand. In ignorance the adulterated medicine, purchased privately for huge sums, is administered to children with meningitis. They subsequently die, but their horrible fate does not worry Lime, who glories in the £20,000 he earns from the medicine purchased before each death. The details of the plot were fictional, but the portraits of the black market and the desperate search for penicillin were movingly accurate. Reality could, of course, be more prosaic: a major crime ring was broken in Berlin in 1947 when a soldier was found dead drunk in a bar, his pockets full of counterfeit penicillin in ampoules ready for distribution.[42] Despite the avalanche of demand, however, this period of scarcity lasted but a short time. In part this was because of growing exports from the USA. Not far behind, however, was local production both by commercial firms which had acquired American know-how and by factories provided by the Allies.

More slowly than recipients would have liked, and with a muddle characteristic of the period, a network of penicillin plants was funded by new international agencies: the United Nations Relief and Rehabilitation

Agency (UNRRA) and later the WHO. The latter, of course, is still a vital force and indeed important in penicillin policy. The former, however, was disbanded in 1948 and its work is not widely remembered. Yet, founded even before the war had ended, it was vital to the provision of supplies in a chaotic time. Linking wartime solidarity to Cold War politics, UNRRA was founded to provide food and medicines by the 'United Nations' when this was still the name given to the coalition fighting the Axis powers.

The new organization was originally formed to help the first European country to be liberated, which was Italy. Through several cycles of development, the Italian experience would be critical to the development of penicillin. First, however, it was seen as a model of suffering as the country was fought over in 1943. In Christmas 1944, the zones now 'liberated' were described by the chairman of American Relief to Italy. Viewing the deprivation around him, he concluded, 'If an epidemic started here it would sweep all before it so low is the resistance of the people. Medicines are very scarce until recently practically non-existent.'[43]

Responding to this challenge, Allied leaders addressed the humanitarian and political challenges posed by civilian deprivation and even starvation. A provision of 1 per cent of the GNP of participating countries was to enable the purchase and provision of supplies. Because the USA was so much wealthier than its weakened allies, it provided 70 per cent of the budget and the director general: first Herbert Lehmann and then the former New York mayor, Fiorello LaGuardia.[44]

UNRRA operated principally in southern and eastern Europe. Working on an enormous scale to prevent starvation and mass epidemics, at its height it employed about 20,000 people directly. In the months after the end of the war, it provided 70 per cent of the food in Italy. UNRRA's success there meant that a feared disaster did not happen. Instead, folk memory would recall the effectiveness of DDT used against malaria-spreading mosquitoes and typhus-spreading fleas, and the provision of penicillin.

The penicillin projects grew out of a marriage of compassion and self-interest in both Canada and the USA. In one move, infection would be cured, disorder prevented, and influence assured. The US government was willing to pay, but private companies were loath to give away hard-won commercial secrets. A solution was found through the support of Lester Pearson, Canadian Undersecretary for External Affairs and head of the UNRRA supply committee.[45] Canada was eager to raise its status as a powerful country independent of Britain and the USA and Lester Pearson offered Canadian assistance. In July 1945, the University of Toronto made its first batch of penicillin using deep fermentation technology in its Connaught Laboratories. Within months, the Canadians had agreed to provide the designs of a plant and train qualified experts from applicant countries.

Canadian support made possible the transfer of expertise from the wartime Allies to the continent of Europe and later to Asia. In the years 1946 and 1947 expertise, and even entire penicillin plants, were provided to several nations. Five countries, each torn by the Cold War, were helped in this way. Italy with its large communist party, two, then, Soviet republics (Belarus and Ukraine), and Poland and Czechoslovakia (both now to become part of the Soviet sphere of influence) acquired factories and advice.[46] Through slightly different arrangements, Yugoslavia and China were also supplied. The plants would later be considered small, but their production capacity of 40 billion units a month could be compared to the total consumption of Canada at the end of 1945, which was just half that. Each plant cost approximately a quarter of a million dollars. Ironically, while, in part, the project had been driven by the Americans' hope that they would win the support of those who might otherwise be tempted by communism, within the USA, UNRRA was accused of left-wing sympathies. In 1948 it was wound up. Its antibiotic responsibilities were then inherited by the newly established WHO.

As the war drew to a close, old alliances were giving way to a jostling for position between the Soviets and the Western Allies, particularly in central Europe. Provision of penicillin would be a part of this competition between East and West. Imports and supplies would be provided by the Americans, and accepted, but not publicized, by governments that increasingly came under Soviet control.

The experience gained by the Czechs in wartime put them in a lead position to draw on Western experience after liberation. The design of the factory they negotiated with UNRRA would determine the character of all other similar plants. Moreover, the country was a prize over which East and West briefly competed. Relatively untouched by the war, Czechoslovakia protruded finger-like into western Europe south of Germany and therefore occupied a most strategic position. Before the Second World War, the country's democratic rule under Masaryk had been unique in the region, and the post-war democratic government of Beneš was also modelled on the Western democracies. On the other hand, there was a most powerful communist party, which had also been influential before the war.

For all Czechoslovakia's relative prosperity, its economy had been damaged by war, and, as elsewhere, food was short. In 1946 it got half a million tonnes of wheat from UNRRA. Not only was food short: so was medicine. Writing in May that year, before the communist takeover, the Minister of Health saw the economy endangered by disease. After the communist takeover, the language was even tougher. Syphilis was no longer to be seen as a personal affliction but a threat to the state, and the individual had a responsibility to endanger neither his own body nor that of the people as a whole.[47]

UNRRA promised penicillin to the Czechs as early as May 1945, with peace in Europe barely a week old. Within less than a month, training sessions for physicians had been set up and an allocation process organized.[48] Their wartime experience was vastly exceeded by the British and the Americans, yet the Czechs had gained valuable expertise. Enthusiastic as they were, they knew penicillin was no magical cure and, before patients were treated, microbiologists examined microbial causes of infections to ensure they were susceptible to the drug.

Ivan Málek, the veteran of the Fragner experiments, and two colleagues were given scholarships to learn about modern penicillin manufacture in Toronto and prepare for the donation of a plant by UNRRA. But travel to North America from Prague early in 1946 was no smooth academic jetsetting. Everything was fraught for the Czechs: visas, travel, and access each presented challenges that were more familiar to desperate refugees. They could not get a ticket on the scarce planes that linked Prague and the USA. Without a ticket, they could not get a visa. Rescue came in the form of a transport aircraft that had brought a consignment of chickens to Czechoslovakia. For lack of passenger insurance, on its return it only took them as far as England. From there a boat that had brought sulphur across the Atlantic took them west to the unlikely harbour of Portland, Maine.

Unfortunately, the plant built in Toronto that they were to emulate was actually in trouble. The penicillium mould was reproducing too fast and genetically changing under the glare of ultraviolet lights installed to kill contaminants. From suppliants, the Europeans became expert consultants and, drawing on their own experience, helped cure the problem. The Czechs stayed four months, travelling to laboratories across North America on overnight trains to save money and time. They knew that their Canadian benefactors, though generous, were well behind such private companies as Merck. But the closest they could get to a Merck factory was a guided tour of a packing facility.

Meanwhile in Czechoslovakia the communist Herbert Gottwald was elected to power. The atmosphere for the Czech visitors in Toronto became noticeably frostier. When it was time for them to leave, they were refused permission to take with them any penicillium spores. Instead the Canadians made a vague promise of a consignment by mail. Now, Málek took matters in hand by shaking a few spores from the cultures he had worked upon into apparently empty test tubes.

Eventually the Canadians did send cultures to Czechoslovakia through official channels, but Málek found that the strain he had already taken was more productive. The problems of the Czechs were not, however, over. The USA was concerned that equipment might be reallocated to biological warfare and refused to allow the export of modern Podbielniak separators from the USA. This would be a running sore between the Czechs and the Americans for a number of years.[49] Nonetheless, the Czechs could benefit from the experience of others because they had not just defined a plant for themselves. They had specified a general UNRRA design. In June 1947 a four-day meeting to discuss the plant design was held in Prague for all the participants (although only the Poles, Czechs, and Belorussians took part), led by the superintendent of Merck's Canadian subsidiary, since the Connaught Laboratories representative was not available.[50] Despite the descending Iron Curtain, the Czechs had successfully converted expertise gained in underground activities during wartime into the basis for a post-war penicillin industry.

As a result of Cold War politics and of the intense suffering on the eastern side of Europe, the only country in the West to benefit from the UNRRA penicillin initiative was Italy, whose conditions had been the original spur for founding the organization. Italy's rapid recovery from wartime desolation, determination to build up a modern industry, and close connections with other Western countries meant it could use UNRRA resources in an unconventional way. Resources destined for small-scale manufacture were diverted into building a world-class penicillin research centre.

Italian ambitions for a great future and their pride in a distinguished past contrasted with present poverty. The Istituto Superiore di Sanita, which was the country's leading public-health institution, benefited from an energetic and visionary leader, Domenico Marotta. Early on, he began to negotiate for a plant from UNRRA, and in April 1946 the offer of a plant was made formally.[51] However, the process of getting the plant built and equipped was almost as chaotic as for the Czechs. Italians, too, went on pilgrimage to Toronto. Yet information on what was to be provided was lacking and delivery was delayed for another year. When equipment began to arrive, it came not in a coherent consignment but through half a dozen ports and was clearly incomplete. The location of the plant had meanwhile to be negotiated: would it be in the industrial heartland of northern Italy or near the Institute in Rome? Looking to the need for ongoing development, Marotta insisted that this manufacturing plant be sited near the research laboratory of his institute on the campus of Rome's La Sapienza University. But when a plot of land was allocated, it was seen to be too small and a new area had to be found. This, of course, all took time and the building did not take place till early 1948. By then the situation had changed. Commercial factories were in the offing. Moreover, Ernst Chain had arrived in Italy.

Chain had been originally invited through the British Council to give a series of lectures on penicillin to the Istituto Superiore di Sanità early in 1947.[52] Perhaps even then Marotta had his designs on Chain as a colleague, for he had already recruited Daniel Bovet, a pioneer of sulphanilamide, from France. During his visit to Italy, Chain learned about the UNRRA plans. Unimpressed by the now old-fashioned and small-scale attempt to compete with private industry, he made a decisive suggestion to Marotta. Rather, he proposed, use the UNRRA-provided equipment as the basis for a pilot plant for future penicillin development. With the funds the Italian government had originally put aside for the factory's full-scale operation, Marotta could establish a laboratory for related research.

Chain's idea was accepted by the Italians. Since the construction of laboratories at the Institute went well ahead of the plant, Chain was invited to stay at first on leave of absence from Oxford and then he was given a ten-year contract to build his institute. This was a wonderful opportunity for a man dedicated to the development of penicillin and fascinated by equipment. Chain and Marotta were both big thinkers. A colleague, Gualandi, remembered them conversing in French, one with a strong Sicilian accent, the other with a German intonation. They thought, however, in similar ways.[53]

Chain built in Rome an enormous institute, far larger than any elsewhere in the world, including the USA: the legitimate offspring of the wartime Wisconsin and Oxford laboratories. Resembling a brigadier in charge of the armoured brigade of the microbiology profession, Chain had a team comprising almost a hundred people. It included twenty chemists and biochemists, three physical chemists, nine microbiologists, two chemical engineers, two mechanical engineers, fifteen mechanics, four electronics technicians, and forty general technicians (see Ill. 15).[54] This 'brigade' could deploy thirty small 10-litre fermenters (these would be large glass flasks), nine fermenters with a capacity of 90 litres (equivalent to a large car's fuel tank), and in addition three fermenters of 300-litre capacity and a full-scale 3,000-litre fermenter. On occasion they could go larger. Gualandi would later recall:

One day, Chain asked me why some certain measurements had not been made in fermenters larger than 12 cubic metres. I answered that that was the largest capacity available in the pilot plant.

'Where are there any bigger?'

'At Torre Annunziata at the Lepetit plant, but they are continuous cycle reactors which cannot be interrupted.'

'We'll see. I'll discuss it with Prof. Marotta.'

Two weeks later, we began a series of experiments in an enormous 100 cubic metre container, graciously lent to the Higher Institute of Health by Livio Zerilli, Chairman of Lepetit, following a phone call from Marotta.... quite unthinkable in any other part of the world or in any other time.[55]

The sceptic might be tempted to dismiss the grandiosity of the Italians' dream and expect that little would be produced. But the sceptic would

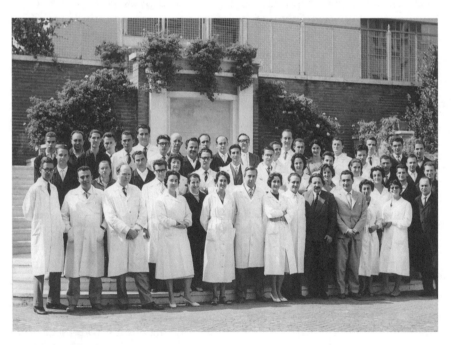

15. 'Chain's babies'. The team of scientists engineers assembled by Ernst Chain at the Istituto Superiore di Sanita in Rome in the 1950s.
Istituto Superiore di Sanita, Rome.

be wrong. It was a research laboratory that investigated the 'cosmos' inside the fermenter and modified the equipment accordingly. The Dutch scientist J. C. Hoogerheide described the fermenters that the chemical engineers had wished upon the first generation of post-war antibiotic makers: 'the converted chemical kettles they offered us invariably led to serious and crippling infections. The engineers then tried to solve this problem with steam seals at every possible point... until we ended up with a hissing and puffing contraption that resembled a noisy old steam engine more than a fermenter.'[56] Online monitoring of the fermentation was developed using the plant, so that, as oxygen was dissolving in the swirling mixture, its concentration could be measured continually.[57] This kind of work took the wartime biotechnological developments forward into a new era. How the work in Rome led to the development of such semisynthetic penicillins as ampicillin and amoxicillin will be discussed later in this book.

Many countries of course did not receive penicillin plants. Yet they too sought independence in controlling a newly vital commodity and expertise in a vital new industry. India, for instance, wished to maintain its independence from restrictions that might be imposed by US companies and took up an offer from the World Health Organization for help, which was delivered by the Swedish company Astra.[58] In Europe too, independent supplies were sought, and private-sector companies helped combine know-how from overseas with local expertise. The Austrian experience would be particularly significant.

The penicillin shortages experienced in Austria were made famous by *The Third Man*. Less well known, but equally significant to penicillin consumers worldwide, would be Austria's response which led to a revolution in the qualities of the drug and the building of what became one of the world's leading penicillin factories. Lying immediately to the south of Czechoslovakia, until 1955 the country was occupied by the British, Russians, French, and Americans. Once the hub of a great empire, the country with just seven million inhabitants had been incorporated in the Reich in 1937. Despite its small size, Austria had a great scientific and cultural tradition focused on, but not exclusively dominated by, Vienna. In the alpine Tyrol region, the occupiers were the French. This beautiful but unlikely mountain area was the scene of a most remarkable story with an even more unlikely outcome. Karl Schroeder, a brewer and pharmaceutical executive who in wartime Prague had discussed penicillin manufacture with Bernhauer, the German penicillin specialist, recounted it in 1979 to a journalist whom he had known for forty years.[59]

In 1945 Richard Brunner who had previously worked with Bernhauer obtained a position in the Austrian brewing company, Oesterreiches Brau. There he found a new partner, Michel Rambaud, an officer in the French army of occupation. Rambaud was a biochemist who had worked in the penicillin laboratory at Oxford. Stationed in the town of Innsbruck near the 500-year-old Kundl brewery, now part of the the Oesterreiches Brau company, he also had the idea of founding a penicillin plant. With the war's end, the brewery had become a food depot. The equipment nonetheless was all in working order, and Rambaud approached its owners full of enthusiasm.

Rambaud and Brunner persuaded the brewers to seek permission from Vienna to convert the Kundl plant to penicillin manufacture. Venereal disease was rampant in Austria, the wonder drug was in short supply, and so Vienna gave permission for the establishment of Biochemie Gesellschaft (Biochemistry Inc.) on the site of the old Kundl brewery, while the money and management came from Oesterreiches Brau. Equipment was drawn from the plentiful detritus of war—remnants of submarines, tanks, gun barrels, and pipelines. Rambaud, who maintained both a personal and a financial interest in the firm, brought a penicillin culture from France. This gift proved to be merely the beginning of a tedious process of selectively breeding a commercially productive strain.

In 1948, the year of *The Third Man*, penicillin was successfully produced by Biochemie to meet some of the needs of Austrian patients. Schroeder, was invited to take over the management of the company. Not just emulating the work of others, in 1951 the Austrians discovered how to make a penicillin that was not destroyed by the acid in the stomach. No longer would penicillin have to be painfully injected. Instead Penicillin V (V for *vertraulich*—German for 'confidential') could be taken as a tablet four times a day.

The development was an accident—resulting from an experiment based on a hunch. The plant was subject to contamination, like all fermentations. Brewers had long combated infestation from the *E. coli* bacterium by adding an acid to their brew. It acted as a sort of pesticide. As it happened, this traditional additive, phenoxyacetic acid, was similar to phenylacetic acid, which was added to the brew in growing penicillium mould to encourage penicillin production—thus providing plenty of raw material for the mould to build an essential branch to the penicillin trunk. Could phenoxyacetic acid be used in its stead, to act both as nutrient and as disinfectant?

The surprising outcome was not just the elimination of contamination but also the building of a different kind of 'branch' on the main penicillin 'trunk'.[60] Although the Eli Lilly company in the USA had in fact already made the resultant penicillin variant some years before, it had not developed the idea. Now, however, Biochemie had developed an oral penicillin that it could not patent. As a result, the two companies, the miniature Austrian Biochemie and the American major, collaborated in building the world market.

Austria's German neighbours also had to build on their own expertise with foreign support. There was, of course, great ambivalence about how to treat the 'villain' of the recent war, and some voices had called for Germany's deindustrialization. Instead, the country was divided into zones whose patrons competed to develop their areas. Moreover, with hundreds of thousands of troops in the country faced by the threat of venereal disease, and the circulation of counterfeit and diluted drugs, penicillin supplies were essential. The British, Americans, French, and Russians each supported the development of penicillin factories in their zones. Quickest off the mark was the Schering company. As well as running its own small fermentation plant, it recycled penicillin extracted from urine in hospitals.[61] By 1950, however, such emergency measures could be dispensed with. The famous pharmaceutical firm Hoechst, based near Frankfurt, opened a large penicillin plant using the latest US technology.[62] In general, German industry did not pioneer in the biotechnology area, preferring its own tradition of chemistry.[63] Nor did Germans, however, take to penicillin therapy as the Allies did, preferring instead their own home-developed sulphonamides right through the 1950s. In western Germany, therefore, antibiotics were not so popular as elsewhere and even in the 1960s made up only 5 per cent of medicines prescribed by doctors at a time when in Britain antibiotics made up 20 per cent of all drugs used.[64] So, many years after the war, such drugs still had not been naturalized in Germany, by either doctors or industry.

By contrast to the German experience, the Japanese had a long tradition of fermentation expertise. Enormous enthusiasm, limited wartime experience, and the post-war guidance provided by a single individual soon enabled the country to make up for lost time and, within fifteen years, to become an international leader in antibiotic development.

In the Second World War, Japan had been cut off from the Allied developments which had occurred largely after relations with Britain and the USA were severed late in 1941. Its scientists had therefore acquired information about penicillin only through the most circuitous of routes.[65] News had trickled in through an article published in an Egyptian newspaper and a spy in Argentina. More information and samples came in a submarine from Germany. Like other communities of experts cut off from Britain and America, the Japanese nonetheless made great progress with limited resources. However, in 1945, crushed by two atomic bombs and with the war suddenly over, they realized how much more progress had been made in the United States.

In Japan, as in Europe, the post-war years were hard and threatening. An American governor, General Douglas MacArthur, ruled the country. The rice crop failed in 1946, and UNRRA had to provide support. Venereal disease was widespread: that year approximately 436,000 cases of syphilis, 556,000 cases of gonorrhoea, and 108,000 cases of chancroid were reported.[66] Again, to maintain public health, penicillin would be needed. In 1947, MacArthur asked George Merck to provide advice to Japanese companies. Merck's response was immediate and remarkably productive. He sent his employee Jackson Foster (who had been a pupil of Waksman at Rutgers, where streptomycin had been found) to Tokyo to teach the Japanese how to make penicillin. Foster spent seven months helping Japanese industry to reorganize. Even heating was lacking in this austere early post-war period. Later, Foster would recall that this was the only time he ever lectured in a coat and hat.[67]

Early in his visit Foster offered Japanese microbiologists an intense three-day report on his experience so far and vision for the future. He behaved like a general in his own right as he urged on his audience. 'It is unthinkable', he said, 'that high success in this mission will not be achieved. Continuing needless tragedy for the Japanese people is the alternative... How successful you are depends on your exploitation of these 3 watchwords: organization, cooperation, and action'[68]

Japanese conditions were very different from the American, and Foster refused to specify the details of manufacture. Rather he introduced his audience to principles, pitfalls, and the American experience, and drew out practical conclusions from homely wisdom. Thus from 'Civilization has learned not to trust human nature' Foster concluded that it was important not to rely on the care of operators to prevent a dangerous vacuum forming in a vessel. Since an error could lead to implosion of the vessel and destruction of the plant, firms should install automatic emergency valves.

On organization, Foster was very direct. He announced there would be a centrally funded pilot plant run by the government, with its own control laboratory, as well as individual plants operated by the manufacturer with their quality-control laboratories. Foster also ensured that engineers, not bacteriologists, would provide the critical expertise. Overturning Japanese tradition, he demanded that the Japanese Penicillin Research Association form special committees for fermentation and for separation engineers.

The Japanese might have regarded Foster's visit as an imposition. Instead, they were immensely grateful. On his departure, ten different companies were able to start manufacturing. A Merck colleague, Boyd Woodruff, would find a decade later when he visited Japan that his own violations of protocol and inadvertent lapses of politeness would be forgiven just because he had had an association with the still-revered Jackson Foster.[69]

Research and production in Japan progressed rapidly. Within three years of Foster's arrival, Japan was self-sufficient in penicillin. In 1950, two Japanese scientists reported the first observation of the core ring of penicillin—the 'trunk' without the 'branches'—though their observations were not followed up at the time.[70] Japanese producers, already world leaders in fermentation technologies, would become globally important in the production of antibiotics. When Foster returned to Japan to do a report in 1960, he found a transformed industry to which even his old company Merck had already turned for help.[71] The Japanese experience showed, once again, the importance of pre-war know-how, wartime experiments, and the value of a personal product champion, transferring expertise about the pitfalls and opportunities of the new technology.

Although pursuing their careers largely in academe, both Foster and Chain maintained close relations with industry. After Foster returned from Japan, he became a professor at the University of Texas, but he remained a valued consultant for Merck. Although Chain was never the employee of a private company, he advised many commercial organizations across the world, most significantly Beecham. These men and the pioneers of manufacturing in such centres as Prague, Delft, Paris, Kunming, Rome, and Innsbruck were dedicated to overcoming shortages, at a time when people were dying for lack of penicillin. Their work supported local manufacturing and the development of penicillin through new technologies, and indeed led to such fundamentally new products as the first oral penicillin, Penicillin V, and the later range of semisynthetic penicillins.

The urgency of early penicillin provision was driven by the health needs of entire communities. In a deprived post-war world, infection still threatened societies as a whole. How to make best use of the new resource was widely debated at the World Health Assembly held in 1948, when the World Health Organization took over from UNRRA. The published discussions highlighted the representatives' acute anxiety about venereal disease, the hopes for penicillin, and the worries that it would be abused until it no longer worked. Concerns over abuse and waste were closely connected with fears of shortages. A specialist committee recommended the use of the purer crystalline penicillin be reserved for the cure of syphilis.[72] Sufferers from gonorrhoea could make do with the more abundant but less pure amorphous penicillin.

Penicillin had travelled very fast from the few centres of the Western Allies to countries across the world, even though it depended on a radically new production technology. This was no mere ripple effect. Instead, the recipients had already been primed by their pre-war and wartime experience. The transfers had also been made with verve and enthusiasm driven by the fear of epidemics and the evangelism of pioneers. Then, as penicillin became cheaper and more abundantly available, the burden of use shifted from protecting society as a whole to treating and reassuring the individual patient.

5

The Carefree Culture and the Third Industrial Revolution

For many in the generation raised after the Second World War, anxiety over infectious disease seemed to belong safely in the past. Between 1900 and 1980, the death rate from infectious diseases in the USA fell more than twentyfold.[1] So, while in 1900 for every 100,000 Americans there had been almost 800 deaths from infection, that had fallen to just thirty-six deaths in 1980. This improvement was widely credited to the emergence of antibiotics which seemed to promise a ready and effective cure for most infections. The hopeful and confident mood of the early penicillin years in just one country was symbolized by the title of a 1958 book: *The Americans: A Story about People, Democracy, Free Schools, Ice Cream, Airplanes, Social Security, Penicillin, Atomic Energy and All the Things that Make our Nation Great.*[2] Even if, at the end of the century, the optimism of such a title might seem facile, it expressed the deeply entrenched appeal of a technical solution to the problem of infection.

The widespread use of the drug was part of a technological transformation of the whole of medicine. Even in the 1950s and 1960s, the deep changes across technology and industry that followed the Second World War were being interpreted as a 'third industrial revolution'.[3] Visionaries such as the British crystallographer and science historian John Desmond Bernal saw the prospect of an escape from the irrational constraints of the past. He described a new scientific industrial revolution characterized by cheap power, automation, the application of biology, and organized research.[4] Wartime electronic and pharmaceutical innovations had been transferred into radically new products that were spreading rapidly across the world through the efforts of new multinational enterprises. The pharmaceutical industry has been seen as providing the very model of such companies, and their products, such as penicillin, and other antibiotics that were developed shortly afterwards, were exemplary.[5] The quantity and pattern of use reflected the drugs' role as much more than chemicals: they came to be essential components of individual lifestyles and medical cultures around the world. This incorporation into the texture of many societies would cause particular difficulty when medical elites tried to limit the drugs' uses, prompted by fears of bacterial resistance.

The enthusiasms of the 'penicillin age' led to large and remorselessly growing consumption. Between 1948 and 1956, the US market for penicillin increased sevenfold to over 450,000 kg, or 2 grams for every person in the country.[6] In western Europe, the growth was similar: Italy, Spain, and France came to be particularly enthusiastic users. If, during the 1960s, the rate of consumption growth then moderated it remained considerable. Thus, in the two decades from 1960, global consumption of penicillin doubled. By 1980, the world's production of 17,000 tonnes of penicillin was enough for a therapeutic course of treatment for every person on earth.[7] The 4 per cent annual growth rate was showing no signs of slowing: by 1990, half as much again was being used.[8]

Other antibiotics were also introduced from the late 1940s. Used when penicillin was not safe, to attack bacteria not susceptible to it, and increasingly to combat germs when doctors did not clearly know what they were, these new drugs greatly extended what has been called 'the therapeutic revolution'.[9] Nonetheless, penicillin and its chemical derivatives would continue to be the most prescribed of all antibiotics. In Europe, even at the end of the twentieth century, they would be specified on approximately half of all outpatient antibiotic prescriptions.[10] The culture of penicillin consumption would therefore colour the whole of antibiotic use and the debates over its control.

Penicillin's public-health effect was to sustain and continue pre-war improvements in mortality and morbidity, but its dramatic effects on the course of many particularly feared conditions also transformed the ways people thought about their lives in the post-war years. Compared to the pre-war atmosphere of self-reliance, self-discipline, and, of course, guilt in the event of failure to maintain health, infection now came to be seen as a technical problem susceptible to a pharmaceutical solution. By the early 1960s, when the industry came under serious criticism, it was chastised as a wayward new example of big business whose practices were inhibiting consumption by making it too expensive. So underconsumption, not overconsumption, was still seen as the main challenge.

Within medicine, the hospital was the iconic centre of the new industrial revolution. Once devoted to a few operations and long convalescence, hospitals came to be idealized as high-throughput health factories offering the prospect of repair by means of new technology and complex operations, in which infection was antibiotically controlled. By 1960, patient admissions to US hospitals had increased 40 per cent since the Second World War.[11] Even in Britain where the shortage of hospital treatment was an enduring political issue, the number of beds had almost doubled since 1938.[12] So the absolute scale and speed of processing grew rapidly; so did the range of technologies used to diagnose and treat, and, again, these benefited from penicillin.

Devices that could monitor the body's working, such as heart and brain function, were based on electronics developed through the wartime radar programme. Kidney dialysis and open-heart surgery also drew upon the new electronics. Antibiotics supported surgeons, who were now confident they could manage infection and were routinely carrying out more ambitious operations. Injections deep into the muscle, and inserting intravenous drips, had once been dangerous procedures risking infection. Now antibiotics could make the process safer. Cancer therapists could also reduce the immunity of patients without the worry of infection.

In general, whereas before strict hygiene had been seen as essential to the avoidance of disaster, now a little less rigour was sometimes afforded. Looking back forty years, a nursery nurse reported this conversation of the 1950s : 'I said, "Dr Silverman, you don't act so particular about your technique now." He said, "Oh, no, Lindsay, we've got penicillin now".'[13] A Harvard professor warned in 1963 that the rapid growth in antibiotic use was due not just to clinical need, but also to understaffing, ignorance, and poor diagnosis.[14] Although anxieties were sometimes expressed about the loss of old standards, the risk of infection in crowded wards prone to infection was even, on occasion, reduced by spraying antibiotic into the atmosphere.[15]

Whether in hospital or beyond it, penicillin was credited widely with ensuring that formerly life-threatening conditions became part of life's natural course, or disappeared from most people's experience. Most incidences of pneumonia, once the 'Captain of the Men of Death', came to be readily curable.[16] In just the fifteen years from 1939 to 1954, the number of deaths it caused in children aged 1–4 years in the USA fell by three-quarters.[17] Similarly, the death rate from rheumatic fever and rheumatic heart disease there fell tenfold between 1940 and 1960.[18] Thanks to penicillin, syphilis was rapidly downgraded from threat to humanity to a vanishing disease. In the USA, by 1954 the incidence of syphilis was just one-quarter of its level between the wars.[19] A historian of the Netherlands has pointed to the falling incidence of syphilis there: for every hundred cases in 1947, there were just two in 1959.[20] A well-known American specialist in the disease, speaking to his British colleagues in 1956, compared their situation to that of a fighter pilot whose plane had been shot from under him.[21]

Penicillin was used to counter day-to-day problems as well as hitherto life-threatening conditions. A detailed British study of GP consultations conducted in 1951 indicated the impact of penicillin on daily life.[22] Out of every thousand patients registered with a practice, just over 700 consulted in a twelve-month period. The most common complaints—common cold (130 patients) and influenza (46.3 patients)—were caused by viruses that were still resilient to agents of destruction. Other complaints, such as bronchitis (77.9), were also often resistant to modern medicine. But pneumonia was diagnosed in 10 patients and could now be generally reliably dispatched within a few days. There were large numbers of other infections that were painful and potentially risky and now easily curable: 31.2 acute otitis media (earache), 22.8 boils and carbuncles, with 10.8 septic fingers and toes and a further 8.9 other abscesses. With over 40 people in every thousand consulting the doctor for skin infections in a single year, over a ten-year period any individual would have a high probability of needing help for such conditions. Now they could be often treated simply with antibiotics, in contrast with the much more traumatic experience of just a few years earlier. In the community, therefore, for conditions ranging from earache to pneumonia, drugs offered effective treatments.

Against the drama of cure, statistical changes in the outcomes of illness were complex and less clear-cut. Much of the overall improvement in post-war health could, for instance, be put down not to drugs but rather to improved nutrition and better, less-damp housing. The pioneer of 'social medicine' in Britain, Tom McKeown, would argue in the 1970s that graphs of deaths from diseases such as pneumonia showed roughly continuous exponential decline through the twentieth century.[23] Nonetheless a 1957 study by the US Federal Trade Commission of the contribution of antibiotics to falling death rates found a difference between those infections that could be treated and those that could not.[24] Whereas the incidence of those infections still holding out against treatment dropped by 20 per cent from 1946 to 1955, the incidence of diseases that could be treated with antibiotics fell twice as fast, by over 40 per cent. There were even more dramatic measures of falling death rates, but it was always hard to disentangle the direct and indirect effects of the many medical and environmental changes occurring at the same time.

Whatever the specific mix of environmental and therapeutic impacts, patients in rich countries were, increasingly, assured wide access to the technologies of treatment. Despite the fierce ideological debates between the proponents of private and nationally funded insurance systems, the very fact of widespread insurance marked a major difference from the past for many people. The 1948 establishment of the National Health Service in Britain made consulting a doctor free of direct cost. By the mid–1950s, two out of three people surveyed had visited their surgery in the past year. Although the British were proud to boast that their system was 'the envy of the world', across Europe schemes of various kinds also came to provide universal coverage. In the USA, private health insurance grew up very quickly, so that by the early 1960s most people were covered.[25] In general, patients in rich countries were being enabled to consult their doctors, if briefly, and to consume medicines.

The promise of modern medicine was also extended to poorer countries, through schemes to eradicate individual diseases totally. Penicillin was introduced during a war being fought for total victory, and afterwards media commentators, scientists, and politicians used the jargon of combat to extol the drug's virtues and world-changing potential. Images of conquest and destruction were used early and often to describe the drug's effects. Nine books with titles similar to *The Conquest of Disease* were published in the period 1943 to 1953. Similarly, distinguished British science journalist Nigel Calder observed in 1958: 'One does not need a crystal ball to predict that, within this generation, medical science will have overcome, and controlled, all man's external enemies.'[26] Such rhetoric was turned into action by energetic public-health campaigners and by the World Health Organization, founded in 1948.

During the 1950s, and into the 1960s, enthusiasts talked optimistically of wiping out plagues that had been feared for generations. By 1963 two of America's top doctors reporting on the 'Philosophy of Disease Eradication' could hardly contain their enthusiasm. They talked of 'the almost boundless optimism which characterises this third and present attitudinal phase regarding disease eradication'.[27] The weapons to hand, along with antibiotics, included vaccines and such new insecticides as DDT. Three diseases—malaria, smallpox, and yaws—were prime candidates for elimination.

Until the late 1960s, the mosquitoes that spread malaria were attacked by means of massive use of DDT insecticide as well as by drainage schemes. However, the insects' ability to develop resistance to the insecticide, and environmental concerns, frustrated the attempt to wipe out the disease. More successful was the attack, by means of vaccination and surveillance, on smallpox, which was successfully eradicated by 1977. Smallpox would stand out as the great success story of the eradication campaigns.

Penicillin was used to address the disease known as yaws, a tropical relative of syphilis. C. J. Hackett, an architect of British yaws policy, describes the disease as disabling—with its ulcers, crippling contractures, facial destruction, and palm and plantar lesions—if not a killer.[28] Unlike the more familiar syphilis, yaws is spread not by sexual but by ordinary skin contact and, typically, infects children. The first use of the drug against yaws had been during 1944, when it was tested separately in Brazil, Fiji, and West Africa. In the post-war years, the World Health Organization (WHO) working with the United Nations International Children's Emergency Fund (UNICEF) made large amounts of penicillin available to complete an anti-yaws campaign that had been fought for thirty years (see Ill. 16).[29] More than 150 million people had been screened for the disease by 1965. Treatment for active, latent, or suspected infection had been given to over 43 million individuals in forty-two countries. In Bosnia, a Mediterranean variant of the disease, bejel, had been eradicated. In parts of Indonesia, infection from yaws was reduced from one person in every six of the population to just a single infected person per thousand.[30] Such dramatic advances in the fight against debilitating infections lent vivid reality to the vision of penicillin as a weapon.[31]

Penicillin was, moreover, just one of many powerful weapons that were added to the doctor's armoury during the 1940s and early 1950s. By 1958, an industry spokesman cited the statistics that an American doctor could prescribe 200 sulphonamides, 270 different antibiotic products, 130 anti-histamines, and 100 tranquillizers.[32] Hardly any of these drugs had been available before the war, and together they represented a transformation of the power of the pharmaceutical contribution to the management of health.

Some older doctors were shocked by this new model of medicine. In 1947, the distinguished bacteriologist Lawrence Garrod commented scathingly in the *British Medical Journal* on his colleagues' practices of pre-scribing penicillin. 'The present enormous consumption of the drug can be accounted for only by a good deal of indiscriminate use,' he complained.[33] An English surgeon addressing an obstetrics conference in 1960 spoke out

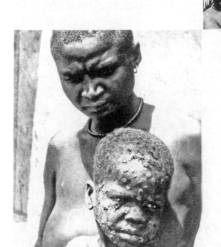

16. Curing yaws. A WHO poster from a 1958 picture set entitled 'World Health Advances'.

World Health Organization.

PENICILLIN CURES THIS DISEASE

This hideous affliction is called yaws. A single shot of penicillin will cure it. By the end of 1958 national teams assisted by WHO and UNICEF had treated 25 million such cases.

against the 'lotus-land of antibiotics'.[34] An American military doctor castigated his colleagues for indulging in 'Antibiotic abandon'.[35]

Among patients, the explosive growth in antibiotic use during the 1950s betokened a profound cultural change in the approach to medicine in general. No longer did patients see drugs as a last resort to be drawn upon when hygiene and morality failed. Instead, infections could be simply cured. The contrast between old and new sources of health was illustrated by Malcolm Muggeridge, maverick British journalist and intellectual, as he parodied the King James Bible in 1962 in an article in the *New Statesman* magazine, 'I will lift up mine eyes to the pills whence cometh my help.'[36] In a 1968 debate, a parliamentarian who was also a doctor told the British Parliament the story of an elderly man who, after the death of his wife, 'consumed what remained of her medicine and tablets before throwing away the bottles and containers. "Why there is nothing the matter with you, is there", the doctor asked. The man replied, "No, but I thought that it might find a weak spot somewhere".'[37]

The change in emphasis from moral control to pharmaceutical cure was even incorporated into social science. In a classic synthesis of 1951, the Harvard sociologist Talcott Parsons portrayed the morality of effective medicine within his total model of society.[38] The citizen, according to Parsons, had just one moral responsibility as patient, to go to the doctor if regrettably he or she did get ill. The new medicine would therefore relieve the citizen of the traditional moral burdens of illness. By means of modern medicines, the doctors and hospitals offered to relieve the patient of the moral blame and guilt traditionally associated with catching an infection.

Direct evidence for the changes in how most people thought about illness as penicillin was introduced must of course be largely anecdotal. A few more systematic studies do, however, pass down to us evidence from that early era. In France, in the early 1960s, the sociologist Christiane Herzlich observed that her older respondents credited antibiotics with elimination of 'real illnesses'.[39] As for blame, they were still willing to apportion it, but they blamed external forces, including urban lifestyles, much more than themselves.[40] For the United States, a later study of older people provided evidence of generational change in attitudes towards blame. In 1989 a team at Brandeis University studied the attitudes of 150 people born between 1905 and 1965 drawn from a range of ages and socio-economic groups in the Boston area.[41] Among the questions asked was whether they felt to blame if they became ill. For all the problems of small numbers in a single location, the results were suggestive. Half (47 per cent) those born during 1924–31 agreed or disagreed only slightly. On the other hand, of those born during 1932–49, only a quarter agreed or disagreed only slightly, and the others instead disagreed or disagreed strongly with such an admission of guilt.[42] The British GP and anthropologist Cecil Helman observed for himself a change in attitudes to illness between the older women with folk attitudes and their younger, less judgemental counterparts.[43] His experience was that a transformation from an anxious moral approach to confidence in the control of illness was due to free medicine and antibiotics.

The reduction of fear had its own social effects. Suddenly, across a wide spectrum of behaviour, 'carelessness'—once condemned—could be afforded. The historian Sue Ellen Hoy begins the postscript to her study of cleanliness with the question and answer: 'Are we as clean as we used to be? Probably not.'[44] The most discussed aspect of moral transformation affected by the new drugs was venereal disease. For the individual, penicillin provided cure both of disease and of anxiety. Diarists recording their thoughts for 'Mass Observation' emphasized their desperation to obtain the drug and even information about it.[45] However the speedy cures offered for both gonorrhoea and early syphilis could also cause moral panic. Licence, permissiveness, and sexual freedom across society as a whole all seemed to follow. Alfred Kinsey's *Sexual Behavior in the Human Female*, widely blamed for polluting innocent minds, suggested that cures for venereal disease had disabled the threat of illness. An official in Britain's Home Office, which was considering censoring the book, was appalled. He accused Kinsey of being 'Monstrously irresponsible' because 'Fear of disease is perhaps the most potent factor in restraining many young people from promiscuous immorality.'[46] Introduction of 'The Pill' in the 1960s helped partners to manage the other risk this could bring. With cures for venereal disease on the one hand and an increased range of contraceptives on the other, all sex was suddenly 'safe'.

Belief in the total safety of penicillin itself underpinned the culture of use. Even though this confidence was occasionally shaken, in most places, patterns of use were not affected. Although most patients could indeed be given massive quantities without ill effect, nevertheless, since the drug's earliest introduction negative reactions in a few cases had been reported by doctors. At first such errant results were put down to impurities and weaknesses in the production process. Yet, even as the purity of the product improved, occasional but consistent reports of skin complaints and inflammations similar to the allergic reactions encountered with vaccinations were still being documented in medical journals.[47] When, in 1951, the US government included penicillin in a list of drugs restricted by federal law to prescription-only access, a key argument put for its inclusion in this category was the danger of allergic reaction threatening unsuspecting users.[48]

In general the symptom of most allergic reactions was a minor skin rash, but, for a very small proportion of the increasingly large number of patients, the reaction could be catastrophic. In 1946 a patient in New York died two days after suffering a fever and a rash apparently caused by penicillin therapy. Three years later, a patient in Detroit died within minutes of receiving a penicillin injection, and by 1953, Henry Welch, responsible for antibiotics in America's Food and Drug Administration, could document twenty-four fatalities that could be ascribed to penicillin.[49] Later, in the mid–1960s, it became clear that breakdown products of penicillin combine with proteins to stimulate the patient to produce antibodies to which they are intolerant.[50] Although, the problems could be reduced by purifying the product of protein which bound easily to the drug, even then the problem was not entirely alleviated. As was pointed out even in 1970, 'There is a fascinating biological paradox in the fact that penicillin, which can be well tolerated in the largest doses, can also cause fatalities in the smallest doses.'[51] Hannelore Kohl, wife of German Chancellor Helmuth Kohl, would suffer an allergic reaction to penicillin in 1993, leading to an intolerance of sunlight, meaning that she could not leave her house; the condition lasted until her death by suicide in 2001.[52]

Such tragedies as Hannelore Kohl's were mercifully rare in the West, and the reputation of the drug seems not to have been affected there, but in the Far East ill effects had a much greater impact. In such countries as Japan and Taiwan, doctors routinely sold drugs direct to patients rather than prescribing them for others to sell. There was therefore a perceived advantage for them to recommend as much penicillin as possible. Early in the 1950s, in both Taiwan and Japan, deaths at the hands of doctors caused by penicillin were reported. Medical men, anxious about legal reprisals as well as concerned for the health of their patients, naturally reduced their use of the drug radically.[53]

By the early 1950s, in any case, other antibiotics had become available. These provided a greater range of pharmaceutical alternatives to the patient, and also new products for an industry that was now coming under great commercial pressure. Because penicillin itself had not been patented, with more and more manufacturers worldwide entering into production, its price fell precipitously. The 100,000-unit dose for which the US government had been willing to pay $20 in 1943 fell to 25 cents in 1951.[54] To the companies involved, this precipitate decline was a threat, but at first reducing costs and exploding markets ensured that profits rose and rose. However, 1951 was the peak year. Production rates kept rising, but the market was saturated and, as the prices kept falling, so did profits. By 1953, the price of that 100,000 units had dropped to less than one cent, and the drug, only recently more precious than gold, was worth less than the bottles it came in.

As the costs of unpatented penicillin fell, the pressure to protect revenues by finding alternative products that could be patented grew intensely. The President of the Bristol-Myers company, a major penicillin supplier, reported to a meeting of the operating heads in 1953 that the industry was sick.[55] The company had specialized in penicillin, and the value of its sales halved between 1951 and 1953, even though production had increased. All the companies had problems. Squibb's profits were also under pressure.[56] The situation was truly ironic: successfully producing high-technology medicines was driving companies bankrupt.

They therefore came under intense pressure to innovate or die, as profits from penicillin manufacture disappeared. Within a few years of the end of the Second World War, US firms had introduced four 'broad-spectrum' antibiotics, which attacked all types of bacteria, not just a narrow range, as was then the case with penicillin, and made themselves extremely profitable.

Pharmaceutical companies found their skills and strengths well suited to the challenges of finding new antibiotics. Following the example of René Dubos in discovering gramicidin, they screened enormous numbers of soil samples for organisms that might produce an antibiotic and carried out numerous tests to find which of the many chemicals produced could be useful as a medicine and would not be toxic. This approach had been proven by Selman Waksman at Rutgers University who, from 1940, with his students had found a remarkable number of powerful antibiotics produced by actinomycetes—including actinomycin, neomycin, and the first effective treatment for tuberculosis, streptomycin.[57] Waksman himself was a visionary, and indeed was responsible for giving its modern meaning to the term 'antibiotic' in 1942.[58] Routine screening of large numbers of soil samples could, however, be better managed and more smoothly conducted by well-organized pharmaceutical companies with the expertise and funds to manage big teams.

The screening process itself was laborious and often fruitless.[59] Thus, between 1949 and 1959 the Lilly company screened 10,000 soil samples and examined 200,000 organisms. From these they isolated 300 chemicals showing antibiotic activity, and just three antibiotics reached the market. Nonetheless, occasionally one could strike very lucky. In 1952 a member of a new family of drugs (a macrolide), which came to be called erythromycin, was announced by Lilly. This drug had been produced from a mould sent to them from the Philippines. Because it was chemically quite different from other drugs, it could be used when resistance had made them ineffective.

Many companies were attracted to the challenge of producing new antibiotics. Thus the Parke Davis company, which had been a pioneer of modern drugs recruited John Ehrlich deputy head of the penicillin programme at the University of Minnesota, where he had screened moulds for high-productivity mutant penicillium strains.[60] In January 1944 the company also gave a grant to the Yale professor Paul Burkholder to seek new antibiotics produced by organisms in soil samples. Over 7,000 samples were collected through the help of collaborators, Parke Davis representatives, and scientists worldwide.

The transport of dirt in the hope that it would contain useful moulds had a certain quirkiness worthy of a Graham Greene novel. In March 1945, a crate arrived at Burkholder's laboratory in New Haven, sent by an expatriate American scientist in Caracas, Venezuela, and containing bottles filled with soil from the compost heap of an émigré Basque vegetable breeder. By March 1946, transparent crystals of a relatively simple compound, chloramphenicol, had been isolated from this compost and in another year remarkable therapeutic properties had been demonstrated. Over the next two years, this compound was shown to cure the feared diseases typhus and typhoid and also had a therapeutic effect on illnesses caused by a wide range of bacteria.

The experience of chloramphenicol spurred the competition. Lederle, a division of American Cyanamide, had entered antibiotics through penicillin manufacture. In August 1945 an interesting yellow mould from a Missouri timothy field was identified. Getting in just before Parke Davis's launch of chloramphenicol, in 1948 Lederle announced its new antibiotic, later called chlortetracycline. Both these drugs had a major advantage over penicillin—they could cure a much wider range of bacterial infections. This meant that doctors could be saved time-consuming investigations of what had actually caused their patients' infections. If it was bacterial, then one of the new broad-spectrum antibiotics would probably knock it out. This not only offered strictly medical benefits: it also made the medical consultation process more efficient, and offered the prospect of a faster throughput of patients.

The most important products of this race came next from Pfizer, which had been the dominant wartime manufacturer of penicillin. It had built its success on fermentation technology, and was not traditionally a pharmaceutical company. Lacking its own links to pharmacists, Pfizer supplied other companies. But it was in danger of being abandoned when, after the war, these began to build their own manufacturing facilities. The company was torn between irritation with its erstwhile customers, who were now competitors, and anxiety about entering a sector in which it had no standing. Left with no alternative, Pfizer decided to enter the pharmaceutical industry itself with its own drug. A fictionalized account of the early 1960s, *In Vivo*, by the writer Mildred Savage captured the mood of the industry at the time. The novel described tension between the visionary scientist dreaming of a new product and the defensive engineer seeking funds for the better production of penicillin, the uncertainty of meetings, the conflicts of personalities, and the waves of optimism and depression before success was achieved.[61]

Pfizer scientists surveyed soils from all over the world. Like all the companies, Pfizer had the problem of distinguishing between similar chemicals that had some effect on bacteria. The compound known as streptothricin, commonly produced by organisms abundant in soil, was already known to be too toxic to use as a medicine. Hopes would rise when soil tests gave positive results, and then laborious tests were conducted, only for streptothricin again to be revealed as the cause, disappointing investigators and wasting their time. The discovery, however, of the technique of chromatography (in which strips of filter paper are used to separate soluble chemicals that creep along them at different rates) was a boon and enabled the rate of selection to be greatly increased. They found in 1949, a sample of soil which turned out to be the 'ore' from which the organism producing the successful broad-spectrum drug Terramycin would be isolated.[62] In 1952/3 Pfizer and Lederle, separately, followed up their first breakthroughs with the even more successful tetracycline, which was related chemically to their two earlier broad-spectrum drugs.[63]

Thus, by the mid–1950s, penicillin had been joined by several dozen other antibiotics and the pharmaceutical industry moved into growth. As a result of its many new products and the booming market, during many of the years in the 1950s the industry was the most profitable in the USA. The shock of this transformation and the unexpected effects of medicine's changing place in the economy were hard to comprehend. The most dramatic indicator of the unexpectedness of growth was the scandal of Henry Welch, the head of the antibiotics branch of the FDA responsible for approving new drugs and batches of antibiotics. He had been himself a pioneer of penicillin, validating batches of the new drug for the FDA during the Second World War.

In 1951 Welch was given permission to edit a new specialist journal dealing with antibiotics, to accept an honorarium, and later himself to act as the journal's publisher.[64] There is no evidence that Welch initially intended to behave corruptly. However, the opportunities his position provided were much greater than his superiors, and probably even he, had anticipated. As well as advertising space in his journal, companies purchased several hundred thousand expensive offprints of articles from him—although these were never distributed and merely kept in a warehouse. A colleague would complain that he had once heard Welch boast that his FDA salary just paid his income taxes. In exchange, he simplified the process of certifying drug batches. As a former colleague remembered, 'Henry would fix up what was needed.'[65]

By 1956, the pharmaceutical industry itself became anxious about Welch's divided roles of profiting from advertising and offprint selling to the industry on the one hand and, on the other, providing impartial rulings. Enquiries were, however, delayed by prevarication, and it took another three years for the story to be revealed. Welch had earned, under the heading of 'honorarium', one quarter of a million dollars. He had been scrupulous about reporting everything except the amount, which seems to have taken aback even the chairman of Merck, who had raised the alarm. Almost certainly he had himself been surprised by the opportunities he found. It was becoming clear that the pharmaceutical industry born out of penicillin represented a completely new ball-game.

As the value of all ethical drugs sold in the USA increased more than tenfold from 1939 to 1958, the industry joined the ranks of big business.[66] 'In becoming a billion-dollar business, the pharmaceutical industry has changed from a small, quiet orderly affair to a fast-moving, noisy fiercely competitive operation,' noted Milton Moskovitz, editor of *Advertising Age*, in 1957.[67] In 1959, the Executive Vice-President of the National Pharmaceutical Council compared the development of his industry with the gold rush, the pioneering days of the railroad, or the oil bonanzas of Texas.[68] Before the war, the ethical pharmaceutical companies such as Parke Davis and Merck had been small and medium-size enterprises. Their scale then may be contrasted with that of the chemical giant Du Pont, which in 1940 employed 53,523. In 1940, the leading pharmaceutical manufacturer, Merck, employed 1,800 and had a stock market valuation of $10 million.[69] Wartime saw the introduction of a host of new drugs, including penicillin and streptomycin. By 1950, Merck had changed league: it now employed 6,000 people and its stock market worth was $130 million. Subsequently it grew so much more quickly than Du Pont that by 1998 the sales of the erstwhile tiddler exceeded those of the 1930s giant.[70]

These companies were not only larger than their pre-war predecessors and more technologically savvy—they were also much more focused on marketing. As well as formerly specialized ethical-drug makers, the industry also included companies which had been active in marketing healthy foods and vitamins before the war. The practice of recruiting a large workforce to systematically visit and brief doctors to prescribe a company's products, developed in the 1930s had come to pervade the entire industry.[71] In the mid–1950s, the US pharmaceutical industry already employed 10,000 to 12,000 'detailmen' who visited individual doctors typically six times a year.[72] The relationship with physicians was friendly, but between company representatives it was more like war.[73]

In the course of aggressive competition, golf balls, more valuable gifts, and free samples were kindly given by generous representatives to grateful doctors. The whole of society, even children, came to be aware of pressures on treatment. An article entitled 'I am a receptionist' in the 1963 edition of an annual for young girls based on the popular medical soap opera *Emergency Ward 10* divulged the shocking news that 'I have heard more than one sulphurous comment about the drug racket.'[74] This marketing effort made the the industry suspect for persuading doctors to prescribe unnecessarily expensive brands.

The growing cost of the industry's products became part of the mainstream debate about the cost of medicine. The mood of regulators and buyers was caught by a November 1959 report to Congress which declared that 'medical care is becoming wonderfully effective and appallingly expensive'.[75] Whereas, traditionally, American doctors had charged just for a visit and included whatever drugs would be necessary, by about 1960, for every five dollars spent on doctors in the USA, four dollars were spent on medical supplies.[76] Drugs, which linked two major political targets—medicine and big business—were therefore a particularly high-profile industry.

In Britain the National Health Service, which began in 1948, was introduced at the same time as penicillin was coming into widespread use. Initially bearing the entire cost of medicines, the Service came under unexpected financial pressure from new demands. In the first year of operation it was expected that 1948/9 expenditure on drugs would be £11.5 million.[77] Instead, the year's costs were more than three times as much, largely on account of penicillin. Between 1948 and 1953 the average cost of a prescription in Britain rose by a half, and they continued to rise despite a host of control measures. When the Labour government felt forced to charge for medicines in a service intended to be free, the Labour Party was split, ministers resigned, and the government soon fell. This was a major event in the country's political history, but it is not often mentioned that it had been caused by the problem of paying for penicillin and other 'miracle' drugs, such as cortisone and streptomycin.

The industry therefore came under assault for making safe drugs too expensive. This attack, which became, in the early 1960s, one of the major political issues in the USA, was not particularly focused on penicillin. It did, however, grow out of the problems and opportunities presented by the drug. Moreover, through the way this attack dealt with the issues of pricing, profits, and marketing, it established the policy concern with underconsumption. In an era just two decades after the Depression of the

1930s, patients and politicians feared an under-provision of pharmaceuticals. They blamed rapidly escalating treatment costs on the industry's excessive prices. In addressing these concerns, economists and politicians passed over the problems of bacterial resistance with which public-health officials, microbiologists, and chemists had been wrestling for a decade.

Throughout the 1950s, the US Congress had voiced concern about the power of large companies in general and about the growing pharmaceutical corporations in particular. To economists, the growth of a major new industry was not a novel phenomenon. It had happened before with automobiles, steel, and oil, and each time a few firms had acquired dominant positions. A group of American economists, addressing the threat of underconsumption in society, now believed that the problems so often associated with a new industry rapidly moving from the margins of the economy to its centre could be pre-empted. They believed that the federal government could ensure that the use of publicity, the licensing of patents, and the setting of prices was in the public interest. Determined to transform America's institutional geography in general, and the pharmaceutical industry in particular, their intervention was crucial to the debates over controlling pharmaceuticals in the 1950s.[78]

The inquiry into the drug industry by the US Senate Sub-Committee on Antitrust and Monopoly named after its chairman, Senator Kefauver, investigated the market in antibiotics and in three other specialities: corticosteroids such as cortisone used by arthritis sufferers, tranquillizers, and oral antidiabetics. The inquiry began in December 1959 and, over the next ten months, 150 witnesses were called to testify. The inquiry's concern over price was expressed in a question put by its Chief Counsel, Paul Rand Dixon (later Federal Trade Commission commissioner), to an industry witness about the cost of antibiotics: 'do you think a cost of $17 to the average mother and father every time their child has a bad cold is down to a point where it can be reached even by the needy?'[79] The detail that antibiotics did not affect colds, and should not be prescribed for them, was swept aside as the committee looked at the plight of the individual patient faced with the power of the corporation.

If not concerned with the use of antibiotics to treat viral complaints, the committee was concerned with the ability of large companies to persuade doctors to prescribe branded and expensive products rather than the cheapest available. Since advertising and marketing were themselves expensive, the committee enquired whether the considerable excess of prices over production costs was due to the need to support that advertising. Companies, the committee suggested, were investing all this marketing effort to persuade doctors to use drugs that differed only marginally one from another. It was demonstrated that spending on marketing exceeded investment in research, and it was argued that, for all the talk of high technology, many of the drugs were merely slight variants of one another. From concern about price, the committee therefore moved to the question of how a patient could tell the difference between drugs and whether differences were substantial or just cosmetic. The committee suspected that many of the innovations boasted by the pharmaceutical industry had been developed abroad or by academics, and therefore the rewards of patenting had not been a significant factor in the pharmaceutical revolution.[80]

As he was concluding the investigative hearings, Kefauver moved from research to action and began campaigning for a new bill to regulate what he considered to be the restrictive practices of the drug industry. There was considerable opposition in Congress, and even from President Kennedy, who had appointed Merck President John Connor as his Trade Secretary. However, the balance of power was changed by thalidomide.

In July 1962 the American Food and Drug Administration (FDA) refused a licence to sell this drug in the USA, although it had been widely sold elsewhere in the world. The examiner, Frances Kelsey, was concerned about the potential effect of this drug intended for pregnant women on foetal development, and, while approval was delayed, damning evidence emerged.[81] The FDA action gave legitimacy to the parents of thousands of German children and the hundreds of parents in the UK, Sweden, Australia, and elsewhere who had blamed the new drug for the handicaps of their children.[82]

The breaking story of how only the vigilance of a single FDA inspector had protected Americans from the misfortunes visited on European and Australian parents dramatically affected public opinion.[83] Suddenly it seemed urgent to contain the power of the companies. On the back of concerns about the safety of thalidomide, legislation that had been intended to increase the ability of patients to obtain medicine was swept through Congress. Ironically, although the catalyst was the fear of the potential danger of one specific drug, Congress acted on legislation that was largely intended to increase confidence in greater consumption of drugs in general.

The thalidomide crisis brought together the issues of corporate trustworthiness, the risks of exploitation, and heedless innovation. The risks of the third industrial revolution had come into sight and, to some, the issues of safety put the use of modern medicines in question. In Britain, the National Antivaccination League had been worrying about vaccines since the late nineteenth century. Now it turned to attacking antibiotics. Its members were still fulminating against the injection of poisons into the bloodstream of naive citizens at a time when there was an outbreak of smallpox. Despite this threat, a session chair at the 1963 annual meeting noted the change since the pre-war days of proprietary drugs: 'These sort of medicines were just ordinary poisons—but the sort of things they give you now—the antibiotics and the other things—are a different proposition altogether. People are coming to the conclusion that these medicines are worse than the diseases themselves.'[84]

Leading this sceptical organization was its President, Joyce Butler, a Member of Parliament and active local politician in north London.[85] Her association with the many elderly members of Antivaccination League might have seemed on the sidelines of history, even backward-looking. But she also had concerns about medicine that made her appeal very modern, and she was an effective politician. For example, later, Joyce Butler would be important in relaxing British legislation on the advertising of health food. She would also pioneer legislation banning discrimination against women. In Parliament she submitted searching questions to government ministers. Her questions to the Minister of Agriculture, Fisheries, and Food in the House during the session October 1962 to 1963 related to toxic properties of chemicals, pesticides in food and antibiotics in milk. To the Minister of Health she put questions on maternity care, thalidomide, fluoridation, oral contraceptives, and vaccination for polio and smallpox.[86] What might have been an old-fashioned disdain for modern medicines was also about to become a modern force.

Whereas Butler was an active politician, the leading prophet of the movement to undo an industrial attitude to the destruction of germs was the Rockefeller Institute's René Dubos.[87] The denunciations he hurled at Western practices were particularly potent because he himself had been an antibiotic pioneer in the 1930s with his product gramicidin. Shortly after that achievement, however, he had experienced a personal tragedy. Dubos's wife Marie-Louise suffered and then died from tuberculosis in 1942. He could not believe that she had suddenly become infected during her new life in the United States. Rather, he saw her death as the result of weakness brought on by worry over the wartime fate of her family left in France. She had become unable any longer to repress the bacteria that had been in her body since childhood. Marie-Louise's illness therefore resulted not just from germs but also from her overall state. Dubos became more than ever convinced that germs alone did not explain illness, and correspondingly that drugs alone could not be the answer to the control of disease.

Instead of germs, Dubos came to be much more concerned with the conditions that made one susceptible to them. Ill himself with a gastric haemorrhage, he was confined to a hospital bed where he read the work of the Chinese sage Lao Tse, founder of Taoism. This praised a calm life as the key to good health. Dubos was intoxicated by this. Later he reported he had read five different translations of Lao Tse's poem 'The Way'.[88] Out of hospital, Dubos gave a lecture to the Association of American Physicians, 'The Philosopher's Search for Health'. Here he introduced two competing Greek gods: Hygeia, who for him stood for hygiene, and Aesculapius, responsible for doctors and surgeons. So soon, he bemoaned, we have forgotten that infectious disease was diminishing long before the antibiotics. Hygeia, he felt, had not had her due. Dubos reported later that half his audience were supportive and the other half thought he was talking nonsense.

In 1959 Dubos extended his earlier lecture to attack further the claims of the medical profession. 'The Mirage of Health' argued that health could only be seen as a symbiosis of organisms. By contrast, he complained that doctors were busily trying to disrupt bacterial ecology. He assaulted the optimism of the medical profession.

The belief that disease can be conquered through the use of drugs fails to take into account the difficulties arising from the ecological complexity of human problems. It is an attitude comparable to the naïve cowboy philosophy that permeates the wild West thriller. In the crime-ridden frontier town the hero, single-handed, blasts out the desperadoes who were running rampant through the settlement. The story ends on a happy note because it appears that peace has been restored. But in reality the death of the villains does not solve the fundamental problem, for the rotten social conditions which had opened the town to the desperadoes will allow others to come in, unless something is done to correct the primary source of trouble.[89]

Dubos was still a lone voice, but an increasingly popular one, and some of his phrases, such as 'think globally, act locally', became catchwords of the environmental movement.[90] He was celebrated but, in the case of antibiotics, not widely influential. In the penicillin age, the technical solution to infection was, instead, embraced, time after time. Even when problems of resistance emerged, at first new products would be easier to introduce than new behaviours.

6

Fighting Resistance with Technology

For all the real and sustained improvements to health of the post-war years, the problems of bacterial infection could not be wholly eliminated. In place of vulnerable strains, weeded out by medical assault, resistant bacteria would often flourish. Microscopic organisms proved almost grotesquely adept at self-defence. Some, for example, produced an enzyme, beta-lactamase, which destroyed the penicillin molecule threatening the construction of cell walls. In a process known as 'efflux', other cells proved able to export those antibiotics that prevent them producing proteins (such as tetracycline) out through their walls, before they had suffered damage, and, it transpired, some bacterial strains assembled the genes for several such defences in a single organism.

The existence of resistant strains was not the result of human antibiotic use, and, although the spread of bacteria might be encouraged by poor practice, even the most careful medical procedures could not prevent bacterial evolution. In any case, with the success of penicillin, it seemed in the 1950s that technology had superseded behaviour control in the management of infection. Rather than dwelling on the issue of practice, most physicians, policy makers, and lay people therefore put their faith in the marriage of professional medical expertise with technological progress—even if the broker was now commercial ambition rather than, as previously, the pressures of global conflict. Notwithstanding the widespread fear at the very end of the twentieth century that existing defences would soon be breached, remarkable technical advances were indeed made, and antibiotics were available to meet numerous infections.

The challenge of resistance was compounded by its patchy emergence and restricted impact. It proved to be an evolutionary process that varied very widely among species and countries. In the 1950s, strains of the bacterium known as *Staphylococcus aureus* were already causing many deaths in hospitals and nurseries worldwide. From the 1960s, outside the hospital too, doctors encountered localized resistance in organisms that could spread through the community. First the gram-negative bacteria of the digestive system such as *E. coli* became the main threat, and then from the 1980s an increasing number of communities encountered resistant strains of *Streptococcus pneumoniae* (known as *S. pneumoniae* or pneumococci). These organisms moved rapidly from developing countries into the developed world, causing a variety of difficult-to-treat conditions ranging from infant 'red ear' to pneumonia.

In the face of such threats, new varieties and combinations of penicillin itself were introduced. Much less well known than the original discovery, the development of the new family was also profoundly important. It made possible new broad-spectrum variants such as ampicillin and amoxicillin, which became some of the world's favourite drugs. Racing to counter bacterial evolution, or at least manage its consequences, chemists also generated other such well-known penicillin products as methicillin and co-amoxiclav, which provided at least a partial vindication of early hopes that resistance could be contained by technology. Nonetheless, the enduring resistance of such feared organisms as MRSA and the rapid global spread of resistant *S. pneumoniae* demonstrated the limitations of this approach.

The experience of combating *Staphylococcus aureus* highlighted the speed with which some bacteria counteracted the threat of antibiotics. From the earliest days of penicillin, bacteriologists had expected organisms to evolve defences, just as bacteria had evolved rapidly to cope with the sulphonamides. As early as 1940, even before penicillin was tested on a patient, Ernst Chain and Edward Abraham in Oxford identified an enzyme produced by the staphylococcus bacterium which was capable of destroying the new medicine. This might have been just a laboratory observation, but in 1945 Australian researchers showed that staphylococci collected from a hospital where no penicillin was used were much more vulnerable to the drug than bacteria collected from a hospital in which the new medicine had already been introduced.[1] It was by then clear that the use of penicillin could favour the spread of bacteria resistant to the medicine.

Occasional observation turned to global public-health threat as early as the 1950s. Within a few years the worldwide spread of resistant strains of *Staphylococcus aureus* caused three separate, if related, epidemics of life-threatening conditions. Bacterial infections of wounds and of the skin beset hospitals, infant pneumonia was endemic in nurseries, and staphylococcal pneumonia affected patients weakened by influenza. *Staphylococcus aureus* is a bacterium particularly common in hospitals, where it infects the weak and the infirm: it is carried by about half of all people on their bodies. A minor cut on the hand of a surgeon or a nurse could nurture a colony, or it could lurk in the noses of staff, in skin infections on their hands, on blankets and curtains, on pencils and light fittings.[2] Even an apparently clean room could be infested.

Stimulated by wartime findings, from 1946 the microbiologist Mary Barber had begun to monitor the adaptation of the bug in London's Hammersmith Hospital.[3] Under the pressure of natural selection, resistant organisms evolved and grew remarkably fast. In 1946, seven out of eight infections the bacterium caused at the Hammersmith Hospital were susceptible to penicillin, but, within two years, the proportion susceptible had halved to three out of eight.[4] So even before the 1940s were out, at the Hammersmith Hospital, penicillin was ceasing to be an effective control of *Staphylococcus aureus*.

The patterns of resistance observed in the USA paralleled Mary Barber's observations of growing resistance in London. Between 1954 and 1958, US hospitals experienced 500 epidemics of antibiotic-resistant *Staphylococcus*.[5] The experience of Seattle in Washington state was typical. In the years 1953 and 1954 there had been just one death attributed to *Staphylococcus aureus*, but in January 1955 lesions on the breasts of new mothers were reported. In March, a mother died of septicaemia.[6] A study of thirty mothers chosen at random that August found that four mothers and seventeen infants had suppurative illness after they had been discharged from hospital. Two of the mothers and twelve of the infants needed outpatient care.

Within parts of the medical profession there were enduring concerns that these outbreaks were the result of excessive use of penicillin and other antibiotics. So bad were the hospital ward infections that in Boston, Massachusetts—arguably the world's scientific centre—the eminent physician Maxwell Finland reached the remarkable conclusion in 1959 that there had been little overall reduction in the death rate from serious infection during the antibiotic era.[7] He suggested that this was because staphylococci had become more dangerous, and organisms not traditionally considered dangerous had become lethal. Other researchers explained the statistics by the use of modern drugs, such as cortisone or cancer chemotherapies, which reduced resistance to infection.[8] The availability of antibiotics had also encouraged surgeons to undertake operations that in the past would have been too risky and even now were laying some patients open to infection. Whichever explanation was preferred, bacteria had clearly not yet been 'conquered'. The Seattle epidemic had serious consequences: almost half the patients admitted with generalized septicaemia studied between 1955 and 1957 died of the infection.[9]

Nurses caring for patient after patient, exposed constantly both to their bacteria and to penicillin, were especially at risk of harbouring and transmitting resistant strains. At a time when childbirth was moving from the home to the clinic, newborn children seemed to be easily infected. They were removed from their mothers soon after birth and kept in large hospital nurseries. These proved ideal places for the circulation of infections between babies and midwives. In Britain, Mary Barber showed how, when student midwives first arrived at her hospital, fewer than three in ten of them were colonized. However, after three months, tests showed antibiotic-resistant bacteria on almost seven out of ten: most nurses had become carriers.[10]

Antibiotic-resistant infections of infants were first reported from Sydney, Australia, in 1952. Particular strains could be classified by their sensitivity to the library of the 'phage' viruses that attack bacteria. Each of these was allocated a number and in turn that number would be used to name the germ. Two similar strains were identified as the most important causes of the 'nursery epidemic' and were labelled as staphylococcus 80/81.[11] Many babies were affected: a British study suggested that the eyes or skin of one child in six carried the bacterium.[12] Within a couple of years, this strain was observed across the world. Reports came in from such diverse sources as Uganda and the United States.

The most dramatic threat caused during the 1950s by the resistance of staphylococcus to penicillin was short-lived but extreme. The bacterium was implicated in complications of the Asian flu that struck the world as a pandemic in the winter of 1957/8. Although the flu itself was caused by a virus, in the community, a wide range of bacteria caused pneumonia complications.

Across the world it has been estimated that a million people died in this epidemic.[13] In Britain almost one in five in the population were estimated to have caught it. Almost daily *The Times* newspaper listed military exercises cancelled, naval ships immobilized, and boarding schools caught up in the epidemic. Like all other viruses, this one was not susceptible to antibiotics. Even though a vaccine had been developed and was available to some it was not universally effective and not generally used, even in the USA.

It is perhaps surprising that the scale of the problems then experienced have not become part of public folklore. Admittedly, the effect of the virus itself was generally just a brief if irritating illness curable with bed-rest, but a small proportion of the victims suffered from bacterial complications that struck quickly and fatally. The death rate for pneumonia caused by staphylococcus—typically contracted in hospital—was 28 per cent.[14] That winter 16,000 extra deaths were recorded in the UK alone. Continental European countries suffered similarly. In the USA, the number of extra deaths was correspondingly higher, 80,000.[15]

Only a minority of the pneumonia cases could be attributed to the dreaded staphylococci. One study suggested they caused one case of pneumonia in eight.[16] Between one-third and one-half of the *Staphylococcus aureus* infecting pneumonia patients proved resistant to penicillin.[17] Nonetheless because overall figures were so large, tens of thousands of people across the world died that year from antibiotic-resistant bacteria that had been nurtured in hospitals, circulated in nurseries, and had then struck down patients weakened by influenza.

In the face even of such challenges, the lay public felt safe in science's hands. Reviewing 1950s attitudes from the standpoint of the mid-1990s, Harvard historian Barbara Rosencrantz reflected that press and politicians alike had given little attention to society's management of resistance.[18] Occasionally, an injunction not to 'waste' penicillin linked the idea of individuals wasting their own money to the community as a whole wasting a medical resource. One of these rare warnings was published in 1953 in America's *Consumer Reports* by a microbiologist at New York's Mount Sinai Hospital. He encouraged his savvy reader-consumers not to waste antibiotics, which he feared were being deployed with no more care, and probably less justification, than aspirin.[19] At a time when the requirement to obtain a prescription for the drugs was still new, the author concluded by explaining how antibiotics worked and reassured his readers that doctors did know best.

The variety of medical professions viewed the unfolding problems of bacterial resistance quite differently. To some, the problem was a question of hygiene and lapses of discipline. Public-health workers and bacteriologists were appalled by what they regarded as increasingly slipshod hospital practice. They condemned the use of antibiotics to cure infections rather than paying closer attention to hygiene, which would have prevented the spread of bacteria in the first place. Repeatedly, they denounced surgeons' frequent use of antibiotics for prophylaxis (treating people with such drugs to prevent infection after operations). In October 1958, a meeting on controlling the spread of infection was sponsored by the leading authorities in the United States. Afterwards, 10,000 copies of the proceedings were circulated nationwide.[20]

In the United Kingdom too, bacteriologists focused on poor hospital practice. In 1959, when Britain's standing medical advisory committee of the Central Health Services Council reported on the control of infection, its first conclusion was, 'The control of staphyloccocal disease depends largely on the application of aseptic methods. The use of antibiotics, either for treatment or for prophylaxis, is by itself unreliable.'[21] One finds the same group of people organizing symposia in 1960, 1963, and 1966, and each time echoing the same messages, increasingly loudly.

Both in the United States and the United Kingdom, surgeons were singled out for criticism. A 1959 novel entitled *The Scientists*, about the development of a drug which countered the resistant staph, quotes its pioneer, 'We've been warning them for years and now these clumsy idiots are beginning to wake up. Surgeons!'[22] Certainly public officers did feel surgeons were inadequately alert to the dangers of resistant organisms. In 1963 Britain's senior Chief Medical Officer, Sir George Godber, complained that a distinguished surgical colleague had even denied there was a problem at all.[23]

Many scientists, on the other hand, could feel confident that a solution to infection from hitherto recalcitrant organisms would soon be found and thus continue the early antibiotic triumphs into new areas. Thus May 1958 brought news of a breakthrough in the treatment of viral diseases that had been untreatable with antibiotics. In London's National Institute of Medical Research, Alick Isaacs and Jean Lindemann had discovered an antiviral substance in the blood which, if concentrated, could boost resistance and fight back against disease. They called the wonder compound 'interferon'.[24] Disappointingly, it was available in such small quantities that its clinical potential would be hard to evaluate, and interferon made no immediate medical impact. Nonetheless, British organizations which had watched penicillin fall to American competitors, hoped that interferon would be to viruses what penicillin had been to bacteria. Off and on, for a quarter of a century, great hopes were held that interferon might have revolutionary implications for viral diseases and even for cancers caused by viruses. In the 1970s it would be one of the first products made using genetically engineered bacteria.

No indication of doubt in eventual success was betrayed by the 1957 conference on the topic of bacterial resistance to antibiotics, which identified the numerous scientific challenges to be overcome.[25] The distinguished Chairman confidently asserted, 'The problem is one of microbial biochemistry, physiology and genetics, and can only be solved by work in these fields.'[26] Five years later, at a follow-up London conference, resistance was also discussed. Participants squabbled over the extent of resistance to be found in different countries. This debate was unresolved, since there were no standardized figures to which one could refer. Though disappointed by the past, however, the conference delegates still had faith in the future. Presenting the introduction, the ebullient penicillin pioneer Ernst Chain himself was unusually downbeat: 'the staphylococcal infections which he thought had been brought effectively under control by the introduction of penicillin therapy had again emerged as a dangerous disease against which he had no effective chemotherapeutic weapon.'[27] Not that Chain himself felt guilty on behalf of his professional colleagues: the process of growing resistance he saw as inevitable and a consequence of natural evolution. In his view, human behaviour had not been responsible for bringing it on, and the solution would have to be chemical.

Against the pessimism of others, the distinguished MIT chemist John Sheehan supported Chain. He rebuked those who were pessimistic, because all they could see was adaptability of the micro-organism, 'How about an expression of faith in the adaptability of the chemist?', he asked.[28] Sheehan was looking forward to a time when new antibiotics would be synthesized at will. Already microbiologists and chemists had found many new products of fungi, such as penicillin, of bacteria themselves, and of a less familiar intermediate family, the actinomycetes. It seemed to enthusiasts, therefore, that the pharmaceutical industry had only just begun to exploit the full range of potential antibiotics.

The two optimists at this London meeting, Chain and Sheehan, were no speculative enthusiasts. They had been the prime movers in the recent development of a new generation of penicillins which had led to success against resistance. Although their personal relations were often uneasy, the work they engendered would ensure the family continued to be medically important. Through the 1950s both had continued obsessions rooted in the wartime endeavour: Chain brought his enthusiasm to the Istituto di Sanita in Italy, while Sheehan, working at MIT, solidly pursued the dream of a full chemical synthesis of penicillin.

Chain's vision of the potential of chemistry would link the observation in 1948 of a sewage outfall in Cagliari, Sardinia, to the development of the new family of penicillins. Despite the importance of the outcome, the events as a whole are not well known and are worth recounting. It was a process that was both inspired, at critical points, by the success of the original penicillin discovery and also reproduced some of its qualities. Success in exploiting an unlikely chain of coincidences followed from carefully wrought connections among early enthusiasts, several academic research institutions, and pharmaceutical companies and the integrated development of fermentation, chemical, and microbiological skills.

As in the original discovery of penicillin, the process could be said to have begun with the efforts of a committed promoter. In 1948, micro-biologist and local politician Professor Giuseppe Brotzu found in the Sardinian sewage outflow a micro-organism that apparently had antibiotic properties.[29] Determined to ensure development of his idea, he went to the lengths of specially founding a journal in which to publish his results, and contacted the British.[30] Thus a sample of his extract was sent to Florey's Oxford laboratory, where it was investigated by Edward Abraham, the penicillin veteran, and his assistant Guy Newton.

Once again, the Dunn school proved its expertise. Three separate antibiotics produced by the mould were identified by the Oxford group. The first component, which they called cephalosporin P, had a structure quite different from penicillin and was without therapeutic value. Much more interest was found in another component of the soup, which Abraham and Newton entitled cephalosporin C. Along with several organizations, the Oxford team developed the traces of this chemical into a new family of broad-spectrum antibiotics, the cephalosporins, chemically related to the penicillins, but with their own highly valued properties. The project proved to be a second triumph for the Oxford laboratory and, because new patenting arrangements were in place, it was very remunerative for both the university and Britain. At the end of the twentieth century, the cephalosporins were the world's most commercially valuable family of antibiotics. Moreover, through the third ingredient of the mould juice, this research project would also spur the development of a new generation of penicillins.

The third component of Brotzu's extract quickly turned out to be a penicillin (alpha-amino-adipyl penicillin) although it had at first been given the codename cephalosporin N. Coincidentally the same chemical was already being investigated for the treatment of typhoid under the name Synnematin. It had a structure similar to conventional penicillin, except that it had a quite different side-chain, with the interesting characteristic that it contained a group which shouted, to the ears of a chemist, 'bond with me'. This was an amino group, easily amenable to other reactions and to the creation of new chains.[31]

In Rome, Chain leapt on the opportunity to develop new penicillin variants suggested by the chemically active cephalosporin N. It had been discovered, after all, in Italy and he had possibly been riled that Brotzu had contacted his old colleagues in Oxford rather coming to him in Rome.[32] While others were already looking at Synnematin, could not other penicillins with an amino acid branch also hold potential? So, attracted by the opportunities thrown up by Oxford and, perhaps, goaded by their successes, Chain turned to research based on another penicillin with an amino group: para-aminobenzylpenicillin.[33]

Meanwhile, in Britain, Chain's growing standing in penicillin technology was on the minds of the management of the Beecham group, the proprietary medicine company that had missed out on penicillin. Now it wanted to find help in developing modern products and manufacturing techniques. Until then, Beecham's research had been short term and practical, addressing questions such as the effect of light on the colour of the company's Lucozade drink. So, as it planned to change gear, Sir Charles Dodds, the company's highly respected adviser, suggested the company seek out the expertise of Chain.[34] Discussions with the new consultant might have begun with the possibilities of a fermentation route to the tartaric acid used in Beecham's long-established product Eno's Fruit Salts, but Chain quickly persuaded the company to look seriously at penicillin.[35] In the era of Britain's newly founded National Health Service, it had already seemed clear to the Chief Executive, H. G. Lazell, that the prescription medicine market would grow faster than the market for proprietary medicines.

The Beecham organization having no experience of fermentation, early in 1956, George Rolinson, a microbiologist, soon joined by the biochemist Ralph Batchelor, both still in their twenties, moved to the Istituto Superiore di Sanita. There, Chain focused their attention on para-aminobenzylpenicillin—the penicillin with a reactive amino arm. In Rome they would produce the penicillin and this would be shipped to England, where the Beecham chemists attempted to make useful products from it.[36]

Indirectly, the development of entirely new and powerful penicillins grew out of the experience of the two English visitors, although their work on para-aminobenzylpenicillin itself proved fruitless. On returning to England, they investigated an anomaly they had observed in Rome. The results of different means of measuring the quantity of penicillin in a broth, while normally the same, occasionally produced quite different results. A chemical method monitored the characteristic beta-lactam ring structure at the centre of the penicillin molecule, while a biological route tested for anti-bacterial behaviour. Occasionally, the biological activity observed within a broth was barely more than a quarter of that the chemical measure would suggest should be the case.[37]

Whereas others had noticed the same anomaly, the Beecham team was the first to ask and then answer the question: could it be that the organism was failing to produce complete penicillin and instead was only making a beta-lactam core? Adding the side-chain apparently missing from the stew could test this hypothesis. The team discussed the issue on a Monday, and by Thursday the matter had been resolved, using simple chromatography.[38] Pure penicillin was allowed to flow down one strip of paper, on a second strip the team put the mystery material, and on a third, the mystery material together with side-chain material. The flow patterns on the first strip with the penicillin and on the third strip were identical. The mystery material had clearly combined with the side-chain to make penicillin. Immediately, the onlookers believed that the compound they had put on the second strip, their mystery material on its own, was indeed the beta-lactam core. They had found a route to the synthesis of new penicillins unknown in nature and possibly able to overcome bacterial resistance.

That was not, of course, the end of the matter, and it took a further six months to obtain crystals of core material, which they called '6-APA'. Because it had a nice amino group handle, it would clearly react with a host of other chemicals without the burden of the benzyl group that had characterized the team's material so far. The inspiration and enthusiasm of Chain and his Rome colleagues had set the Beecham group on their route to success. So, the names of Ernst Chain and three Italian collaborators led the list of authors of the 1959 scientific paper describing the work on para-aminobenzylpenicillin, though they were not involved directly in the subsequent development.[39] Chain's role here, as elsewhere, had been as a spur to penicillin development.

By itself, producing 6-APA was in any case not sufficient for the development of new drugs. Similarly, earlier reported sightings of the same chemical by Japanese teams in 1950 and 1953 had not proved fruitful.[40] Possibly because of the unpopularity of penicillin in Japan at that time, following reports of harmful allergic side-effects, or possibly because the experiments were hard to repeat, there had been no attempt to follow up the initial observations. In addition to the observation of the chemical, for new drugs to be developed there needed to be that vision of building

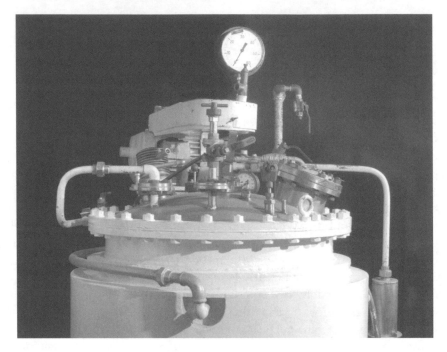

17. Fermenter built to a design developed in Rome by Chain's team and used in early work on semisynthetic penicillins by Beecham at Brockham Park. In the collection of the Science Museum, inventory number 1984–477.
Science Museum/Science & Society Picture Library.

a family of penicillins with which Chain had inspired his Beecham colleagues.

This represented a scientific breakthrough, but it was still on a laboratory scale, and technological challenges of production remained to be overcome before new penicillins could ever be made for the mass market. Although the company had built a replica of the Rome research-scale fermentation plant at its English research centre, the scale of a manufacturing facility would be much greater and Beecham still had no large-scale fermentation facilities (see Ill. 17). So Beecham did a deal with an established antibiotic manufacturer, the Bristol-Myers company in the USA. In his autobiography, Lazell said he felt the Bristol brothers were 'gentlemen'.[41]

Bristol also had its own stake in new penicillins. The company had been supporting the work of the MIT scientist John Sheehan, whose career had been devoted to the complete chemical synthesis for penicillin. In March 1957, Sheehan succeeded in his drive to synthesize penicillin, although the cost of his process meant it could not be used directly to make commercial products.[42] He also asserted at a 1958 meeting that he had prepared 6-APA even before the Rolinson team. The competing claims gave work to patent lawyers for more than a decade. Stretching into the 1970s, this argument became increasingly of private rather than public significance.

Meanwhile the two companies, Bristol and Beecham, collaborated and established a formal partnership in April 1959. By using the 6-APA starting point, new chemicals could be synthesized relatively easily, and by 1959 200 different penicillins had been made in the Beecham laboratory alone.[43] The Americans were particularly anxious to get a product out onto the market, and in October they launched, with Beecham, the first semisynthetic penicillin, phenethicillin.

This breakthrough offered the chance for the original penicillin story to be replayed. On the one hand, the triumphant successes of the earlier breakthrough—the integration of science and technology, industrial-scale research, the use of the most advanced biotechnology and the collaboration between organizations—were each repeated. On the other hand, the marginalizing of the British, and indeed the concentration on just a single product, did not recur. However, one problem, it was discovered, could not be overcome. Even now the emergence of resistance could not be prevented.

Beecham, sought to take full advantage of what, in chemical terms, was a major breakthrough. Even at the launch it broke with the reticent tradition of the ethical pharmaceutical industry and announced the new product not within the traditional, closed medical circles, but at a press conference held at a well-known restaurant. This raised the hackles of traditionalists such as Lawrence Garrod, who denounced the company in the *British Medical Journal*, but it pleased the daily press.[44] In the *Daily Express,* still owned by Fleming's defender Lord Beaverbrook, the leading science correspondent Chapman Pincher used the opportunity to refight an old war and link Beecham's work with a newly defiant Britain:

Even Britain's share of the prestige for the basic discovery is being ignored in the American write-ups. The only way that British firms like Beechams can compete with this US hogging of the credit is by adopting the American method of banging the drum at a press conference. British doctors consider this unprofessional and the *British Medical Journal* has publicly attacked Beecham's for doing it. They may be right, by old-fashioned standards but the alternative is to hand all credit to the Americans on a plate.[45]

The timing of Beecham's move proved to be unfortunate, and the launch brought little publicity in the mass media. The day before, the

Soviet Union had flashed around the world pictures taken by the Luna 3 satellite of the far side of the moon, seen for the very first time. This had been an enormous media event that quite eclipsed the launch of the first semisynthetic penicillin.

More products were however being developed, even as the first product was being launched. Scientists such as George Rolinson were anxious to tackle the challenge of antibiotic-resistant staphylococci.[46] A new member of the penicillin family that would cure staphylococcal pneumonia and ward-acquired infections caused by bacteria resistant to existing penicillins would make a genuine difference to humanity and a rewarding achievement for the researchers. In October the team tested the compound that would become methicillin.[47] The molecule's shape gave it protection from the enzyme penicillinase used by the staphylococci to attack traditional penicillin G.

If methicillin provided a future to the use of penicillin, the testing technique rather evoked medicine's heroic past. The Beecham medical director, Knudsen, and the microbiology research director, George Rolinson, approached each other with syringes filled with the drug. First Knudsen injected Rolinson—should the product be poisonous, Knudsen, the doctor, needed to be conscious. After half an hour and no immediate ill effect, Rolinson injected Knudsen. Both survived. By September 1960 the product that would be called methicillin was on the market.[48] In this period before the elaborate testing that would be required in the wake of thalidomide, the company had gone from discovery to launch in just a few months.

Methicillin did require a new production technology. The first semisynthetic penicillin, phenethicillin, could be made without accomplishing the difficult step of isolating 6-APA. Making methicillin, however, required the pure core compound by itself. In principle, this isolation had been achieved at Beecham, but in practice their process was laborious. How much easier if an enzyme could just snip off existing side-chains from ordinary penicillin to reveal the core! In October 1958, Beecham managed to find an E. coli bacterium that made an enzyme able to produce 6-APA from the Penicillin V that had been developed in Austria. Going one better, however, within a few months, the Bayer Company in Germany found how to do the same from the cheaper relative, the original Penicillin G.[49] This technology was in turn licensed by Beecham, who were able to develop it further. The chemists were therefore given a cheap source of reactive 6-APA on which they could build to assemble new penicillins. The dream of chemical control which had inspired the wartime synthetic enterprise had now been partly realized. As in the original penicillin development, a host of scientific and technological resources had had to be assembled for success to be achieved. It had come out of a chain of events linking work in Sardinia, Oxford, and Rome, and the Beecham, Bristol, and Bayer companies.

The technical triumph had complex consequences. On the one hand, certainly, methicillin was a revolutionary drug, as was shown in an early and dramatic victory on the set of the movie blockbuster *Cleopatra* in 1961. The star, Elizabeth Taylor, was filming when she became ill with pneumonia.[50] She almost died before she was treated with methicillin. This celebrity achievement got the drug into the *New York Times*. But in retrospect the achievement was double edged. The public had won legitimate faith in a working drug. The achievement had, on the other hand, sustained hopes for endless antibiotic solutions to the problem of infection that could not be fulfilled.

Standing slightly outside the heat of this battle, leading geneticists and virologists were convinced that such antibacterial success could never be total. At a 1962 meeting in London entitled 'The Future of Mankind', some of the world's most distinguished bioscientists reflected on the war against infection. Agreeing that the total eradication of diseases was not even desirable, they rejected the military model and favoured instead an ecological interpretation. Humankind had to learn to live with even the most virulent of germs. If we defined the contest with bacteria as one of total war, then we would only lose.

Hilary Koprowski, an expert on viruses from Philadelphia's Wistar Institute, had been working on a polio vaccine and was particularly worried. If humans eradicated a disease without addressing the conditions causing it, then, he warned, another micro-organism would fill the niche left vacant. His talk ended with an ironic note 'to my great grandson if he intends to become a healer'. He wrote: 'if a universal antibiotic is found, immediately organise societies to prevent its use. It should be dealt with as we should have treated, and did not treat, the atomic bomb. Use any feasible national and international deterrents to prevent it falling into the hands of stupid people who probably will still be in the majority in your time as they were in mine.'[51]

The justice of the sceptical arguments aired at the CIBA meeting was being demonstrated at the very time of the conference through the evolution of *Staphylococcus aureus*. In a dramatic demonstration of the link between the history of methicillin and its nemesis, it took just one year before a resistant bacterium, later to be known as a 'superbug',

MRSA (methicillin-resistant *Staphylococcus aureus*), was encountered in a hospital. The bacterium's effect was recognized because of the care taken by a pioneer of methicillin, and himself an enthusiast for the drug's potential, the Scots doctor Gordon Stewart, to challenge his own confident assumptions. Beforehand, he had been reassuring his colleagues that the danger of bacterial resistance to the new drug might in principle be a concern, but in practice it would prove a mere formality. He was soon to alter his opinion. Taking place in a closed community, the first epidemic of MRSA provided a preview, in miniature, of what would come to happen on a global scale.

During the Second World War, Stewart had dispensed some of the first penicillin to be given to patients. Now he was a pioneer of the most modern development. The first warning that something might be amiss came almost immediately the drug was launched. Mary Barber, the doyenne of antibiotic resistance studies, published a paper showing that organisms resistant even to the new methicillin did exist.[52] The next year, even more worrying news came from Patricia Jevons working in a laboratory at London's Public Health Laboratory Service. Doctors across the country sent samples of infectious organisms to Dr Jevons. Occasionally, she was finding, even in these clinical samples, small quantities of a bacterium able to grow despite the methicillin. At first Stewart was tempted to dismiss the importance of such findings and indeed wrote a letter to the *British Medical Journal* arguing that Mary Barber's results were immediately of laboratory rather than medical significance.[53]

Stewart was, however, soon to encounter the limitations of methicillin himself, in a setting that could have served as an appropriate movie set for the story. He worked in Britain's largest children's hospital, Queen Mary's, near London, with over a thousand patients spread over a large campus.[54] The hospital environment encouraged the spread of bacteria. In an era in which it was still common to inter the mentally and physically infirm for long periods in institutions variously called asylums, sanatoria, and long-stay hospitals, this was a hospital that took children out of society. Some were protected, and indeed subsequently remembered Queen Mary's with fondness and gratitude, going on to success in later life. Yet, while the medical and surgical wards were hygienic, in the long-stay wards children with Down's syndrome mixed with the mentally ill and the physically handicapped. Many were incontinent. They were potted in long lines. Hands and faeces came into frequent contact. The staff struggled to cope, but their numbers were few and often they were restricted to maintaining order. This remarkable campus offered a strange caricature of wider human society and a bizarre setting through which future possibilities could be first seen.

With the rise of antibiotics, infectious diseases had become a steadily less terrifying force at Queen Mary's. Where once children died at the rate of three a week from rheumatic fever, which caused heart failure, from tuberculosis, and from infections caused by malnutrition, patients were recovering. Even the dreaded polio, whose treatment included the incarceration of children in iron lungs, could now be prevented. The hospital was, however, not complacent. It was, for instance, testing a new vaccine against measles on its patients (in conditions which were themselves to become highly controversial).

After the launch of methicillin, and despite his confident dismissal of the first sightings of resistant organisms, Stewart had been checking for their emergence in the throats, nostrils, and skin folds of his patients. In May 1961 a child with a navel infection of *Staphylococcus aureus* was admitted. The illness was minor, but the bacterium appeared to be insensitive to methicillin. Within fourteen months, Stewart had followed the spread of the infection to seventy-five children, including fifty-five newborns. In June 1962 a child with the challenging birth abnormality spina bifida was operated upon but became infected and gravely ill with septicaemia.[55] Caused by *Staphylococcus aureus*, the infection did not respond to methicillin. The child became more and more ill. The treatment was changed to another antibiotic, erythromycin, but even this did not work and the child died. He was the world's first fatal victim of MRSA.

There was much wringing of hands but little action when, in February 1963, Stewart reported his case to the *British Medical Journal*. Correspondence from other hospitals in Poland and Denmark suggested they too had already encountered the resistant bacterium.[56] The *Journal* published an editorial arguing that, with proper management, methicillin could still be enormously useful.[57] Against this measured caution, many hospitals still used increasing quantities of antibiotics to replace the disciplines required to maintain hygiene. At first the threat of MRSA spread slowly and was not reported in the USA until 1968. Its fortunes also fluctuated, with a decline in the 1970s, but within thirty years this bacterium proved a routine and serious threat to health worldwide.[58] First found in hospitals, it also came to be endemic in the community. There are several varieties of it, but much of the MRSA found in the twenty-first century can be traced back to this single Queen Mary's strain.[59] The hope that the evolution of bacterial colonies resistant to antibiotics could be beaten by the chemist developing ever-more powerful penicillins had been dashed.

Despite the emergence of MRSA, technology and better hygiene seem to have been responsible for bringing the epidemic of *Staph. aureus* 80/81 under control. Methicillin was certainly important; so was a renewed emphasis on hygiene in the wards. Many hospitals introduced infection-control officers and required hierarchies of approval for the use of antibiotics by junior doctors.[60] Leaving newborns with their mothers, rather than mixing them with other children, in part controlled the nursery epidemics. If patients became infected, nonetheless, methicillin could now be used to save them.[61] In addition, the bacterium itself may have evolved further, vanishing as mysteriously as it had arrived. By 1970 Robert Williams, who in the 1950s had been a leading critic of antibiotic misuse, was reflecting on the resistant staphylococcus outbreak as history and warned of bandwagons overemphasizing particular microbial threats.[62] By then he felt that there had been too much focus on just the type 80/81 bacteria. Concern merely with this one organism would distract attention from the general problems of hygiene and the diverse infections to which patients were susceptible.

Methicillin itself was but a step in the development of the semisynthetic penicillins. Although it continued to be a powerful counter to most antibiotic-resistant bacteria, compared to other penicillins, it was not particularly active in the test tube and, moreover, needed to be injected. The Beecham team was particularly interested in finding compounds that were biologically active and also stable in the presence of acids. These would be suitable for taking by mouth rather than having to be injected. At the end of the twentieth century, such successful products of this project as oxacillin, cloxacillin, and flucoxacillin were still in use, while methicillin itself was withdrawn in 1993.

Penicillins with a wider spectrum of action were a second range of products coming out of the work on the 6-APA nucleus. The first to make a major difference was ampicillin, marketed as Penbritin by Beecham and as Polycillin by Bristol. Illustrating Beecham's confidence, ampicillin's price was initially set as twice the price of its nearest competitor, the broad-spectrum drug tetracycline.[63] Like the tetracyclines, ampicillin also addressed a much wider range of bacteria than traditional penicillin, including such bacteria as *E. coli*, salmonella, and *H. influenzae*, whose outbreaks would make their names familiar even to the lay public.

Such so-called 'gram-negative' bacteria were quite different from the staphylococcus. At the microbiological level, the differing structure of the cell wall made them immune to conventional penicillin. At the medical level they, too, were clearly distinguished: while staphylococci were a threat mainly in hospital, salmonella, for instance, was contracted in the community. During the post-war years, it was painfully evident—to victims of food-poisoning as well as to statisticians—that infections from such bacteria were multiplying. They were taking advantage of changing social habits. People travelled more to exotic locations, ate more fast food, and much more meat. Even the biologists travelling to international conferences suffered problems. At a 1981 conference held in the Dominican Republic, half the scientists suffered 'turista' gastro-intestinal problems.[64] Staying at home was also proving more risky. Cases of salmonellosis in the USA tripled from 2,000 in 1950, when statistics began to be kept, to 1960 and tripled again by 1970: that meant practically a tenfold increase in just two decades.[65] Moreover, as cases of salmonella in human victims rose remorselessly, so resistance to the hitherto effective antibiotics began to be detected.

Some of these 'gram-negative' bacteria caused only mild diarrhoea, and in general, infections of the digestive system were discomforting rather than lethal. Other consequences, such as typhoid fever, could, however, be fatal. Even dangerous variants of common *E. coli* and salmonella sometimes threatened the lives of babies and the sick and elderly. In 1955 a Swedish report told of an outbreak of salmonella that had killed ninety people.[66] The development of the new penicillin, ampicillin, which could attack such bugs, was therefore of great importance. It was also convenient for doctors, who could prescribe for an infection without knowing what kind of bacterium was the cause.

Further penicillins based on 6-APA also made possible assaults on other bacteria. The Beecham laboratories alone could generate twelve derivatives a month. Although most proved clinically useless, by the 1980s Rolinson could list thirty in several related families.[67] Some, such as methicillin and its successors, were effective against resistant gram-positive bacteria, while others, such as carbenicillin and ticarcillin, were used against particular species of bacteria (pseudomonas). In 1972 ampicillin would be followed by a chemical relative, amoxycillin (which came to be known as amoxicillin and was branded by Beecham as Amoxil). This was better absorbed by mouth than ampicillin, giving higher blood levels, and had a higher degree of bactericidal activity, enabling dosage to be reduced. (see Ill. 18).

Both bacteria and chemists proved capable of yet further 'wily' moves. Gram-negative bacteria also proved able to develop resistance to the new penicillins. Some produced large quantities of the enzyme 'beta-lactamase', the chemical that destroyed the beta-lactam ring at the drug's core. In principle, the penicillin could be protected by introducing another

18. Box of Amoxil, produced by a Beecham subsidiary, mid-1980s. In the collection of the Science Museum, inventory number 1987–311/448.

Reproduced by permission of the GlaxoSmithKline Group of Companies. Science Museum/Science & Society Picture Library.

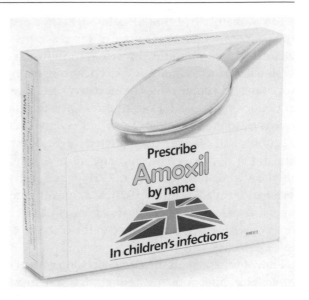

sacrificial chemical that would mop up the destructive enzyme. The approach had been conceived as early as the 1950s. Thus the discovery of a fabulously successful (if fictional) inhibitor lies at the heart of the 1959 novel *The Scientists*.[68] Methicillin, which was immune to beta-lactamase, made this approach unnecessary for the gram-positive bacteria. However, with the emergence of penicillins attacking gram-negative bacteria and the growing resistance of such bugs, realizations of this early dream were sought.

New projects were set in hand at a number of companies to find an appropriate molecule that could be blended with penicillin.[69] At Beecham, in 1967, Rolinson's team started systematically screening broths in search of an inhibitor.[70] Testing a culture recently used to produce a new cephalosporin, in 1968 they found this also produced a quite different chemical. Resembling a penicillin, it had its own beta-lactam ring and displayed weak antibacterial properties. At the same time, the compound known as clavulanic acid proved to be a powerful inhibitor of beta-lactamase.

A combination of clavulanic acid with amoxicillin (co-amoxiclav) was launched in September 1981 to the enthusiastic headline in the London *Daily Mail*, 'Doctors get the "superbug" drug'.[71] The new penicillin was a powerful counter to the resistant *H. influenzae* common in complaints such as earache, sinusitis, and bacterial bronchitis. This bacterium was often implicated, along with others that, at the time co-amoxiclav was introduced, were still considered to be universally vulnerable to amoxicillin, although resistance was emerging. Where clavulanic acid led the way, a few others followed. In the 1980s, two other inhibitors were introduced, sulbactam and tazobactam.[72]

The new penicillins were convenient to use and often successful as cures for infection. Their widespread deployment may also, however, have promoted the worldwide spread of resistance of key bacteria during the last forty years of the twentieth century. By the 1980s there were fewer new antibiotics but more new resistant strains. The most unexpected, but widespread and clinically significant, growth in such bacteria was resistant *Streptococcus pneumoniae*. Against this organism there was no new penicillin, but much better surveillance was deployed than ever before.

For a quarter of a century after penicillin's introduction, this organism showed no sign of resistance. At the time that resistant *Staph. aureus* was breeding rapidly in the 1950s, driving out its more susceptible cousins, just one ten-millionth of a gram of penicillin in a millilitre of blood would kill *S. pneumoniae* in the test tube.[73] Like salmonella, *S. pneumoniae* is transmitted by people in the community. Of the one in ten people who harbour the bacterium, most do not even know it, and a further proportion are merely inconvenienced.[74] Yet this bacterium was also responsible for many of the incidences of the acute respiratory tract illnesses such as pneumonia that, at the end of the twentieth century, together still killed four and a half million people every year and caused more deaths than any other category of infectious disease.[75] Across the Western world, typically three-quarters of antibiotic prescriptions addressed such complaints.[76]

Because the very young are vulnerable to getting sick from pneumonia, this one organism cuts off more years of life than any other. It is responsible for a variety of other infections of the respiratory tract, including coughs, sinusitis, and bronchitis. *S. pneumoniae* has also been a common cause of the painful form of ear infection known as acute otitis media (AOM) typically characterized by a red and very painful eardrum and fever, affecting perhaps around seven out of ten infants. This bacterium, whose most common effect in the USA was short-term pain, could also be life threatening where levels of general health were poor and appropriate medication was not to hand. There, AOM—so common and self-limiting in richer countries—could be a dangerous hazard. A study of eleven developing countries found the legacy of the illness in the one-third of the population with hearing impairment.[77] The effectiveness of penicillin against this bacterium was therefore, around the world, one of its greatest benefits.

Unlike the quickly resistant staphylococcus, the enduring susceptibility of these germs to penicillin was a 'fact' of medical practice into the 1960s. When the phenomenon of resistance was occasionally observed, as in Boston in 1965, it was therefore ignored.[78] A group led by Maxwell Finland was investigating the response of bacteria to tetracycline, and it reported without comment that two out of 200 strains they were studying, while still ultimately vulnerable to penicillin, did require rather more than the normal dose to inhibit their growth.

Two years later, however, a new observation of a strain of resistant bacterium was reported, and this time it was reflected upon. A team from the children's hospital in Adelaide, Australia, under Dr David Hansman, had found that a patient in Sydney who had been treated with a variety of antibiotics was now infected with a pneumonia-causing bacterium resistant to both penicillin and tetracycline.[79] Searching out further cases, Hansman and his colleagues found their next examples of resistance not in Sydney, nor elsewhere in the developed world, but, in a foretaste of the new era, in Papua New Guinea. Soon they reported similar findings from the even more remote Trobriand Islands.[80] Early in the twentieth century, these islanders had been taken by anthropologists as the model of 'primitive people'. Now, because their bacteria had been exposed to penicillin too, they were at the forefront of global trends.

The global saturation of penicillin meant that it was again in the southern hemisphere that the drip of observations of resistant *S. pneumoniae* became a shower. South Africa, where gold was extracted from deep mines and miners were prone to contract pneumonia, had long been a centre for the study of the disease.[81] Even before the First World War, Sir Almroth Wright, Alexander Fleming's boss, had experimented there with a vaccine. Shortly after, the South African Institute for Medical Research (SAIMR) had been founded. This continued the hunt for a vaccine. Half a century later, the hunt was still on, and Dr Robert Austrian from Philadelphia was testing vaccines in the early 1970s under the aegis of SAIMR.[82]

It was in 1977 that a degree of antibiotic resistance was reported from Durban on South Africa's Indian Ocean coast. A year later, another group found bacteria, again with some resistance, in two very different hospitals in the Johannesburg region at a time of the social turmoil of riots in Soweto. Although the country was still politically and economically divided by apartheid, one resistant case was in a rich middle-class area, the other in paediatric wards serving poor black children in the large Baragwanath hospital. From then on, antibiotic-resistant *S. pneumoniae* was known as a widespread phenomenon.[83] Worldwide, it was concentrated in a few widely distributed areas. In Europe, Hungary was the first country in which more than 20 per cent of infections were resistant. Across the now-rusting Iron Curtain, Spain emerged as the country of greatest concern.[84] In 1979 no streptococcus found there was resistant to penicillin, but, by 1989/90, almost one in six of the infections observed were insensitive to all but the highest doses of penicillin.

Spain was specially important because it was a favourite holiday destination. Its sun-baked beaches and historic sites were so popular internationally that its germs had exceedingly good access to human populations around the globe. Soon microbiologists were tracking descendants of the Spanish strain of *S. pneumoniae* carried across the world, from Iceland to the USA to the Far East. Iceland proved a most interesting example, since resistance to *S. pneumoniae* emerged there suddenly between 1989 and 1992.[85] The genetics of the bacterium suggested the outbreak had been caused by the naturally bred clones of a single microbe that had been brought onto the island, most likely from Spain. This global migration of a resistant bacterium highlighted the communal nature of resistance and the need to watch movements on a worldwide scale.

Early in the 1990s, pharmaceutical companies began to sponsor worldwide surveys of the changing patters of resistance. This would inform both drug development and recommended dosage. Thus the global dynamics of resistance to *S. pneumoniae* were monitored in the so-called 'Alexander Project', early in the 1990s.[86] Bacteria isolated across the world were flown back to London, where they were tested in a laboratory. There, microbiologists mapped the spread of the antibiotic-resistant bacteria into niches across the globe. By 1995, ten nodes had been identified. These included such countries in the southwest of Europe as Spain and France, a group in the centre and east of Europe including Hungary and also Israel, northwest Russia and South Africa, two Asian nodes in Japan/South Korea and Papua New Guinea and four nodes in the Americas from Alaska to the cone of South America.[87] This distribution from the north-west of Russia to the southern tip of Argentina, and including both Israel and Papua New Guinea, was a remarkable indication of how interconnected was the human and also the bacterial population at the end of the twentieth century. Social trends in one country could lead to the evolution of bacteria spreading across the globe.

Resistance was not, however, absolute, and many apparently recalcitrant organisms could be managed by more adroit use of existing products.

Destroying colonies of bacteria is not like throwing a switch, and similarly resistance is not 'on' or 'off'. Some antibiotics kill bacteria by massive concentrations in the blood. With others, including penicillins, the length of time bacteria are exposed to particular doses is critical. Most resistant *S. pneumoniae* could be fought successfully by increasing the dosage of penicillin used as treatment. By increasing the dose given in the first place, doctors could often ensure that the critical concentration of penicillin was in the blood long enough to destroy even resistant strains of bacteria. Many 'resistant' cases of pneumonia would succumb to large doses that increased the initial concentration twentyfold and ensured penicillin would be present in the blood for sufficient time.[88] This was not a solution which would last for ever. By itself, of course, savaging, but not destroying, colonies of bacteria that showed merely 'intermediate' resistance would in the long term just select for the more resistant strains. Increasingly, resistant *S. pneumoniae* would be fought with vaccines rather than antibiotics.

'Wily' chemists, to use Sheehan's term, may not have kept up with bacteria, but they had enabled a commercial success. Following the lead of Beecham and Bristol, many other companies had made similar drugs. The Beecham team, at least, during the 1960s, 1970s, and the early 1980s had, however, proved to be the world's leading innovator of penicillins.

In these terms, just as Lazell, Beecham's chief executive, had hoped when he first contacted Ernst Chain, the problems of Beecham itself were cured by penicillin. At the end of the 1960s, the company's pharmaceutical sales alone exceeded £32 million or approximately $100 million—fifteen times their value in 1961 and approximately twice the group's entire turnover in 1952.[89] For three decades, the former proprietary-medicine maker was one of the major pharmaceutical manufacturers, until it was involved in a global network of mergers, which led to its name being subsumed within the pharmaceutical conglomerate GlaxoSmithKline in the year 2000. Similarly its American partner, Bristol-Myers, would grow until losing its separate identity within the new Bristol-Myers Squibb company.

The development of semisynthetic penicillins had replicated some of the features of the original pioneering of the drug. If it had not led to the eradication of infection, the tenacity of individual scientists, their multi-institutional collaboration, and the drawing together of diverse areas of expertise had made for technical success and medical relief for many. The new developments ensured, too, that this family of chemicals would continue to dominate the antibiotics. US consumption of semisynthetic penicillins increased tenfold in the two years after 1962. By 1964, therefore, the value of the US semisynthetic market at $41 million was already half as great as that of penicillin G.[90] The new products ensured that the consumption of penicillins there went on to double between 1965 and 1971, continuing to grow until the early 1990s. At the end of the century ampicillin and amoxicillin were still the most popular antibiotics for outpatient care in America.[91] Powerful chemicals as they were, however, such use owed as much to society as to bacteria.

7

Doctors, Patients, and the Brand

Lying at the heart of the 'tragedy' of penicillin has been the divide between the logic of the chemical and the logic of the brand. From the 1960s, particularly, medical specialists argued that new antibiotics alone could not vanquish infection and that the problem of resistant organisms would have to be controlled by restricting antibiotic use to cases where it was biologically essential. Meanwhile, antibiotic consumption grew remorselessly until the end of the twentieth century, at rates that could not be explained by any narrow criterion of therapeutic need. Even at the beginning of the next century, there were reports that only half of all antibiotic prescriptions could be justified on microbiological grounds alone.[1]

The escalating use of penicillin could seem 'irrational' when seen just as the administration of a chemical. It was explicable and even 'rational', however, as the pattern of consumption of a brand associated with a variety of hopeful expectations, reassuring personal experiences, and reputed benefits. Both in richer countries and in the developing world, penicillin would often be prescribed to sustain patients' trust in their doctor, whatever its effect on microbes. With little time allowed for traditional caring, a doctor would use a prescription to provide moral reassurance as well as infection control. Decisions over when and how penicillin and other antibiotics should be used were therefore locked into complex relationships among patients, doctors, insurance bodies, and the state. So, in decoding the pattern of penicillin use, we need to follow particularly the radical shifts in patients' attitudes to doctors that took place during the years after the Second World War.

As early as the 1950s, rich information about the incorporation of antibiotics within diverse local medical cultures was being collected by sociologists and health-care workers. While most such work would focus on Britain and the USA, studies of countries on the European mainland also provided, for instance, surprising comparisons of Catholic and Protestant communities' attitudes to antibiotics. Although material conditions in the developing world were often very different, there too social scientists and policy analysts found a rich vein of cultural meaning in a shot of penicillin. The act of taking penicillin was inexpensive, and its significance within a variety of medical traditions meant that practices came to be well entrenched within local cultures. Even as the World Health Organization promoted better health care, it found difficulty in defining a policy for 'rational drug use'.

The prospects for scientific rationality had looked so promising in the wake of the biomedical triumphs of the Second World War, when governments had decided to rely on physicians to protect the public interest.[2] A doctor's prescription for most antibiotic uses was required in the USA from 1951. In Britain, supply was placed firmly in the hands of the doctors even sooner.[3] Until the early post-war months, the government in London could use the excuse of shortages to justify rigid limitations to penicillin's use. With supplies growing, however, that quickly ceased to be an acceptable basis of rationing. Because only poisons were then limited to 'prescription-only' purchase, legislation and thus discussion and debate would be required if penicillin access were to be similarly restricted. This was not done lightly: at a time when Britain's population increasingly resented the heavy regulation of post-war life, yet more regulations would have a political cost.

Early in 1946, British civil servants sought advice on whether they needed to prevent lay access to penicillin, in order to stop bacteria developing resistance. 'This', wrote Alexander Fleming to such an enquiry, 'has happened with other drugs and it will inevitably happen with penicillin if everyone can buy it and use it with and without adequate knowledge.'[4] Without controls, he and other leading doctors warned, sufferers of syphilis and gonorrhoea in particular would consume small quantities of ineffective penicillin pills to avoid the embarrassment of seeing a doctor and the pain of injections. To thoroughly destroy infecting bacteria, and not just diminish their number, patients needed instead the injection of massive quantities of penicillin. The consequence of misuse would inevitably be that shortly penicillin would be rendered useless. Perhaps surprisingly, the pride of ownership of the brand, and the threat of loss of a vital medicine, drove British ministers to act with unaccustomed speed.

Introducing the 'Penicillin Bill' measure to the House of Commons in 1947, Aneurin Bevan, Minister of Health, put the case that: 'It would

141

be an appalling thing if, as a consequence of its misuse, the population might, in a period of years, receive no advantage at all from it because it would have developed resistance in those who take it.'[5] The debates were energetically argued in both the House of Commons and the House of Lords, with opponents denouncing the minister for removing the right to buy a medicine of choice. Nonetheless, arguments that the potency of penicillin had to be protected carried the day.

Ordinary patients would be prevented from wandering into pharmacies and buying small quantities of the drug whenever they felt it might be needed. Instead, doctors would be depended upon to make wise decisions, good for both individual and society, on when patients would use penicillin and how much they should take. This model of delegation was entrenched in the rights of the personal physician. Accordingly, when a dozen years later the Hinchliffe Committee investigated drug costs, it recommended that the government should not seek to control doctors' prescribing behaviour.[6] The privacy of the consulting room had been protected and the government's continuing confidence in the medical profession demonstrated.

Against this theoretical model of the godlike doctor, in practice later twentieth-century societies became, increasingly, critical of bodies such as the medical profession which were claiming to act on behalf of the public good and arbitrate on behalf of society as a whole. From the 1960s humanity's use of technology and of nature in general was being harshly debated. We were charged with taxing the environment excessively in many ways, whether it be through the use of insecticides such as DDT or the dumping of chemical waste. The short-term interests of the individual and the common good of society seemed to be pitted one against another, often without a resolution. Providing an eloquent catchphrase for the era, demographer Garrett Hardin entitled a 1968 essay 'The Tragedy of the Commons'.[7] Using the metaphor of medieval common land, he contrasted the interests of the community as a whole, in the sustainable and measured use of the land, with the self-interest of each inhabitant who sought to benefit personally by exploiting resources to the utmost.

It was, however, difficult to find respected and powerful arbitrators who would manage the 'freeloader'. In his influential *Bowling Alone: The Collapse and Revival of American Community,* published at the end of the century, Harvard professor Robert Puttnam argued that 'social capital'—the forms of solidarity that sustained trust—had reduced radically since the early 1960s.[8] In particular 'thin trust', the automatic bestowal of credibility on others, had declined. Statistics assembled by the sociologists

Seymour Martin Lipset and William Schneider support his argument. In the early 1980s they used poll data to document the widening of the 'confidence gap' in the United States over the previous twenty years. Between the 1960s and the 1980s, the proportion of interviewees expressing confidence in the leadership of the country's leading institutions halved. The proportion of Americans with faith in the leaders of the executive branch fell from 41 per cent to 24 per cent, and Congress did even worse: faith in its leaders fell from 42 per cent to 16 per cent.[9] With these parallels the fall in confidence in the leaders of medicine from 72 per cent in 1966 to 37 per cent in 1981 might be dramatic, but not out of the ordinary.[10] Polls and public discussion demonstrated similar trends in Europe.[11] Such large shifts framed public perception of medicine not just at the very end of the century, as many might assume, but throughout the post-Second World War era. They would also strain the balance of public and private welfare in the administration of penicillin.

A singularly useful interpretation of the concept of trust has been formulated by the sociologist Barbara Misztal. One of a number of models she uses to interpret its meaning is a cultural space cohabited by the partners in a relationship. This conception, well suited to the medical profession, provides a means of visualizing relationships among the ways in which trust is maintained.[12] In some societies, occupancy of that shared space is constantly in question and needs to be earned, while in others it is taken for granted.

The tradition of a caring and respected 1920s doctor was, for instance, portrayed in the books by the Scottish physician and writer A. J. Cronin which underpinned the popular post-war BBC television series *Dr Finlay's Casebook*. In an era of small communities and hierarchical class structures, doctors in western Europe and the USA often were the authoritative community leaders described by Cronin. Early in the 1950s, the sociologist Earl Koos reported attitudes to health and doctors in a small town in the middle of the state of Pennsylvania, which he represented as Regionsville.[13] Koos found that, as an educated man, the doctor was still automatically looked up to by patients and fellow-citizens.[14]

Even as Koos was writing, however, America was changing. The deeply knowledgeable expert on rural society Charles Loomis warned in a 1950 study that bureaucratization of the medical system would bring a less personal, communal feel to medicine. It would be replaced by a more 'secular, rational, efficient, planned and impersonal' relationship.[15] The industrial revolution in medicine described in Chapter 5 brought enormous benefits, but also a shifting attitude to care.

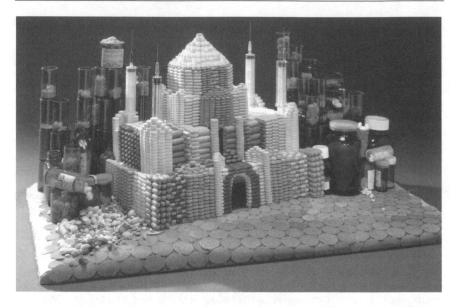

19. Castle of pills built as part of an attack on the commercialization of medicine in a campaign to prevent the closure of a London hospital by the East London Health Project in the late 1970s. It expresses the doubts about the purveyors of medicines that grew up from the 1960s. It is now in the collection of the Science Museum, inventory number 1982–486.

Science Museum/Science & Society Picture Library.

This transformation in medical practice from the 1950s onwards was reported and examined systematically, particularly in Britain and the USA. Groups and centres of social scientists, or 'social observatories', following the French usage, documented the responses of doctors and patients to changes in medicine. In such areas as Bethnal Green in London's East End (the Institute of Community Studies run by the inventive sociologist Michael Young), and in Chicago (the more-established National Opinion Research Center), social scientists watched the culture of an old and isolated working class wither and new cultures emerge.[16] From the 1980s, the increasingly rich literature included many studies of the use of antibiotics. These provide graphic descriptions of the negotiation, both explicit and implicit, between doctor and patient over appropriate prescribing of drugs. On the overall outcome for the profession as a whole of half a century of change there is still dispute.[17] Nonetheless, the significance of the individual forces at work, both challenging and supporting confidence in the doctor, has been widely recognized (see Ill. 19)

144

Many of the early social 'astronomers' of medicine were starting out in academic careers, but, even in the USA, networks of academics did not have a monopoly on research. The medical profession used market researchers to find out what the public thought of their politically contentious industry. Above all in the USA, they used the Institute for Motivational Research run by Ernest Dichter, Vienna-trained psychoanalyst and market-research pioneer. Known as 'Mr Mass-motivation', Dichter trained as a psychoanalyst in Vienna and, as a refugee in New York, pioneered the use of focus groups, which he called 'psycho-panels'.[18] For his advice, Dichter's rates were $500 an hour, a fortune at the time.[19] His insights were, literally, highly valued.

As early as 1950, Dichter explored, for the California Medical Association, how broad social changes were translating into new relationships between doctors and patients. Focus-group discussions easily elucidated the challenges to the traditional deference to authority. A doctor complained to one of Dichter's interviewers about the slovenly dress in which patients were now attending his surgery. They didn't even bother to change before coming to a medical appointment after a day in the steel mill: 'Those patients don't seem to have any respect for the doctor so I treat them with as little respect as possible. They do not deserve anything else.'[20] While Dichter concluded, 'The patients of 1950 are no longer the patients of 1914 or 1920', he warned his client that, rather than welcoming the changing expectations of patients, 'many doctors regret this'.[21] He suggested that such conservative physicians were fighting against powerful social forces. In explaining the greater participation being demanded by patients, Dichter compared the period around 1950 to the religious Reformation 500 years earlier, when parishioners had demanded direct access to the Almighty. 'It is', he said, 'comparable to a period where the Bible was being translated from Latin into English.'

While, even in the 1950s, patients were therefore becoming more demanding, doctors in the United States also had less time to give a consultation. In 1960 the average American saw the doctor twice as often as a counterpart in 1930, although the total number of physicians providing the service in America was unchanged.[22] The typical US doctor was working sixty hours a week, with one-third of the profession working seventy hours a week. Such were often the conditions in which prescribing antibiotics became a part of a medical culture. Academic sociologists who studied a practice in North Carolina in 1956 observed overwork and short cuts, scarcely ever a history taken, and massive amounts of antibiotics prescribed in lieu of diagnosis. Two-thirds of the doctors who were presented with an upper respiratory tract infection, such as a cold, gave antibiotics 'indiscriminately to all patients or to most patients'.[23] For half a century, antibiotic use associated with pressure to increase efficiency, growing demands, and prescribing without careful bacteriological diagnosis would be reported time and time again.

The medical profession as a whole was experiencing widespread criticism in the 1950s. In February 1958, the respected American *Business Week* magazine, reflecting on the profession's recent press, reported an overwhelming impression of wealth, greed, and laziness.[24] The advanced level of modern medicine was being explained by citing the wonders of drugs, not physicians. The solution to such criticism of the profession in the USA would come to be an attempt to reconstruct what was known as 'comprehensive medicine' through promotion of family practitioners.[25] Their new title indicated a wish for a new start in primary care. On the other side of the Atlantic, the situation of general practitioners was better, but also problematic. In 1950 the often squalid facilities of British general practitioners had been systematically studied, and roundly condemned, by a visiting Australian physician.[26] Within the profession, this evaluation engendered shock but also recognition.

Social scientists' publications in the 1950s and 1960s recorded the decay of patients' taken-for-granted trust in doctors. A review of British medical services, reporting in 1962, found that a quarter of patients did not feel they could confide in their general practitioner.[27] Even an anthropologist of the time could be surprised by the changing status of the GP. Starting her incisive study of social networks in a British urban community during the early 1950s, Elizabeth Bott initially assumed that a doctor's introduction would quickly get her accepted by local people.[28] Instead she heard doctors described as 'superior plumbers'. That was not just a snobbish put-down of professionals as 'tradesmen', but the translation of medicine to the world of anonymity. Mildred Blaxter, studying three generations of British women in the 1970s, found her oldest subjects, born before 1930, still idealizing 'their' doctor.[29] She cited the pride in consulting a distinguished man and shock if he made a medical mistake. On the other hand, the younger British women whom she studied, typically born around 1950, had very different and much more pragmatic attitudes.

As early as 1949, the report of a study of British doctors by the polling agency Mass Observation had quoted the typical complaint, 'Then he objects to the dictatorial patient who know just what he or she wants and comes to the doctor to demand it. The doctor for them is merely a convenient agent who provides them with a bill of exchange.'[30] A study of pharmaceutical advertising carried out by Dichter in 1955 found that '"Give me a penicillin shot" is one of the most frequently referred to and most hated expressions of "do your own doctoring" trends among patients (see Ill. 20).'[31] Similarly, an American physician made the telling comment, reported by sociologists in 1966: 'Nowadays you give a shot of penicillin for pneumonia and cure the patient, but that's no credit to the doctor; all credit goes to the drug. An old doctor wouldn't have had so many patients; he would sit at the patient's bedside until the fever broke.'[32] Within a few lines he had captured the shift away from the world of the caring old-style physician to a new drug-centred system. At the extreme, doctors were beginning to seem more or less interchangeable agencies by which canny customers obtained a desired medicine.

Early in the 1960s, the impact on patients of long-term trends in the place of medicine in society was accentuated by coinciding crises, each of which raised further doubts about placing trust in doctors. Thus the thalidomide scandal emerged in 1962, and it transpired that doctors were

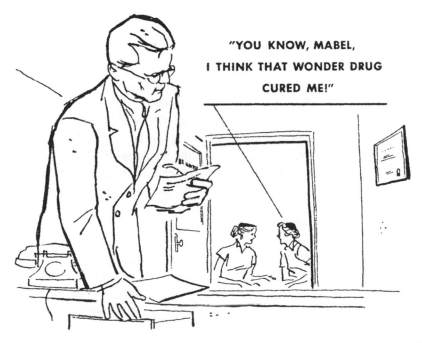

20. Cartoon used by the Institute of Motivational Research early in the 1950s to evoke doctors' views on patients' attitudes. It was shown to doctors who then gave their responses to the characteristic scene it portrayed. Many were very hostile.
Healthcare Marketing and Communications Council Inc.

147

prescribing a drug that maimed unborn children. At the very same time, doctors and pharmaceutical companies were accused of experimenting on patients, a charge that resonated with contemporary images of Auschwitz and the activities of the inhuman Dr Mengele. Those associations were very much alive when Maurice Pappworth, a respected physician, published an article in the British magazine *Twentieth Century* warning the public that experiments with new drugs were routinely carried out on unsuspecting patients and giving twenty-two examples of specific cases. He went on to write the book *Human Guinea Pigs*, which gave several hundred more examples.[33] The resulting debate about the trustworthiness of doctors led to the formation of a lobby for the users of Britain's National Health Service, the Patients' Association.[34] Internationally, stories of indiscriminate experiments on hospital patients led to an agreed code of ethics requiring consent to medical treatment. But all this was too late—the damage to the standing of medicine had been done.[35] Thus, in its aftermath, we find rising concern about water fluoridation as a form of medical experimentation.[36]

The opening-up of detailed academic study of trust in medicine was an interesting indicator of growing questioning by the general public. Again this dated from the early 1960s, when the distinguished American economist Kenneth Arrow published what would prove to be a classic paper. In his treatment of 'uncertainty and medical care' he homed in on the contradiction between the necessity for total confidence and scepticism about its possibility.[37] He argued that, with military defence and legal help, medical care is one of those services the individual needs rather rarely and unpredictably, but when it is needed the requirement may be desperate. With lack of experience came the need for that special kind of reliance put on doctors. 'One consequence of such trust relations', Arrow proposed, 'is that the physician cannot act, or at least appear to act, as if he is maximizing his income at every moment of time. As a signal to the buyer of his intentions to act as thoroughly in the buyer's behalf as possible, the physician avoids the obvious stigmata of profit-maximizing.' Even 'the very word, "profit," is a signal that denies the trust relations'. At that critical moment of doubt, Arrow was pointing his readers towards the public questioning of the private interests that might lie behind a doctor's behaviour.

Studies of regions as diverse as North America, Britain, Australia, Italy, and East Africa have explored the general and local challenges to the traditional standing of the doctor and of medicine in general that multiplied from the 1960s onwards.[38] A 1987 study in the USA found that almost two-thirds of people agreed with the statement, 'people are beginning to lose faith in doctors'.[39] There were many continuing forces for change. Across the world, the women's movement protested against traditional medical behaviour and attitudes. There were also local factors. In the United States the cost of medicine was a continuing issue, while in Britain the National Health Service was accused of imposing unacceptable delays on patients awaiting treatment. The proportion of people expressing dissatisfaction with the Service increased from about a quarter in 1983 to almost a half in 1990.[40] About a quarter of the respondents in this period were dissatisfied with the medical services of the general practitioner. The totally disenchanted were still a minority, but the general shift from passively supplicant patients to an active customer mentality came to be widely commented upon.[41] We see, therefore, over the half-century that followed the Second World War, the working-out of Dichter's 1950 diagnosis of a veritable 'reformation' in the relationship between lay person and expert. It had proved challenging to the professional authority that had achieved control by means of prescriptions.

Yet, in general, patients were of course continuing to consult their physicians in the hope they would get well.[42] The frequent success in maintaining confidence, at an individual level, was testimony not just to the sick person's need to believe in their carers, but also to doctors' commitment to sustaining social relationships within their practices and to their medical success in dealing with acute conditions. The two were connected: as the distinguished British general practitioner Marshall Marinker explained, 'in the medicine of general practice the physical, the psychological and the social components of the diagnosis are valued together; that the response of the doctor must take them all into consideration'.[43] Late in the 1950s a survey conducted by the University of Chicago's National Opinion Research Center showed the new-found authority that the power to prescribe penicillin and other antibiotics bestowed on the doctor. Despite the already widespread criticisms of the profession in general, the survey came to the conclusion that American patients' respect for their own doctors had never been higher.[44] Even though as many as one-third of the respondents believed that doctors took a 'little' or a 'lot less' interest in their patients than thirty years before, almost all the respondents to its study felt that it was easier to have good health than it had been thirty years earlier. The availability of 'wonder drugs'—of which penicillin was the model—was singled out as the most important factor for such progress.

The personal meaning of such statistical evidence was graphically illustrated in a 1954 article published in *Parents Magazine*, which reported

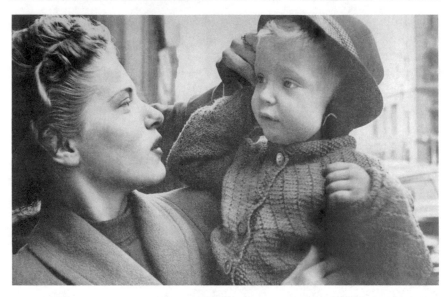

21. This photograph illustrated the article 'What We Know about Young Ears' by Louise Fox Connell in *Parents Magazine* in March 1954. It supposedly depicted the anxious mother tending her child about to be relieved by a doctor armed with penicillin.
Fernand Fonssagrives Archive/As seen in *Parents Magazine*.

a mother's experience of relief when a doctor prescribed penicillin for her child suffering from earache.

A SCREAM from her baby waked a mother in the middle of the night. She found her small son pawing his ear and shrieking in agony. He had had a cold for several days but no fever. Now, however, he felt hot. In terror the young mother phoned her pediatrician. Within half an hour the doctor was there and examining the baby's ear. 'Germs from your baby's cold have infected his middle ear', he said. 'It's full of fluid and gas which are pressing against his ear drum. Lucky you called me at once. I hope that antibiotic treatment will relieve the pressure by morning. A few hours can often make all the difference; so don't worry.' He gave the baby an injection of penicillin and also a pain-killing drug.[45]

The doctor had prescribed penicillin and the story goes on to tell how the child soon recovered (see Ill. 21). Whatever the patient's perceived problem, the doctor could now often provide the solution. The power of the prescription to which the doctor was the point of access had given him (it was still largely him) a new basis for authority. Its effectiveness meant that, while deference to other educated professionals was declining, the standing of doctors was maintained and even increased with their personal patients. Rather than the abstractions of public health and public good,

150

it was a standing reflecting the benefits medicine could bestow on the individual.

In the face of perceived patient expectations, the doctor's use of the prescription to prove his or her continuing trustworthiness to the patient has repeatedly come up in the studies of antibiotic use conducted by social scientists. For instance, a British study in the 1990s reported the prescribing behaviour of doctors: 'many were concerned to preserve and build relationships with their patients, and it was not worth jeopardising this "for the sake of a prescription for penicillin V".'[46] Another general practitioner was quoted, 'In a way it would be better for the community that so many people would not take antibiotics. So here is a little bit of conflict of interest in a way ... now antibiotics are cheap and no harm is done if antibiotics are prescribed once or twice a year for an upper respiratory tract infection or a little bronchitis. Now why should I deprive my patients?' These sentiments, quoted in an article published by the *British Medical Journal*, promptly elicited considerable support, which indicated that the phenomenon was not one just of the 1990s. Thus a retired general practitioner wrote: 'Butler and colleagues are to be congratulated on illuminating one of the most important reasons for GPs' apparently irrational behaviour in their inappropriate prescribing of antibiotics, i.e. their need not to endanger the doctor–patient relationship. My thirty years in general practice endorses this view.'[47] This comment highlighted the deep entrenchment of such considerations in medical culture.

Whereas overt demands from patients were disliked by doctors and often proved counter-productive, subtlety could bear results in the shape of a desired prescription. Anthropologists shadowing patients found complicated word games in the consulting room worthy of a master playwright. For instance, a Southern Californian study of parents of children with acute symptoms found that half wanted antibiotics for their children when they went into their physician's surgery. Only one in a hundred actually asked.[48] There were, however, smarter ways of getting round to the issue and a third of the doctors felt that, even though patients were not asking outright, they were expecting antibiotics. A patient would, for instance, point out how bad she felt. An example is given in another article:

The patient was sitting up on the table, and right away he told Dr Lamont, 'I just can't shake it. I feel like the back of my throat has raw hamburger hanging in it.' Dr Lamont checked the patient's throat well, and the patient said, 'This has lasted 4 days and it has been getting worse today.' Dr Lamont checked the patient's ears, glands, and lungs. 'I'm going to give you a shot of penicillin, slow release. It's some kind of an infection. It may be a virus.'[49]

Alternatively, a patient might suggest a diagnosis to the doctor, such as 'strep throat', which immediately would imply an antibiotic cure. For many patients the past experience of receiving a prescription for a viral condition suggested that antibiotics would be useful in the future. A British study conducted in 1999 found that more than a third (39 per cent) of respondents believed that bad colds and 'the flu' could sometimes be treated with antibiotics, and one in twelve people believed that these treatments were always appropriate for such conditions.[50] A study of Italian doctors, who were prescribing large amounts of broad-spectrum antibiotics, suggested that social mores rather than medical textbooks explained their behaviour: the diagnosis was an 'alibi' rather than the explanation for a prescription.[51] Again, the antibiotic prescription was seen to be just part of a complex conversation between doctor and patient, which might itself have powerful therapeutic consequences.

Such frequently non-verbal negotiation was, of course, not conducted in ideal circumstances. Rushed communication between doctor and patient, at a time of increasing demands on the surgery, could lead to false assumptions and misreading of patient wishes. The British sociologist of medicine Nicky Britten has studied the numerous reports of patient pressure on doctors to prescribe antibiotics.[52] Distinguishing between doctors' perceptions of patient expectations and what patients themselves expect, she found that over one in five patients who were not expecting a prescription received one anyway.[53] Meanwhile, many a patient might have preferred careful attention to a quick prescription for amoxicillin. If patients came with an unspoken hope not to be given a pill, sociologists found that caution often went unnoticed.

As penicillin became a commodity, its deployment became a decision in a new economy in which there were many pressures. Prescribing an antibiotic was not just prudent: it was also useful in the practical business of medicine. At a time when employers and insurers were seeking economy, and demand from the public was growing, pressured doctors could speed up patient throughput by writing antibiotic prescriptions. Increasingly, doctors worried about litigation from below, pressures to cut costs from above, and guilt from within. '"How do you doctors know that an antibiotic would not help me?"' asked a patient when her physician refused to prescribe a course to cure a cold.[54] Two Harvard

Medical School doctors described the consequences for the prescribing of antibiotics:

A prescription for an antibiotic is often seen as the quickest way to end the visit of a patient with possible infectious symptoms. The number of patients seen per hour is increasing, and such 'increased productivity' is frequently commended in the same management memorandum that criticizes out-of-control drug expenditures. Ironically, managers' desire to reduce the use of diagnostic tests (cultures) and prevent return visits also creates pressures that favor heavy antibiotic use.[55]

Accounts of doctors themselves told of how the existence of powerful drugs increased their own self-expectations, and, in the event of failure, anxiety about their patients' and communities' anger and blame. Whatever the probable diagnosis, were something to go unexpectedly awry, then other people, and perhaps even they themselves, would ask why antibiotics had not been tried. The distinguished British physician Lord Winston was unusual only in his frankness when he described his trauma as a young doctor as a patient died:

It is true that an antibiotic almost certainly would not have helped—in fact, the post-mortem did not show any evidence of bacteriological infection—but that, for a young doctor, does not make any difference. You wonder whether you should have given that antibiotic.[56]

In the event of disaster, the decision not to use antibiotics therefore could lie heavy on the professional conscience.

Strictly social factors did not, of course, exist in isolation from the strictly medical. There was genuine uncertainty both over the medical dangers of not prescribing antibiotics for an infection and over what small risks might be acceptable in different cultures without undermining the trustworthiness of the doctor. The combination of social, medical, commercial, and political issues in penicillin use was illustrated by the debate over prescribing penicillin for the ear condition known as acute otitis media (AOM) which had been so graphically represented in the 1954 *Parents Magazine*. It is typically caused by *S. pneumoniae* and, in 1990 in the USA, AOM accounted for almost 25 million visits to doctors.[57] Between 1982 and 1996, prescriptions to treat the condition in the USA increased by 150 per cent.[58] This community of doctors clearly felt justified in using antibiotics, yet a great debate on the value of such prescription for AOM had been raging over this period.

As recently as the late 1940s, AOM had been much feared: it had often caused severe infections deep in the head, and one in three of untreated patients suffered from infection of the mastoid bone known as mastoiditis. Combating it had come to be a major cause of penicillin use. However, improved health and nutrition meant that, although intensely painful to the patient and worrying for the parents, by the 1980s in developed countries with better good health AOM was generally a short-term condition even without medication. In 1981, two teams of European doctors independently published reports suggesting that, in the vast majority of cases, a treatment with nose drops and painkillers was quite adequate and that the condition cleared up in three or four days. Only then, they concluded, was it worth moving to penicillin.[59] This advice led to a radical change in practice in the Netherlands. By the 1990s, only a third of AOM patients were considered to require penicillin there, while elsewhere it was prescribed in almost all cases.[60]

The issue of how to treat AOM was complicated for doctors by vitriolic debates over the credibility of the underlying medical data in a context of large medical expenditures, contested professional self-esteem, and endangered commercial interests. Conflict erupted in 1987, for instance, at the University of Pittsburgh, where a group was exploring the effects of reducing antibiotic use.[61] The widely reported and long-running dispute involved claims that the results of the study were being manipulated to make the use of antibiotics look more beneficial than in fact it was. Because the public interest was at stake, the issue grew beyond a professional disagreement and the university and even a Congressional Committee came to be involved. Beyond this case, in the absence of agreement on acceptable levels of risk, statistics could not determine a clinical conclusion. The evaluation of what constituted a legitimate risk and the balance between communal and individual benefit continued to be struck differently in the Netherlands and the USA.

The issues of control, trust in doctors, and trust in medicines were therefore balanced differently in each medical culture. Although great divides were evident between the medical cultures of richer and developing countries, even within the apparent coherence of western Europe there have been great variations in the willingness to trust doctors and indeed in patterns of antibiotic use.

A 1983 study showed that Spain was then the largest user of antibacterials, with the UK (and the USA) consuming about half as much, with Germans' consumption at half their level.[62] More detailed studies of Europe in 1997 showed startlingly different uses of penicillins in particular. The Germans used fewer than three daily doses for every thousand people.[63] The Dutch and Scandinavians were also low consumers.[64] On the other hand in France and Spain, for every thousand people, over eighteen doses of broad-spectrum penicillin (ampicillin and amoxycillin) were prescribed daily.[65]

A Spanish team has argued that Catholicism was a key marker of high antibiotic use. According to its calculations, predominantly Catholic European countries used approximately twice as much per head as predominantly Protestant countries.[66] A telephone poll of 1,000 Spanish households found that two out of five had at least one antibiotic packet in their medicine cabinets, and in general these supplies were remainders of past prescriptions.[67] Explaining how the drug was used, the Spanish researchers suggested that in Catholic countries there was less willingness to trust the doctor than further north. They used this model reflection to express the views they found: 'A similar (mild) infection (or any other illness) to that I am now suffering from was successfully treated on a previous occasion with a particular drug. As I have such a drug stored at home, I will start with it, or try to get more of it at the pharmacy, or ask my doctor for it.'[68] Certainly, the Eurobarometer surveys, conducted by the European Commission since 1980, suggested that people in southern European countries such as Italy, Spain, and Portugal were much less trusting of each other than their counterparts in northern European, predominantly Protestant countries.[69]

The differences in attitudes to antibiotics between Protestants and Catholics were explored in a remarkable study comparing the use of medicines in two nearby towns, Middelburg in Protestant Holland and Bruges just 65 km distant in Catholic Belgium.[70] Four types of attitude to antibiotic were identified, ranging from the most positive, 'better safe than sorry', to the slightly less positive, 'antibiotics, if there is no alternative', to the more negative 'rather not, but accepting', and finally 'very sceptical'. The authors found that Dutch-speaking Flemings in Belgium tended to take the two rather more positive attitudes, while the Dutch themselves took the more sceptical approach. These different attitudes to the taking of antibiotics were linked to distinct approaches to seeking medical help in general. Not feeling well, the Belgians would diagnose bronchitis and go to the doctor in search of medicine. With the same symptoms, the Dutch would stay at home and hope to recover by themselves. The analysts found that the Protestant Dutch had a greater faith in the body's ability to heal itself, while the Catholic Belgians favoured the ritual benefits of attending a doctor's surgery and taking a medicine. Interestingly, Catholic Dutch people had an intermediary position.

So, even in developed European countries, the use of antibiotics reflected local values and the unspoken qualities of the 'life worlds' of the patients and their doctors rather than the abstract imposition of the public sphere.[71] Willingness to trust medical judgements, as the Spanish researchers had shown, could lead patients to access antibiotics directly. Similar issues could be seen underpinning the search for antibiotics in countries beyond western Europe. Different, more anxious, but still very respectful attitudes were found by a study of mothers in Turkey and Colombia. There, antibiotics are 'strong', they undermine the body's immunity, part of a course can be saved for future use, great concerns regarding children with respiratory infection are expressed, and the demand for medical support is high, even though many mothers think they are better judges than their doctors.[72] In developed and developing countries alike, penicillin was assimilated into local cultures or life worlds without the regulation that medical scientists would have wanted to associate with it. Instead, across the world its use was widely governed by pre-existing rules. These rules, however, were neither antique or simple.

Thus, in Africa, penicillin first acquired its reputation in the anti-yaws campaign of the 1950s, and its reputation even in later years grew out of that early encounter. In the 1920s, injections of arsenical preparations such as Salvarsan had been employed, and these had been followed by campaigns using a compound of bismuth. Even these inter-war measures had been fairly successful, particularly in East Africa. However, penicillin, with its broader spectrum, greater effectiveness, and safety, was much quicker to act and therefore more attractive, reducing the length of the campaign from a generation to a few years.[73] The success of the yaws initiative seems to have given the use of penicillin a special mystique and even had the surprising legacy of lending special power to administration by injection. C. J. Hackett, the British pioneer, tells the story of arriving in Dalao in the Ivory Coast, at the end of a campaign to eradicate sleeping sickness. The public had lost interest in that endeavour, but when Hackett offered a free penicillin injection, attendance at vaccination clinics was the largest for years.

Injections themselves could be a statement of autonomy and of personal control. The anthropologist Susan Whyte has suggested that the use of Western medicines represents a shift in the meaning of therapy in many countries.[74] Reflecting a change of emphasis from the manipulation of relationships to the administration of substances, injections are the ultimate private individualistic medical experience, whereas pills can still be shared. Penicillin injections therefore fulfilled the needs of a newly developing local culture.[75] In the early 1980s, Dianna Melrose, a British Oxfam worker, reported the enthusiasm in Upper Volta for injecting antibiotics to treat conditions ranging from nappy rash to concussion.[76]

However applied, medicines as a whole have typically been an expensive burden on the formal medical systems of developing countries and this made their proper control all the more difficult. Whereas in developed countries at the end of the twentieth century medicines constituted 20 per cent of the costs of medical care, in developing countries the percentage could be twice as high.[77] Much of this expenditure benefited relatively few people. In former colonies, which had inherited elaborate hospital systems intended for the treatment of Europeans, what has been called 'the three-quarters rule' long endured.[78] Three-quarters of health expenditures went on facilities that benefited just one-quarter of the population, while the remaining three-quarters have had to share the quarter remaining. Instead of certified doctors controlling medicines, commonly a wide range of experts from different traditions have been available to sell their advice more cheaply, and, in addition, customers could buy the drugs without any intermediary.

Thus numerous studies reported a mixture of antibiotic prescriptions from doctors where available, and, where they were not, patients self-administering pills or obtaining them from other healers. A study of Nigerian patients conducted in 1987 found that two-thirds of the patients attending government hospitals had been prescribed ampicillin.[79] Those attending private clinics took a wider range of penicillins, but the general impression of overuse was the same. In this study, 500 randomly chosen members of the public were also quizzed. All had previously medicated themselves with antibiotics. A 1993 study of a suburb in Mexico City presented a similar picture.[80] About one in twenty of the people living in over a thousand randomly chosen households had taken an antibiotic in the previous two weeks alone, often without medical advice. Over half the treatments had been given for assumed infections of the respiratory tract, and about half the treatments were penicillin.

That infection in developing countries caused half of all deaths, rather than the one in ten deaths in richer societies, gave special significance to the power of antibiotics. Two anthropologists summarized the situation: 'pharmaceuticals have the dubious distinction of being as popular and available around the world as Coca-Cola. In the smallest villages in many countries, one can purchase an antibiotic capsule as easily as a bottle of Coke.'[81] During the early 1980s, the British Oxfam worker Dianna Melrose reported on the attraction of gaily coloured capsules sold individually in markets of countries such as Upper Volta to people neither minded nor able to buy entire courses of treatment.[82] Incomplete treatments might mask the symptoms, but they would also favour the growth of resistant strains of bacteria.

In societies where the medical community could exert very little control, the use of drugs could become divorced from the practice of Western medicine almost entirely. Particularly from the 1970s, therefore, students of anthropology became interested in how antibiotics came to be so widely used in societies that had been much less touched by Western medical theories. No single agency could be blamed for what was widely criticized by public-health workers as excessive use of antibiotics. In a wonderful prize-winning essay published in 1996, J. P. Loefler, a Vienna-born Kenyan doctor, blamed these consumption patterns on 'the unholiest of alliances': consumer demand based on misinformation, mercantile interest, and the insecurity and cynicism of the middlemen.[83] Although the pharmaceutical industry was widely criticized for excessively promoting drugs to developing nations, that, in part, reflected the shortage of doctors as well as the low cost of salesmen. In any case, unofficial channels for obtaining drugs and their significance within popular culture meant that industry's tactics were just one cause of 'irrational' patterns of antibiotic consumption.

The power, mass production, and relative cheapness of penicillin had made the drug itself much easier to import across the world than the entire structure of Western medicine, or even the doctor or Western-style pharmacist. Thus one analyst has distinguished between the indigenous provider of medicines who will use Western medicines without adopting Western theories of how diseases are caused, and practitioners of traditional indigenous medicine.[84]

In the absence of practitioners of Western medicine, the antibiotics could be assimilated within other traditions. As early as 1955 a striking contradiction between total confidence in antibiotic injections and the lack of commitment to a germ theory of disease was reported among Mestizo coastal communities in Chile and Peru. 'It is important to note that these modern remedies are utilized mostly for the illnesses whose aetiologies fall within the categories of gastrointestinal obstruction and hot or cold. Moreover, the modern cures have not replaced popular remedies but have simply been added to the popular repertory. They are regarded as alternative cures, not necessarily as better ones, and are used along with household remedies.'[85] Similarly in mid–1950s Greece, anthropologists placed penicillin between oil of mouse and ground hedgehog in a list of commonly used 'praktika'.[86]

Penicillin and other antibiotics had entered cultures well used to finding ways of coping with and interpreting new medicines. There are reports of penicillin being translated into Ayurvedic medicine in India by a practitioner who incorporated it in his repertoire of traditional medicines.[87] This emergence of such pharmaceutical equivalents to world music had problems distinctive to medicine. Anne Ferguson, studying the use of drugs in El Salvador, Central America, described some of the difficulties in blending medicines in her report of a tragedy.

An infant had suffered from recurring bouts of upper-respiratory infections since her birth and had been treated by a physician for bronchitis. So, when the child experienced difficulty in breathing, relatives at first sought help from the government-supported health post. Ferguson describes how after several hours' wait, the family instead went to an idómes (pharmacy clerk) who provided an injection and recommended the exclusive use of ampicillin and cough syrup, warning that any other medicine would cause a 'clash'. Although the child seemed to recover initially, by the next day she found difficulty in breathing and thereafter passed away. Critically, the family had not sought any other treatment, because of trust in the 'strength' of the idomes' injection and for fear of the 'clash' with other drugs.[88]

Such problems were frequently the result of the failure of basic health care and the shortage of both antibiotics and knowledge of how to deploy them. Early in the 1970s this led to a criticism of international agencies, particularly the WHO, which had, until then, been most focused on eradicating killer diseases.[89] Its success against smallpox could be seen as a vindication of this concentration, but the organization was seen as effectively prosecuting three competing strategies: the single-disease campaigns, together with its promotion of hospitals, and of basic health services.[90] In response to such criticisms, a greater focus on primary care was introduced to the WHO in the mid-1970s by the new Director General, the Dane Halfdan Mahler. Increasingly he made it into a campaigning organization. His fifteen-year tenure would see the WHO become the central player in a debate about the global provision of such drugs as penicillin and their rational use.

Rather than concentrating on high-technology solutions to single dramatic diseases, Mahler focused upon the simple but often fatal ailments. These could be cured by means of basic primary care and greater but managed access to such common medicines as penicillin. Calling in 1975 for 'Health for All by 2000', he hoped not for a utopian end to illness, but for the creation of a new and appropriate infrastructure of health.[91] Thus, rather than endeavouring to give all countries access to all drugs, he drew upon pre-Second World War Scandinavian social security systems and promoted the concept of a limited list. This approach promised to cap the unaffordable drugs bills of countries encouraged to buy the latest medication for a few, while the many could not afford even clean water to wash down their pills. The publication by the WHO in 1977 of a list of 220 essential drugs intended to meet 90 per cent of developing countries' needs proved most controversial, with the manufacturers in Western countries blamed for fighting it tooth and nail. Naturally penicillin was one of those key drugs.[92] Nigeria, the Philippines, and Bangladesh introduced national policies based upon essential drug lists. They were supported by a new international lobby, Health Action International (HAI), and opposed by the pharmaceutical industry concerned that such limitations in albeit small markets would spread to richer countries.

In Tanzania, the Chinese had promoted the model of the locally trained provider of basic health care, the 'barefoot doctor', and this attracted attention from developing countries across the world. At a time of international tension, the Soviet Union was vying for status with China and offered $2 million for a major conference on the topic of primary health care to be held on its own soil.[93] Accordingly, in 1978 the world's representatives (excluding the Chinese, who boycotted the conference) met in Alma Ata, capital of Kazakhstan. Out of that meeting, held just before the onset of AIDS, came the institutional support for 'Health for All' and a new focus upon primary health care.

Complementing 'Health for All', scientists opposed to the apparent chaos of the market were attracted to 'rational drug use', through which the physician, rather than trying out various treatments in the hope of finding one that worked, would go from scientific diagnosis to scientifically chosen treatment. It did not apply only to antibiotics or penicillin; its application to such drugs would, however, be particularly apt. Embodying more than clinical theory, this approach also expressed a hope that commercial pressures and personal predilections would be superseded by good medical practice.

The 'rational drug use' vision was discussed at a conference held by the WHO in Nairobi, Kenya, in November 1985.[94] Vivid in the memory of its participants, it became a seminal conference, and the atmosphere there would be recorded in memoirs more lively than the formal proceedings. Briefing papers were written and circulated in advance, with little time allowed for discussion at the meeting. Such an organizational structure minimized open dissent and drove debate to the corridors. It clearly proved difficult to reach a consensus. A briefing paper written by two American consultants on rational drug distribution was extensively edited.[95] While the authors promoted the role of private industry in the improvement of what they saw as a corrupt system, the final paper emphasized the significance of government measures. Beyond the wide appeal of 'rational use', fundamental disputes over how it would be achieved still remained.

The Nairobi conference's concern with rational use of medicines was not reserved for developing countries. Ironically, whereas the problems of shortage in such countries were desperate, they were relatively easy to solve—in principle at least. In subsequent years, the relations between private industry and lobbies for developing countries improved.[96] New systems of distribution through state dispensaries, which could charge for drugs in order to buy more supplies, may have encouraged use of antibiotics and fostered resistance as well as improving health.[97] Underconsumption therefore could be addressed through improved distribution, but overconsumption would prove a much more recalcitrant problem.

In developing and developed countries alike, antibiotic use had become a key part of social life as well as of strictly medical practice. Its growth reflected the many valuable roles it played in maintaining diverse medical systems and also the weakness of professional control. In particular, doctors had come to use prescriptions as powerful tools for the maintenance of trust, in a period in which trust was increasingly endangered. Such processes defied redirection through the action of individual professionals alone and, until the end of the twentieth century, their dynamics evaded public scrutiny. In most settings, medical practice was still too private a topic to be examined as policy. Moreover, the threats from infection were still generally low compared to past experience and other current threats.

The problems of infection were described, by one analyst at the turn of the millennium, as 'serious, but not yet desperate'.[98] A rise from the 36 deaths per hundred thousand they caused in 1980 to 63 deaths in a hundred thousand in the United States in 1995 represented a shocking growth rate, but still to a small number. Cancer death rates were more than twice as high and heart disease was taking ten times as many victims. Resistant bacteria were not yet causing such a torrent of deaths that the public were calling for action which would override the privacy of the consulting room or the normal economics of the market. MRSA was still a threat restricted to hospitals and not widely familiar to the public.

Resistant pneumococci could generally be addressed, for the moment, by means of increasing doses of penicillins and other antibiotics. *Salmonella typhimurium* came in waves but was only life threatening to the weak or elderly. So, instead of human uses, it was the less taboo topic of antibiotics in agriculture that would first become controversial.

8

Animals, Resistance, and Committees

We shift our attention, in this chapter, from the surgery to the farmyard. Over several decades, both in Britain and in the USA, debates over the threat posed by animal-borne resistant organisms spreading to humans served as a surrogate for debate over human uses. Antibiotics had become a high-technology solution to the problems of newly intensive farming, and the economic stakes were therefore very high. So, it was feared, were the medical stakes.

In terms of the penicillin 'brand', there has of course been an enormous difference between drugs used to preserve human life on the one hand and, on the other, the treatments administered to animals to make them grow faster and more healthily. The particular chemicals used have, however, been identical. Since the 1950s, at least a quarter of the antibiotics made have been administered to animals, and many drugs such as ampicillin used on animals were exactly the same as those used to treat human diseases.[1] Nevertheless, the link between the bacteria infecting people and animals was, and has remained, much less clear, and the debate over its importance has therefore proved to be particularly heated and long lasting.

Risks heightened by the increasing consumption and production of meat lay behind the public concern. Both stomach infections and the selection of resistant bacteria could be linked back to animals. Thus, whereas poultry had been responsible for an insignificant proportion of human infection in Britain during the early 1950s, by the end of the 1960s it caused more than half the increasingly frequent outbreaks of salmonellosis in humans.[2] Strains of bacteria that had developed resistance to ampicillin in the animal gut would also be resistant to the same penicillin in the human patient. Even more worryingly, resistance genes might be transferred between separate organisms infecting animals and humans, creating 'superbugs' immune to many different antibiotics.

Blame and recrimination between veterinarians and doctors would characterize the debate over antibiotic resistance. Medical campaigners have regarded as narrow-minded, self-serving, and wrong those who did not see the implications for human health of the widespread agricultural use of low doses of antibiotics. As early as 1959, 94 per cent of a sample of 900 Swiss doctors believed such medicines should not be administered to animals at all.[3] Farmers and agrochemical companies countered that speculative and defensive blaming by doctors should not justify the undermining of two generations' achievement in modern agriculture. This relationship was summarized at the end of the twentieth century: 'In the past, the medical profession has delighted in blaming the veterinary profession for all aspects of antibiotic resistance. The veterinary profession, feeling under siege, has done likewise with the medical profession.'[4]

Although the debate therefore pitted major professions and indeed major companies and institutions against each other, a few individuals managed to win significant personal influence. In part they worked through friends in the media, but they also drew upon the power of committees, often the key actors of late twentieth-century science. Committees may have been impersonal, but their findings gave political weight to the judgements and knowledge of their scientist-members. Though little attention has been given to their role, their conclusions have frequently determined what is agreed to be 'true'.

The question of animal uses of antibiotics has been particularly problematic, because human illnesses are generally quite separate from infections in live animals. Few strains of gram-negative bacteria cause infections in both humans and animals. It is therefore not obvious that the use of antibiotics to cure diseases of livestock could breed disease organisms resistant to treatment in a human population. In 1953, the distinguished chemotherapist Lawrence Garrod assured British Agriculture Department officials that any loss of health to animals through infection from antibiotic-resistant bacteria would be insignificant compared to agricultural benefits and have no implications for human medicine. His advice informed a meeting between civil servants on the use of antibiotics in animal feed, summarized thus:

Neither of us is inclined to pay any serious attention to the possible danger of encouraging the development of antibiotic-resistant strains of *Salmonella* by including antibiotic supplements in food for pigs or fowls. As you know, none of the food-poisoning group of samonellae are very sensitive to any of the known antibiotics, so that they hardly affect the picture. The only *Salmonella* that is relevant to this problem is the typhoid bacillus, which is susceptible to chloramphenicol and Aureomycin. This organism does not affect either pigs or fowls, and is therefore not likely to come into contact with antibiotics given in animal food.[5]

Doctors would come to oppose bitterly such reassuring judgements, but would find it difficult to assemble compelling data convicting animal uses of promoting the spread of resistant bacteria widely threatening to humans. Microbiologists endeavouring to prove their case against animal uses of antibiotics found it tantalizingly difficult to 'prove' linkages between animal infection and widespread human problems. By the time an epidemic occurred, the infected animals had been slaughtered and evidence of their medical condition was circumstantial. An American professor reported to a 1982 British symposium: 'In 1978, when we needed to enter the official FDA argument into the Congressional record, we found no convincing evidence that antibiotic resistance arising in animals fed on or injected with antibiotics had caused great problems in human medicine. So we simply stated in the Congressional record that there was a theoretical chance of a compromise of human therapy. In fact we labored for almost a year over the choice of the term "theoretical", or the alternative of providing direct evidence.'[6] Such lack of evidence created deadlock in US debates over the use of antibiotics in animals for more than two decades.

Certainly antibiotics were useful to the farmer. They prevented infections spreading through crowded animal enclosures and accelerated the growth of young animals to slaughter size. Tetracycline was a popular antibiotic with farmers, while ampicillin, the new semisynthetic broadspectrum penicillin, and cloxacillin, effective against antibiotic-resistant bacteria in mastitis, quickly became popular too, after their introduction early in the 1960s. To many veterinarians and farmers such drugs seemed to be a key to the assurance of a plentiful food supply. The use of penicillin and other antibiotics on animals sustained the growth of intensive agriculture that so dramatically changed diets and, through its increased efficiency, also released labour in the 1950s. The use of penicillin therefore sustained the evolving culture of the post-war world not only through its medical impact, but also through the vast meat supplies it guaranteed to the newly prosperous citizens of western Europe and the USA.

The use of antibiotics on animals had dated from the earliest days of the drugs. Although the first antibiotic, gramicidin, developed by René Dubos in the late 1930s, had proved too toxic for internal use, it could be used to treat such local but painful and dangerous cattle infections as mastitis. The potential of this new therapy was demonstrated when it was first tried out on an entire herd in the very public arena of the 'Foodzone' of the 1939/40 New York World Fair. In the dramatic presentation of the Borden milk company entitled 'The Dairy World of Tomorrow', a herd of 116 cows was automatically milked using the modern 'Rotolactor' (Ill. 22).[7] Not to disappoint children longing to see 'Elsie', Borden's recently launched trademark cartoon figure, which appeared on the labels of every product, one of the specially recruited 'Gotham herdsmen' identified a cow in the herd named 'You'll do Lobelia' as the real-life Elsie.[8]

Enthusiasm over Elsie made the Borden exhibit the fair's second most popular attraction. Unfortunately, the herd was afflicted with mastitis. In a short time, sixteen cows suffered and the entire exhibit was threatened. At first sulphonamides were tried, but they were not sufficiently successful. Then the vet turned to gramicidin. René Dubos was brought in to work with a US Department of Agriculture team. They experimentally used the new drug on the highly controlled herd so visibly on show. In May 1940, sixteen cows were treated. Of these twelve were saved, and with the

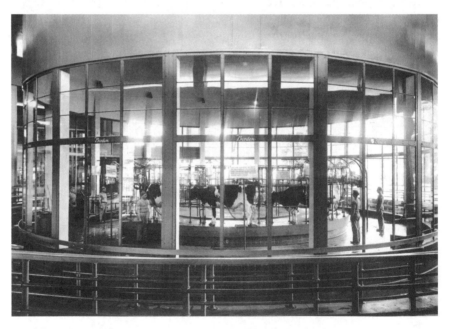

22. Rotolactor on display. Cows milked on this high-technology milking machine at the New York World's Fair caught mastitis but were cured with the early antibiotic gramicidin.

Plainsboro Historical Society, NJ, USA.

loss of just four cows both the herd and its public image were preserved. According to Dubos, interviewed in 1955, the lucky patients included Elsie. Even if the Gotham herdsmen themselves (and surviving records) cast doubt on Dubos's claim that Elsie herself had been infected, she was in the herd and benefited from the containment of the infection.[9] Following this dramatic demonstration on the most high profile of herds, gramicidin became an accepted and successful treatment for mastitis.[10]

Enthusiasm for the technology tested on the Borden herd reflected the new hopes for an industrialized and more productive agriculture. Just as the regulation of antibiotic provision to people was framed against the background of historic underconsumption of drugs, so debates over animal husbandry have been coloured by memories of underconsumption of food in the past, and fears of underconsumption in the future. At the beginning of the twenty-first century, the press in both Europe and America voiced fears of obesity rather than of starvation, but that overabundance for almost all is recent. Just as memories of the Depression had cast their shadow over post-war drug regulation, so memories of deprivation lived on, long after the experience had finished.

The urgency of increased production meant that, in the USA and increasingly in Europe, the culture of small-scale farming was replaced by the logic of industry. Even if small farms were supported by subsidies, they were often put out of business by the economies of scale of larger enterprises. Between 1940 and 1980 the number of US farms raising livestock fell by 80 per cent, but the number of animals doubled.[11] Prosperity depended on both deploying the opportunities available and deftly avoiding numerous threats. Farmers faced many challenges, notwithstanding the generous subsidies that sustained them—declining workforces otherwise attracted by the delights of cities, ever more demanding supermarkets, and greater awareness of competition. They needed every help they could get, and that included drugs. Sometimes these complemented improvements in husbandry, and sometimes they compensated for decline in good practice. Three types of animals in particular were affected: cattle, chickens, and pigs, and each presented their own industrial problems to which antibiotics contributed solutions. To appreciate the eagerness with which these solutions were grasped, it is necessary to recognize how pressing the challenges seemed to the farmers themselves.

It was in the USA that consumption of beef grew first and fastest, but such tastes spread through the world by means of such cultural changes as the new-found popularity of the burger. By 1963, for example, McDonald's had opened 500 restaurants and sold a billion burgers.[12] For many years a sign over the golden arches on each store would inform eager eaters of the number of billions they had helped consume.

Production of beef to meet growing demand was being transformed by the use of cattle-feed lots for final fattening. Increasingly holding more than 2,000 head of cattle, these lots made possible rapid weight gain at low cost.[13] Historically, infectious illness had been a defining problem of the mass raising of animals. Allowed little exercise, prevented from instinctive feeding practices, and kept in close quarters, animals easily became ill, and epidemics swept through the early intensive-breeding centres, making them unviable. Had antibiotics not been available, the animals would have succumbed to the infections that the drugs successfully kept at bay.

In Europe it was the transport of cattle that particularly benefited from antibiotics. European consumption of beef has been lower than in the United States, and farmers have been less dependent upon income from it. Instead, the raising of cattle for meat has been a by-product of milk production, because cows only give milk if they also have calves. This was fine for the 'girls', who could be used to produce more milk, but their brothers were superfluous to the dairy industry. They were therefore removed from their mothers and reared for the production of beef and veal in separate farms. Demand for veal from calves led therefore to a wholesale transport of young animals around western Europe, mixing healthy and infected individuals.

Britain was a particularly important source of these young animals. By the late 1950s, each year a million 'bobby calves' (the unwanted male calves) were born there. Young animals bred in the dairy centres of Devon and Cornwall in the country's south-west were sent, barely weaned, across Britain to wheat- and barley-growing areas hundreds of kilometers away for fattening, and to the Continent, where they were consumed as veal.[14] They would be sold in markets, mixing with animals from different herds as they were traded on. This was an ideal context for the spreading of infection, which could be contained only by the mass use of antibiotics. In the mid-1960s, one major farm would send its calves to market with little bags of antibiotic swinging from their necks.[15]

Not only could antibiotics cure animals of infections; more mysteriously, they also helped stock grow faster. This property was discovered by accident shortly after the Second World War. Farmers raising pigs on concrete floors rather than letting them root in muddy sties had found that their animals were suffering nutritional deficiencies.[16] A 1946 experiment had seen pig farmers feed their herd waste products from the production of vitamin B to boost their nutrition. Surprisingly, the animals grew faster. At first, the farmers assumed that leftover vitamins in the feed had caused this boost. Instead, however, it was found that the waste containing strep-tomyces sludge had been producing small quantities of antibiotic, and it was this that for some reason encouraged growth. Adding small quantities of pure antibiotics such as penicillin to the feed proved to have the same effect. Animals were fed a tablespoonful of antibiotic in every tonne of feed, a much smaller dose than that used to cure an animal of an illness. Typically cure (and the total destruction of bacteria) required between 5 and 28 times as much antibiotic as growth promotion. Correspondingly, the doses given to promote growth would challenge rather than destroy populations of disease-causing bacteria.

The antibiotic growth promoters seemed like an unlooked-for boon to US farmers, who responded enthusiastically to energetic marketing by pharmaceutical companies and the evangelism of Lederle's nutritionist Thomas Jukes, whose long life would span almost the entire twentieth century.[17] The business magazine *Fortune* reported in March 1952 under the headline, 'Here is good news for both farmers and meat eaters. Antibiotics provide more meat with less feed.'[18] Animals were growing 5–10 per cent faster on 10 per cent less feed. The discovery was described as 'Just about the biggest news in the country (if not in the city)'. The first recipients were American pigs and also chicks. The use on calves, with their different digestive systems, was never so widespread. Many European farmers were impressed and followed suit. Others, however, worried that the improved growth merely resulted from antibiotics helping animals cope with dirty conditions. There were indeed enduring doubts about whether the growth promoters offered any long-term benefits at all to farmers.

Meanwhile the pressure to produce more for less was remorseless. While Americans doubled the amount of beef they each consumed, on average, between 1940 and 1975, they tripled their average chicken consumption.[19] Again this was made possible by intensive industrialized rearing sustained by the use of antibiotics. Many producers found these speeded the growth of individual animals and prevented disease that otherwise would have laid low the huge flocks now assembled. The low-price, low-fat meat had once been a minority taste: in the pre-war years, the average person ate three times as much beef as chicken. By 1990, however, chicken consumption had almost caught up with beef. Whereas historically chickens had been used to lay eggs until they died and were then eaten, the post-war industry had divided. Chickens were raised specifically for eating so they would grow faster and could be killed younger. In the USA, consumption exceeded two billion 'broilers' by 1961.[20] They too had become an industrial product dependent on antibiotic use.

In other countries, following the American example, meat consumption boomed too: in the UK, the number of broilers increased twentyfold in just seven years from five million birds in 1953 to 100 million in 1960. After that, growth there slowed down somewhat; elsewhere, however, it continued at a hectic pace. Thus, Brazilian production of chicken meat increased fiftyfold in the last four decades of the twentieth century.[21] The mass assemblage of chicken cages as 'batteries', introduced in the United States in the 1920s, had sustained the doubling of egg production between pre- and post-war America and quickly spread worldwide. Whether for meat or eggs, graphs of chicken use in the West resemble the trajectory of an aeroplane leaving the runway. Even if antibiotics did not power this flight, they did sustain it.

The economics of that other industrially bred animal, the pig, traced a rather different pattern. Rather than soaring away since the Second World War, demands for pork chops, ribs, sausages, bacon, and ham have instead varied cyclically, and farmers have had to cope with ferocious competition. Thus in the United States from the 1940s, many farmers turned away from raising pigs in muddy sties with the expense of dealing with parasites, water provision, and fencing, to concrete lots and centrally provided nutrients (see Ill. 23).[22] This turn to industrial conditions from the chaos of the pigsty was not a new attraction. As early as the 1890s, the Hungarians—intending to 'catch up' and indeed to overtake more industrialized societies—had experimented with the intensive rearing of pigs. In 1894 the Kobanya pig-fattening plant on the outskirts of Budapest handled 622,000 pigs.[23] This intensity was not then sustainable, and disease ended the experiment. When, however, post-war US farmers encountered similar problems, they were armed with antibiotics. Again, those same drugs given in small quantities could speed the growth of animals, bringing closer the day of sale.

Beyond the consumption of meat, there were the benefits to the output of other products, above all milk. Mastitis was not just a public-relations problem at a World's Fair. Because losses to farmers in both milk production and cows' lives were substantial, victory over what was a serious economic challenge was of enormous benefit. As early as 1943, Florey offered a recycled extract from a human patient's penicillin-rich urine to a veterinary investigator, who used it experimentally to treat two animals.[24]

As supplies of penicillin increased, so the drug came to be administered routinely to cure the cattle disease.

Penicillin did, however, have one problem as a mastitis treatment: while it controlled bacterial infection very quickly, it took days to clear from an animal's system. Veterinarians therefore recommended that milk from a treated cow should not be used for a period of up to eighteen days afterwards, depending on the cow's lactation cycle. On the other hand, farmers had drums of penicillin stored in farmyards and these were used with, but also sometimes without, the assistance of veterinarians. Moreover, a small illicit addition could prevent spoilage in milk waiting too long in the sun to be picked up by a tanker arriving late. A little corruption was perhaps inevitable, but its results were not healthy. Low-level mass consumption of penicillin could sensitize unwitting milk-drinkers to the drug, so that when they needed it medically they might suffer allergic reactions. Those people already allergic could suffer skin complaints from drinking a glass of milk.[25]

Concerns were first raised in the mid-1950s in the USA, when it was found that milk was not curdling into cheese. First the FDA and then the British found that a full 10 per cent of milk was contaminated with penicillin. In 1963 a World Health Organization report revealed the worldwide levels of penicillin in milk.[26] The wonder drug had become a pollutant.

With wholesale use of preservatives, and the increasing ability of sensitive chemical instruments to detect trace impurities, more than ever before customers were becoming aware that the foods they were ingesting were far more complex than they had ever imagined (see Ill. 24). A contribution to Britain's *Guardian* newspaper complained, 'Time was, when the Hatter's phrase "I see what I eat" might have passed for tolerably good sense, today it would be madness indeed. With benzoic acid in orange juice, sulphur dioxide in sausages, polyphosphates in ham, toluol in fats, chlorine dioxide in bread, and penicillin in milk, it is now no easy matter.'[27]

News of penicillin in milk resonated with worries about pollution of both air and water by the radioactive element strontium-90.[28] Nuclear bombs tested in remote areas released this relative of calcium into the global atmosphere. It was concentrated in cows' milk and from there got into human bones. Radioactive strontium was even found in the bones of babies fed on cows' milk. So great was the public outrage that the testing of bombs above ground was prohibited in the first of the test-ban treaties. Kubrick's 1964 film classic *Dr Strangelove* linked poisoned food

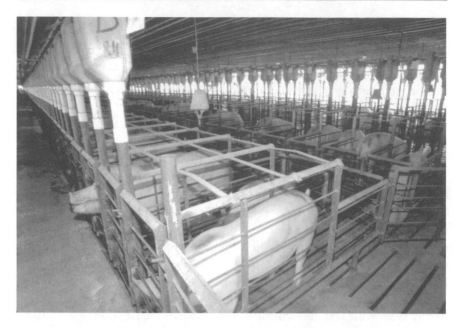

23 *(above)*. Modern pig husbandry.
USDA, photo.

24 *(right)*. Anxieties about penicillin in milk
entered public consciousness in the early
1960s. This cartoon by 'Jon' was published in
the *Daily Mail* 31 May 1963.
Daily Mail.

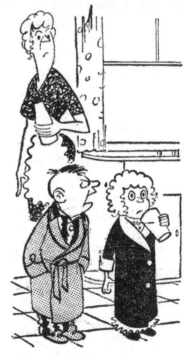

" **Drug addict** "

to the work of cold-hearted weapons scientists. Mad General Jack Ripper, responsible for initiating an attack on the Soviet Union, was inspired by fear of 'fluoride'. He warned that fluorides were not only polluting water: he had heard of intentions to add such chemicals to all manner of foods, including *'Ice cream*, Group Captain, *children's* ice cream!'[29]

Milk was turning into poison because of penicillin and that was an economic as well as cultural threat. By 1962, with public anxiety about to break in Britain, a senior civil servant in the Department of Agriculture was reflecting, 'We now have the opinion of the medical experts in the Ministry of Health that no penicillin ought to be tolerated in milk and, unfortunately, we are still not able to suggest any satisfactory remedy.'[30] While penicillin had become a feared pollutant of milk fed to children, for people at the other end of life milk was already implicated in heart-disease fears. The fat in the milk was being widely linked to the dangers of coronary thrombosis and, from being a good thing, it looked as if milk too was becoming seen as a danger.[31] Fear of encountering penicillin, it seemed to Ministry of Agriculture officials, would compound this anxiety.

As the public became aware of the problems of penicillin residues, the concern of professionals was already leading to action. Anxiety about antibiotics in food put paid to their experimental use as preservatives by reputable manufacturers. Simple-to-use techniques, developed over the next few years, enabled regulators and farmers alike to carry out simple and speedy tests for antibiotic pollution. Using the same principles as Alexander Fleming had employed when he deduced that something strange was stopping his bacteria growing, new instruments, such as the so-called 'Delvotest', could monitor traces of penicillin. This device could give a positive and simple traffic light-like indication to the farmer or regulator: use or don't use. Still on the market at the time of writing, it uses the acid produced by some bacteria when they grow: this reacts with a dye to change its colour. If the colour of test paper in the device changes from purple to yellow, bacteria are growing and there is no penicillin.[32]

While the introduction of better controls reduced anxieties of food pollution, bacterial resistance became an ever more urgent problem. A study conducted during the late 1990s of the scientific literature since 1970 showed that 585 scientific papers had been published on the problem of antibiotic residues. In the same period, ten times as many papers were published on antibiotic resistance and human health.[33] Resistance was proving the major challenge to antibiotic use.

As in the original work on penicillin, now Britain was in the vanguard of developments. Although everywhere medicine was a more powerful lobby than agriculture, nowhere else was the difference between the two sectors so marked. Not just the home country of penicillin and the site of a powerful public-health agency, Britain was also the site of agricultural politics' weakest link: the economic importance of agriculture was low there compared to most countries, and sensitivity to animal welfare was relatively high. This distinction would give particular power to a public-health officer questioning the human cost of agricultural practice.

'Factory farming' was also a continuing issue for public debate in Britain through the 1960s. A denunciation of the practice published in 1964 by Ruth Harrison in her book *Animal Machines* had enormous impact. The parallel with Rachel Carson's *Silent Spring*, which had denounced DDT, was evident in its tone—and made explicit in the preface by Rachel Carson herself.[34] In discussing the use of antibiotics on the farm, British medical and farming interests played a game of chess through intricate but very public and indeed bad-tempered manoeuvrings, which would affect perspectives across the globe. Those negotiations are worth following in detail, because for the first time they translated medical and public unease about the use of penicillin and other antibiotics in the farmyard into legislative action.

In Britain, concern about the unnatural feeding of animals was very widespread and deeply rooted. In March 1961, an MP had passed on to the government the 'resolution of the Shropshire Federation of Women's Institutes representing 8,599 countrywomen'. Normally associated at that time with jam and cake sales, the Women's Institutes expressed their anxieties about the use of new chemicals. They resolved 'That such substances as hormones and antibiotics should not be allowed to be offered for sale commercially, for the fattening of animals for human consumption, until the full implications of the use of these substances has been subjected to adequate study by a suitable body appointed by the government'.[35] The number of signatures elicited in a rural area from an organization normally associated with country people testified to the depths of public concern.

Responding to such anxieties, the government believed that science could establish safe, acceptable boundaries for the use of antibiotics as growth additives and the results would shut the issue down. So, in 1960, the Medical and Agricultural Research Councils had been asked to elicit the facts and win the support of farmers. They convened a joint inquiry, which sat until 1962, consisting of two bodies: a scientific committee dominated by medical scientists and a supervising policy committee. The inquiry as a whole was referred to by the name of its chair, the President of the National Farmers' Union, Lord Netherthorpe.

At this point it still seemed that the problem of bacterial resistance in animals could be kept separate from the problems in humans. A briefing paper from the Central Veterinary Laboratory described the lack of control of antibiotics, but 'The remarkable feature of what can only be described as a chaotic position is the few ill-effects that have resulted.'[36] The committee's final report recommended that permission to broaden the use of antibiotics as growth promoters to calves be given and that no action was needed to curb existing applications in chicks and pigs. Even if animals did harbour organisms that had become resistant to antibiotics, that cost could be set against the benefits of using these drugs. It was assumed that even if bacteria became resistant to the few drugs permitted for such uses, penicillin, oxy-tetratracycline, and chlortetracycline, they would remain susceptible to other antibiotics. This report therefore broadly reassured farmers and the public that it was safe to continue to use antibiotics in animal feeds. Often cited as the first report of the animal-antibiotic crisis, the 1962 report of the Netherthorpe Committee was, in fact, the last of the previous era of reassurance.[37]

The assumptions on which the Netherthorpe report were based were, however, being actively undermined even as they were published. During the early 1960s the belief that bacterial resistance in animals could have no direct consequence for human health was proven wrong. In 1955 a Japanese team had noticed that bacteria causing dysentery (shigella) that were resistant to penicillin were also resistant to tetracycline, which they had never encountered.[38] A few years previously it had been shown that bacteria could share their genes. Their proclivity to do this had been dubbed their F-factor, where F stood for fertility. Such F-factors turned out to be circular pieces of DNA now known as plasmids, which could be exchanged between bacteria. The Japanese scientist Watanabe showed that these plasmids, then still called 'episomes', could explain how bacteria 'caught' resistance. It seemed that episomes could contain genes, which came to be called 'R' (for 'resistance') factors, responsible for creating enzymes protecting the organisms against antibiotics such as penicillin. Such R-factors could then be transferred to certain other bacteria, including those of a different species. These Japanese results were not well known in the Europe and USA of the early 1960s. However, the specialist on the genetics of microbes Naomi Datta, grappling with an outbreak of salmonella at the Hammersmith Hospital in London, had her attention turned to these results by her distinguished colleague, a nephew of J. B. S. Haldane, Denny Mitchison.[39] Drawing on them for a paper on the transmission of resistance to the typhoid-causing bacterium, she made the Japanese work become known in the English-speaking world.[40]

The link between animals and people was made not just by publications, but also by an active campaigner. At the Central Public Health Laboratory in Colindale, where Patricia Jevons had already found the first staphylococcus resistant to methicillin, E. S. Anderson (known as 'Andy'), Director of the Enteric Reference Laboratory, was investigating diseases among calves. In 1965 he announced that two years earlier he had found salmonella resistant to streptomycin and sulphonamides in calves, and now he had identified salmonella bacteria that were resistant also to ampicillin and to chloramphenicol. Moreover, and most worryingly, the very same strain of this resistant *Salmonella typhimurium*, type 29, had been responsible for human illness. He reported that 590 people had suffered and six had died from type 29.[41] The fear that a chloramphenicol-resistant strain of typhoid would spread through the human community drove the campaign forward.[42] Anderson also applied the new episome concept to explain for the first time how this multiple drug resistance cumulated in bacteria.[43]

Anderson ensured that debate over the use of antibiotics on animals, inspired by anxiety over resistance spreading from bacteria infecting animals to those affecting humans, would provide the first serious discussion about the limits of use of the new drugs. He was, of course, not the only person working in the field. At the Animal Health Trust, H. Williams Smith carefully demonstrated the tendency of antibiotic use to breed resistant *Salmonella typhimurium* in the gut of animals.[44] It was, however, Anderson, a powerful character despite his cuddly 'Andy' nickname, who was particularly anxious that public-health concerns be heard. His efforts were amplified by the press through a campaign that drew upon the general public's new scepticism of the 'benign' care provided by the authorities. By means of his remorseless persistence and the inspiration he gave to key journalists, Anderson managed to convert the public concern about the use of drugs in agriculture into fear of untreatable epidemics among humans. Instead of limiting himself to the more traditionally private discussions about resistance, he engaged the public in the debate. In the era of Rachel Carson's warnings about DDT in *Silent Spring*, and soon of recombinant DNA, ordinary people's distrust of the establishment could be harnessed by the canny campaigner, and public engagement could come to be a critical part of the scientific process itself. Not that Anderson was a conscious, or even a likely, pioneer of such a world: he was more akin to the innovators of modern science who were metaphorical 'sleepwalkers', then recently characterized by the writer Arthur Koestler.[45]

Anderson's findings forced the prompt recall of the scientific subcommittee that had only recently permitted the continuing use of antibiotics in animal feeds. Now, the subcommittee was alarmed, and called upon the government to institute a major inquiry into the use of antibiotics.[46] It was this second, 1966, report of the Netherthorpe Committee, rather than the first of 1962, that could be seen as launching the new age of investigations, reports, and discussion of legislative control. However, from a broad governmental perspective, the issue of antibiotic resistance even now ranked low. Politicians had other concerns as British agriculture confronted quite another catastrophe: foot and mouth disease, a virus-caused infection of cloven-footed animals such as cattle, sheep, and pigs. An epidemic started to spread across Britain in October 1967. In response, the government imposed the same measures it had used for a century: it eradicated the disease by sacrificing all stock in infected herds and flocks. By the end of the epidemic, in June 1968, almost 450,000 animals had been slaughtered and rural life violently disrupted.[47] This major crisis dominated the concerns of the Ministry of Agriculture and Fisheries and Food.

Meanwhile, despite the distraction of other issues, in a newly inquisitorial era specialist journalists had become interested in the agricultural use of antibiotics. In the liberal *Guardian* newspaper, the science correspondent Anthony 'Phil' Tucker began to write articles condemning government inaction in the face of the second Netherthorpe report.[48] At *World Medicine*, a new journal established to inform doctors of recent developments, a bacterial biochemist, Bernard Dixon, became interested too.[49] He was shocked to discover Anderson's fears of impending disaster. Dixon wrote an article about the antibiotic issue and then, to prevent any conflict of interest, submitted it to the *New Scientist* rather than his own journal. Published in October 1967, the article 'Antibiotics on the Farm: Major Threat to Human Health' would be constantly referred to thereafter by journalists in the more popular press and politicians, for whom the primary scientific literature was too esoteric. Although factually rich, the article was clear and the tone passionate. It concluded: 'The facts are that multiple infective resistance was unambiguously described in 1965, that it has increased at an alarming rate in recent years, that the evidence for its association with the misuse of antibiotic in husbandry is compelling, that research workers in this field have issued repeated warnings. And that no action is to be taken.'[50] A few months later, Dixon moved on from *World Medicine* to a post at the *New Scientist*.

Dixon was no enemy of the drug industry, but he was of a generation that was newly aware of the social relations of science. The use of nuclear power in Britain had already become a major issue, and the abuse of antibiotics, it seemed to Dixon, might be of the same order. His power to bring it to the public's notice was soon increased when he was unexpectedly himself promoted and offered the editor's chair at the *New Scientist*.

The analysis of Anderson, the interpretation of Dixon, and a newly critical media redefined the context of animal and human antibiotic use. They framed the single event that brought into the public domain the fear that animal use of antibiotics was beginning to compromise human health, and led to the first legislative action limiting the use of antibiotics in husbandry. It was the winter of 1967, a period of frayed emotions, high expectations, and frightening drama. In the USA, controversy over the Vietnam War was at its height and the 'credibility gap' between public anxieties and government reassurances had never been wider. In Europe, students were already revolting and challenging the traditional relationships between teachers and the taught. In Britain, as in the rest of Europe, new attitudes to abortion were being given a legal framework. Christiaan Barnard performed the first heart transplant in South Africa. This was the moment when it was reported that British children in Middlesbrough, in England's industrial north-east, had begun to die from infections of bacteria resistant to antibiotics.[51] Medically, the Middlesbrough outbreak may have been unexceptional; politically, it was an epidemic of enormous importance. The case was made in the press that this resistance had possibly been bred in farms. The government was forced to act.

During November 1967, young children began to be admitted to West Lane hospital in Middlesbrough suffering from gastroenteritis caused by *E. coli* bacteria, and others contracted the infection there. The numbers, amounting to a few dozen, were not huge, and the children were given the standard treatment of neomycin. Rather than recovering, however, they declined rapidly. In less than two days, their condition deteriorated. The bacterium was resistant not just to neomycin, but also to ampicillin (the broad-spectrum penicillin), streptomycin, tetracycline, chloramphenicol, kanamycin, and sulphonamides. This local situation was worsened when children started being transferred from West Lane to other local hospitals. Most of the casualties, ten of the children, were already so handicapped that they might have been expected to die prematurely. One normal healthy baby whom the consultant paediatrician would have expected to survive did, however, also succumb. Although by medical standards, and indeed so far as the subsequent official report was concerned, the event was merely moderate, neither public nor politicians were aware that in the 1960s, in the era of heart transplants, children were still dying in hospital of infections contracted after they had been admitted. The deaths of these infants shook the country. They could have been anyone's children. From such small beginnings do avalanches start.

The hospitals communicated the problem professionally, but in a routine manner.[52] Previously, one might have anticipated a meeting to discuss the press statement to be attended just by reporters from the two local newspapers. Instead a large number of journalists fired a barrage of questions and the television cameras were there too. The tone of reporting is captured by the summary provided a few months later in the local newspaper, 'the diary of a tragedy'—'the day-by-day account of death and the battles for life fought on Teesside during the grim period that brought a new word, an awful addition to the vocabulary of anxious parents—Gastro'.[53]

In the new world of 1967, the press was now routinely inconsiderate of authorities. On 21 December the BBC current affairs programme *Twenty-Four Hours* investigated the outbreak and suggested a link with the feeding of animals.[54] That was followed up by an inundation of telephone calls from media who, the official report would complain, were less than helpful. One bereaved family engaged a lawyer, who questioned whether the children should have been admitted to a hospital known to be infected and demanded a public inquiry.[55] This was not how community outbreaks of moderate proportions had been dealt with in the past.

The hospital board commissioned a report which found that, while the outcome had not been unusual, a litany of errors had been committed.[56] Perhaps worst of all, these errors were not exceptional and grievous, but the typical failures of a system in which people were overloaded with work and unaware of the potential dangers. Nursing practices had been inadequate to prevent infection. Doctors had been slow to communicate between hospitals. A single infected child had been admitted to a ward from which the patients were later distributed to a number of other wards and then to other hospitals, taking the infection with them. When the Health Ministry refused to release the report in its entirety on the grounds that it included the personal names of medical staff, the irritation of a worried population was exacerbated. There was a debate in the House of

Commons in which the popular press and editorials in the *New Scientist* magazine were extensively quoted. Members of Parliament expressed outrage.[57]

Public anxiety was stoked by the concerns of 'Andy' Anderson, who confirmed that the infections had been caused by two virulent strains of the *E. coli* bacterium commonly found in the gut. Critically, Anderson warned that this strain of bacterium had also been found in animals. He could not say whether it had been caught from animals, but he did warn that the problems would not stop with tummy bugs. Here was a demonstration of the dangers of transferable resistance. What would be next? Suppose, Anderson worried, the agent of typhoid fever, *Salmonella typhi*, had become resistant to chloramphenicol.[58] What then for the confidence of a modern country that such diseases were no longer to be feared? Within a few years this fear was realized in a nationwide epidemic in Mexico which affected 10,000 people, and also found victims in the USA.[59] Of the bacteria tested during this time, almost all were resistant to several key antibiotics, including chloramphenicol, tetracycline, and streptomycin, though they were still susceptible to ampicillin. The British press and parliament did not wait for the Mexican experience. Teesside had been bad enough. The popular tabloid newspaper the *Daily Mirror* demanded action on behalf of its frightened readers.[60]

There was now an urgent political need to protect confidence in antibiotics. Government ministers were themselves becoming concerned about bacterial resistance. A civil servant reported that the junior Minister of Education, Shirley Williams, had been alarmed: '(possibly in the light of recent press reports that transferable resistance may have been a factor in the Teesside deaths of babies) about a press article which appeared recently recommending what looked like large-scale and indiscriminate use of antibiotics in the treatment of 'flu.'[61] With the press demanding some action to protect the benefits of antibiotics, the Ministry of Health therefore revived the recommendations of the Netherthorpe Committee, now two years old, and insisted on a formal inquiry into the use of antibiotics for animal feeding.

This decision to call an inquiry raised new questions about whether to include human uses of antibiotics in its remit, or whether to focus just on agricultural uses, as the earlier Netherthorpe Committee had done. The Agriculture Ministry argued that, if antibiotic resistance was the real concern, then human as well as animal uses should be explored. This suggestion worried the Health Ministry, conscious that doctors treasured their autonomy from political interference and that the introduction of new drugs was already about to be controlled by a new Medicines Act.

To support their case, Medical Research Council officials pointed to the exact wording of the Netherthorpe recommendation, which referred only to agricultural uses.[62] That nicety had been the result of a last-minute intervention by a committee member, the same Lawrence Garrod who had once denounced his colleagues for misusing antibiotics. Originally the committee had suggested an inquiry into 'the use and control of antibiotics and kindred substances in animal husbandry and in animal and human medicine'. Only at the last moment had Garrod suggested a critical change to 'the impact of antibiotics on animal husbandry and veterinary medicine and its implications in the field of human health'.[63] There is no record of why Garrod did this. Whatever the trigger for Garrod's change of heart, the consequence was that, as an Agriculture Ministry official put it, 'Originally it was intended that the enquiry would cover the use of antibiotics in humans and animals but this was later dropped by the main committee, and I shall be surprised indeed if the medical side accept it.'[64] The writer was completely correct: the Health Ministry would not accept an investigation of the use of antibiotics on human patients. The opportunity to review thoroughly the full range of uses of antibiotics was therefore lost. Instead the spotlight was shone just upon the agricultural context.

Moving from defence to attack, the medical side had strong views on the make-up of the committee. The choice of chairman proved unproblematic, and Michael Swann, Rector of Edinburgh University and Chairman of the BBC, was chosen. However, bearing in mind the prominence of 'Andy' at the Public Health Laboratory, it seemed clear he should also be a member. If he were not, the Health Ministry officials warned, he might be so irritated that he might not even testify, threatening the authority of the findings.[65] For its part, the Agriculture Ministry was outraged because Anderson's strong views on the culpability of farmers were already well known, and the Ministry would have to convince its agricultural constituency of whatever the committee recommended.

In the end, a compromise was found: the committee would look only at agricultural uses, but Andy would not be a member. The exclusion of the person raised more interest than the formal limitation of the brief. There were complaints from a wide spectrum about Anderson's non-membership of the committee. Naomi Datta, the geneticist whose findings on the transferability of resistance had prompted Andy's work, objected.[66] Nonetheless, the government stuck to its decision, and the so-called Swann Committee began sitting in March 1968.

The final report linked concerns, now twenty years old, about antibiotic resistance in general to the much more recent findings about transferable resistance and the use of growth promoters in agriculture.[67] The Swann report distinguished between high-dose therapeutic uses of antibiotics and growth promoters, which were administered in doses too low to kill bacteria. The former were not considered a threat to the efficacy of antibiotics; the latter were. The prophylactic or preventive use was apparently overlooked, and there was no pressure to transform husbandry and marketing practices in general, as Anderson had urged. Nonetheless, the report recommended that low dose application uses of the antibiotics most important to human health, the penicillins and tetracyclines, should be forbidden. Going beyond its narrow brief, it also recommended that a new and powerful committee should advise on the use of all antibiotics in both animal and human health applications.

Although the committee's report was at first apparently pigeonholed, once more campaigners, led by Bernard Dixon of the *New Scientist*, went into action to urge its implementation. At least one pharmaceutical company entered into a bitter, personal, and very public row with Dixon.[68] Nonetheless, the Swann Committee's recommendations were implemented in part by the new Conservative government, which came into power shortly after the committee reported. The use of penicillins and tetracyclines as growth promoters was banned in Britain. That did not mean the use of these drugs in veterinary contexts was prohibited—they were still allowed in large doses to cure animals of infection. The recommended committee was established, but only as an advisory body to advisory bodies. It reported to the Veterinary Products Committee and to the newly established Committee on the Safety of Medicines, which was focused upon the effects on individuals of medicines, and in practice neither of these clients turned to it often. The committee had no power to police veterinarians who might distribute antibiotics nominally for therapeutic purposes, but knowing full well that a drum of penicillin could as well be used to enrich some feed as to cure mastitis. Nor was there any power to insist that industry pass over any information it might have about the effect of drugs. This group, the Joint Committee on Antimicrobial Substances (JCAMS), was eventually abolished in 1980 during a cull of advisory groups conducted early in Prime Minister Margaret Thatcher's first administration.[69]

JCAMS was born sickly and died young, but the ban on the use of key antibiotics as growth promoters following the Swann Committee report was cited around the world. Its influence spread just like an infection in its own right. The report was particularly influential in Europe. During the 1970s, the Common Market, the forerunner of the European Union, devoted a majority of its funds to agricultural support, and trade in agricultural goods spread risk across borders. So the British rules were quickly adopted by several countries, including the Netherlands, Denmark, and Germany. Across the Iron Curtain, a first international meeting on infectious antibiotic resistance was held in Czechoslovakia in September 1971. The 'preface' to the *Proceedings* took but a few lines to reach a testimonial to the Swann report.[70] Czechoslovakia and Sweden soon also prohibited the use of penicillins and tetracyclines as growth promoters.

The Swann experience had been a remarkable demonstration of how science worked in the modern age. 'Andy' Anderson, an individual scientist and civil servant, had managed to mobilize a new generation of journalists sensitized to the politics of science. They had been able to communicate the sense that big issues, the penicillin brand itself, were at stake behind the discussion of molecules. An old report and an outbreak of an infection had been converted into a crisis to which the British government had had to respond by means of an authoritative committee. The findings created an international precedent and a new boundary in the history of penicillin: its value as a human medicine was not to be endangered by applications to animal nutrition.

Ironically, the epidemic of infections caused by multi-resistant salmonella that had galvanized Anderson at Britain's Public Health Laboratory Service and had driven him on his campaign had actually ended some time before the Swann report was published. Anderson himself attributed the epidemic largely to a single farmer he blamed for sending out calves with bags of antibiotic hanging around their necks and it had stopped after the farmer had died.[71] However, relief was temporary. In 1980 John Threlfall, Anderson's successor at the Public Health Laboratory, reported on a new epidemic. He showed that two types of antibiotic-resistant salmonella identified in cattle since 1977 could now be blamed for 290 cases of human infection.[72] He could also link the emergence of yet another strain to a new antibiotic given to calves. However, other strains of salmonella that had also caused epidemic outbreaks, such as *Salmonella dublin*, were apparently not able to acquire resistance to antibiotics.

The immediate result of the new regulations was to halve the amount of antibiotics administered to British animals. However, within a few years, use started to climb and by 1977 it had reached pre-Swann levels and kept rising.[73] The new regulations could therefore be said to have failed. The continued outbreaks of infections caused by resistant strains, despite the Swann regulations, highlighted the complexity of talking about bacteria and resistance exclusively in terms of animals. In a well-known letter published in the *British Medical Journal* in 1980, the distinguished microbiologist Sir Mark Richmond addressed the question, 'Why has Swann Failed?'[74] He concluded that too often farmers had increased their use of therapeutic antibiotics and, more importantly, that human uses had not been managed. Controlling antibiotic use for growth promotion alone would not, he concluded, reduce the spread of resistance. The next year, a conference was convened to review a decade of the regulations. Instead of celebrating success and ten years of pioneering legislation, the meeting was downbeat, as speakers reviewed the causes of failure and the lack of medical, government, and agricultural support for the limitation of resistance.[75]

But what about the United States, the world's foremost agricultural exporter as well as the country that spent most on medicine? With powerful and opposing lobbies, the debate there would be more prolonged and even more bitter than in Britain. For a decade, the Food and Drug Administration, advocates of control, contested for influence with the President and Congress against industrial interests and such lobbies as the Council for Agricultural Science and Technology (CAST), which were vehemently opposed to limiting the use of drugs in agriculture. Founded at the State University of agriculturally based Iowa in 1972, CAST was intended to be the 'voice of agricultural science on the national scene' and to combat an 'increasingly difficult' professional environment.[76]

The Food and Drug Administration was pondering restrictions on agricultural antibiotic use from the mid-1960s. The Swann Committee's report encouraged the agency to pay the matter greater attention, and it established a task force to look into the same issues.[77] This recommended, in 1972, that companies demonstrate that the use of their drugs would not damage human therapy. Although it was impossible to prove current danger, and the requirement was soon withdrawn, by 1977, the FDA felt confident that it should ban the use of penicillin and restrict the use of tetracycline for the purposes of growth promotion. The reasons were twofold: the evidence that bacterial resistance had been enhanced and the weakness of record maintenance. The move was resisted by industry, which made Congress aware of its concerns. The House Agriculture Committee made the FDA wait to implement any new rules on agricultural uses of antibiotics until an elaborate scientific audit of the evidence on transferable resistance had been conducted by the National Academy of Sciences.

Between 1977 and 1985 many academic scientists supported the FDA in an unsuccessful campaign to persuade Congress and the executive branch to control the use of antibiotics as growth promoters. The debates were often personal and bitter between, on the one side, those concerned that resistant strains were being spread unnecessarily by bad agricultural practice, and, on the other, those for whom the medical focus on animal sources of resistance was unproven. It was characterized in 1979 as an arena in which 'opposing advocates usually seek to make their case or ridicule their opponents in the most exaggerated terms'.[78] The issues were polarized at a time when American society was already divided. In 1979 President Carter warned that the United States was experiencing a crisis of confidence that struck 'at the very heart and soul and spirit' of the nation's will. Shortly after, he lost the election to Ronald Reagan, who promised a massive relaxation of regulation.

The US debate over the use of antibiotics in agriculture was precipitated not by journalists, but by the FDA's move to regulate growth-promoting doses of antibiotics. In any case, during the late 1970s science journalists in the USA were more concerned with the debates then raging over biotechnology. So, in general, the debate was not conducted in the public media but within the broad scientific community.

The highest profile of the scientist-protagonists questioning agricultural uses of antibiotics during the late 1970s debates was Richard Novick, chief of the plasmid biology department at the independent Public Health Research Institute in New York City. Despite this long title he was no bloodless bureaucrat, but rather a distinguished microbiologist and an active campaigner.[79] During the protests against the US policy of defoliation in the Vietnam War, he had fought against the military use of biological and chemical agents. Novick's concerns extended to the dangers of the bacterial menace at home. In 1975, he came to public attention as an organizer of the meeting at Asilomar, California, which recommended a delay on scientific experiments on recombinant DNA until suitable regulations were in place. The anxiety of the time was that genetically mutated organisms against which no antibiotics were effective might escape unregulated laboratories and play havoc within unprepared ecosystems.

Novick had been involved in the study of antibiotic resistance since he had been a post-doctoral student in London in the early 1960s. Then he had been looking at the mechanisms by which staphylococcus became resistant to penicillin.[80] While in London he had written an angry letter to the medical magazine *The Lancet* criticizing experiments in spraying methicillin in hospitals to prevent infection.[81]

In the 1970s, Novick was again ready to criticize doctors of human patients who abused antibiotic prescribing. Thus he penned a prominent *New York Times* article explaining the way their behaviour could lead to bacterial resistance.[82] Early in 1977, he was caught up in the debate over the proposed FDA constraint on agricultural uses when he was recruited to a CAST subcommittee on antibiotics in feed chaired by Virgil Hays of the University of Kentucky. Not having hitherto heard of the organization, he entered into the issues with energy and enthusiasm.[83] Nonetheless, at the end of the year Novick and other distinguished academic biologists who had been recruited to the panel resigned, complaining that unfavourable evidence had been neglected. This very public move was covered by a two-page article in *Science*, the key magazine of the US scientific community, and was followed by recriminations when CAST loyalists and the resignees blamed each other, as if in a marital break-up.[84]

Unpleasant as it was, the lively debate between Novick and Thomas Jukes, founder of the antibiotic growth additive field, had a high profile and offered bystanders a sense of the stakes. Jukes wrote a letter to *Science* accusing Novick and his colleagues of misrepresentation.[85] Responding in June 1978, Novick suggested he had been mistreated.[86] Another year later, he published an article in the popular magazine *The Sciences* entitled 'Antibiotics: Wonder Drugs or Chicken Feed?'[87] The argument was summarized in the strapline, declaring that the unrestricted inclusion of antibiotics in feed promoted the spread of illness in humans. Again Jukes responded vigorously, dismissing Novick's articles as overly rhetorical and partly misinformed and, in any case, the work of a relative newcomer to the field.[88] Whereas Novick had, he claimed, only been involved in the subject since 1977, Jukes cited the debates of the 1950s over animal uses of antibiotics in which he had been central.

As controversy was playing out in the scientific community, personal resentments adding to the heat of debate, a study of 'Drugs in Livestock Feed' was conducted by Congress's own 'think-tank', the Office of Technology Assessment (OTA). The final report presented options rather than a decisive recommendation, but it implicitly supported the FDA in its bid to restrict the use of penicillin and tetracycline in animal feed.[89]

The account in *Nature* of the report's public launch indeed cited the deputy head of OTA expressing her belief that subtherapeutic uses needed to be controlled.[90] So the OTA effectively encouraged Congress to follow the European route. Once more, it seemed, agriculture was in the dock.

However supportive the OTA was, the strong opinions of FDA were not backed in the critical and long-awaited National Academy of Sciences report, which appeared in 1980.[91] The academicians refused to back the growing condemnation of agricultural uses, and said there was just not enough evidence for a judgement to be made. Consequently the FDA was unable to act. The committee was doubtful of the claim that only veterinarians and farmers were misusing antibiotics. Guilt had to be shared by those who treated people as well as animals, and it was difficult to decide whether therapeutic or subtherapeutic uses were the more responsible for the growth of resistance.

The National Academy of Sciences had transformed the debate over how to manage antibiotic resistance. No longer could the issue be dominated by castigation of agricultural abuse of valuable human drugs and regulation proposed solely of agriculture. The 1980 report was, however, far from marking the end of moves to restrict the subtherapeutic uses of penicillin and tetracycline. Thus when a 1984 study seemed to prove that an outbreak of *Salmonella newport* in cattle was linked to infection in the neighbouring population, an environmental lobbying group, the National Resources Development Council, claimed that there was an 'imminent danger'.[92] This was a technical term and, if accepted, the government would have been forced to ban the use of subtherapeutic doses in animals. However, the proof was again not considered compelling and the bid was rejected the following year.

In any case, by 1985 the debate was becoming slightly less polarized. Despite the National Academy's refusal to recommend a ban, the beef industry, alarmed by adverse publicity about the use of antibiotics, as well as anxieties over the link between cholesterol and heart disease, announced a voluntary withdrawal from the use of penicillin and tetracycline feeds.[93] On the other hand, the 1960s British model of controlling just one factor, the low-dose use of antibiotics in animals, had been proved to fail as a means of limiting agricultural uses of popular antibiotics and managing the resistance of the bacterial population. Instead, an increasing number of public-health officials and biomedical scientists were looking at the variety of contexts in which antibiotics were employed and in which antibiotic-resistant organisms were bred.

The scientific interest shown in plasmids also moved on the discussion about the transfer of resistance. These circular pieces of DNA which lie outside the main genetic material in the chromosomes had been explored as part of the explanation of antibiotic resistance, but in the 1970s they acquired a quite different significance. Because they could be used to transfer genes from one organism to another, their study lay at the heart of the DNA revolution. From an esoteric byway of microbiology they became a central avenue to money-making biotechnology. Thousands of scientists worldwide were studying this area, hailed as a new industrial revolution. By increasing our understanding of bacteria, this work could also help map the development of antibiotic resistance. The molecular biologists involved in such work were not committed to either animal or human medicine. They did, however, in one very important respect, have a special interest in antibiotic resistance. Penicillin resistance was a usefully visible quality to transfer intentionally into a bacterium by means of a plasmid. By adding penicillin, the biologist could then easily see if a bacterium had been affected by a genetic experiment. If it had, it was insensitive and would survive—and if it had not, it would succumb to the penicillin. Intentionally provoked resistance was therefore used as an indicator of success in the planned transfer of genes into bacteria.

The shifting focus of scientific interest in richer nations converged with the concerns of physicians in the Third World. Whereas in developed countries the salmonella bacterium is always present in the animal population, and only spasmodically reaches out into the human community, in many poorer regions the human population has acted as a reservoir of such infections. The implications for antibiotic resistance became clear in Europe during the 1970s, through an outbreak of a resistant bacterium known as *Salmonella wien*.[94] In late 1969, a new epidemic of infections caused by this organism began in North Africa. A group of children in a ward in Algeria suffered severe diarrhoea caused by an aggressive strain resistant to four different antibiotics. From Algeria, the bacterium next moved to France. Within seven years this antibiotic-resistant organism was the dominant cause of gastrointestinal infection in Europe and had caused outbreaks of illness in Yugoslavia, India, Iraq, Italy, Austria, Great Britain, and Ireland. This epidemic was the result of the mismanagement of antibiotics in human medicine, not animal husbandry.[95]

The experience of developing countries informed a meeting organized in the Dominican Republic in January 1981 on a topic of interest to students of both antibiotic resistance and the new science of recombinant DNA.

Its subject was 'Molecular Biology, Pathogenicity, and Ecology of Bacterial Plasmids'.[96] It was co-organized by the physician and microbiologist Stuart Levy, whose physician sister had married a citizen of the Dominican Republic. Although Levy had made his name through the study of transferred resistance between animals and humans, he had become both fascinated and worried by developments in poorer countries.[97]

Participants at the 1981 conference were drawn from both the new community of biotechnologists whose expertise increasingly focused on modifying and deploying plasmids to make useful products from bacteria and those whose main concern was antibiotic resistance. The two communities were meant to sustain each other. The enormous interest in plasmids of the molecular biologists had led to new techniques and devices, making research much easier for those whose main interest was resistance and not plasmids. This unlikely sounding meeting might have had all the hallmarks of a failure: two different communities could easily talk past one another. Yet instead it saw the birth of a new consensus.

During the proceedings, Stuart Levy met informally with like-minded scientists worried about the growth of antibiotic resistance caused by excessive use in either humans or animals. Collectively they issued a 'Statement regarding worldwide antibiotic misuse'.[98] This emphasized the variety of misuses of the drugs, the danger of advertising them as 'wonder drugs', and the error of using them in place of good hygiene. Use of clinically useful antibiotics as growth promoters was included among the misuses but did not dominate the listing. The first steps urged on governments were globally uniform standards of prescription and distribution, and agreements on means of advertising and dispensing.

Subsequently Levy sought to create an international advisory group that would issue guidance around the world. In August 1981 he struck with simultaneous press conferences in Santo Domingo, Rio de Janeiro, Mexico City, and Boston. They each warned of three interrelated threats: indiscriminate prescription by doctors, the use of antibiotics in animal feed, and the uncontrolled use of antibiotics in the Third World. Again, animal use had been integrated into a mesh of concerns. Rather than blaming farmers, the statement criticized abuse at all levels, by consumers, prescribers, dispensers, manufacturers, and government regulators. The concerned scientists formed a worldwide network under Stuart Levy's leadership, APUA, the Alliance for the Prudent Use of Antibiotics.

Tremendous publicity was given to the announcements. The *New York Times*, *Washington Post*, *Newsweek*, *Time*, and *Nature* each gave generous coverage to the Boston event.[99] They were all impressed by the celebrity signatures that had been gathered. Walter Gilbert, then known as one of the founders of the leading biotechnology company Biogen, and Ananda Chakrabarty, who had obtained the first patent to be granted for a living organism, had both attended the recent meeting and were signatories to the statement. Two days after its initial news coverage, the *Washington Post* ran an editorial as well. It commented not just on the concern of doctors about 'a worldwide public health problem', but also that 'their statement will come as a surprise to many Americans—including most doctors'.[100] The awareness of citizens who had grown up with antibiotics that they might lose them was just beginning to take hold.

A few months after the 1981 Boston press conference, the public-health worker Dr Marc Lappé published a popular but serious book entitled *Germs that Won't Die*.[101] This book, which had taken two years to write, pioneered the genre of campaigning polemics that flourishes to this day. The argument, through framed separately from the APUA appeal, was perfectly in tune with it. As a public-health worker with a scientific rather than a medical doctorate, Lappé was outraged by the use of antibiotics as growth factors, but also by the attitude of physicians who prescribed drugs for their patients without thought of the consequences for the community.

Concerns about animal use did not go away. In the 1990s, a new multiply resistant strain of *Salmonella typhimurium* DT104 would arise and sweep the world. Again Britain was in the vanguard of the epidemic. Between 1992 and 1995 the number of British victims of this bacterium, which had been found in chicken, burgers, and sausages, tripled to 3,500.[102] Using DNA fingerprinting techniques John Threlfall, a successor to the now-retired Anderson at London's Public Health Laboratory, would be able to show for the first time how the gene for antibiotic resistance within this strain had evolved to protect the bacterium from more and more assaults. Increasingly, the problem would be seen from the point of view of resistant genes and plasmids, rather than doctors or veterinarians. With this high-technology laboratory science came a recognition that bacteria containing such resistance genes could have reservoirs in either animals or human beings.[103]

The fundamental problem was to prevent cross-infection between susceptible and non-susceptible strains. As Alan Linton, the Bristol University microbiologist, pointed out in 1981:

I believe that Swann succeeded by being a failure. The report focused attention on the growing problem of antibiotic resistance and, by its failure, has forced the opinion that the control of infection by multiply-resistant pathogens must be pursued along conventional epidemiological lines and not solely by imposing more stringent restrictions on antibiotic use.[104]

In the 1990s, as the British and then the Europeans and organizations across the world revisited the control of antibiotics, the implications of this observation would become clear.

9

In Face of Catastrophe

The threat of a 'post-antibiotic' age became first a public and then a political issue across the Western world at the very end of the twentieth century. Fifty years after the introduction of penicillin, the danger of regressing to a world without its benefits entered political debate. Already the limitations of medicine's ability to control infectious disease were made manifest by the epidemics of AIDS and then the cattle disease BSE. Despite their many differences from antibiotic-resistant bacterial conditions, these disasters created an environment in which the best use of antibiotics was discussed with a new intensity.

Across the governments of the developed world, and the community of international agencies, forests of reports confirmed there was a risk and led to programmes to measure both the use of antibiotics and the spread of bacteria able to withstand them. The editor of one medical journal wrote of the 'politicization of antibiotic resistance'.[1] Whereas someone in his position might once have been expected to condemn such a development, he welcomed it. This process of politicization would involve changing public opinion, professional practice, the political agenda, and even the reappraisal of economics.

In consequence, the world's governments, medical associations, and private organizations attempted to work with their publics to reform attitudes to antibiotics in general. In the past, the fear of infectious disease had been successfully treated with the balm of news of antibiotic development, but in an age of slower drug innovation and the global spread of resistant bacteria this was no longer possible. Instead, the use of drugs such as penicillin was fundamentally reappraised and the accolade 'miracle drug' was confronted directly in public information. Rather than itself the nemesis of penicillin, this engagement with public perceptions of infection represented an attempt by medical authorities to preserve its distinctive benefits. The entire process could be seen as a collective attempt at 'rebranding'.

The chapter explores media frenzies over terrifying new conditions, and the professional and increasing political anxiety about the problem of how to change patterns of antibiotic use. Ironically, these were set against the background of a revolution in biotechnology which, for a time, seemed to offer hopes for a new generation of rationally designed drugs that would destroy bacteria.[2] As key tools in the transformation of genetics, the use and study of bacteria were at the centre of the practice of biotechnology. *E. coli* bacteria, for instance, were often used as the template within which genes were swapped and DNA modified and reproduced. Understanding of bacteria was also radically enhanced through the techniques developed during the 1990s for sequencing the human genome.[3] Thus, biochemists used the automated sequencing of nucleic acids to decode the relatively small number of bacterial genes. Pharmacologists hoped that they could translate this genetic understanding into new means of destroying bacteria. By 1997, fifty projects to sequence various bacterial genomes were under way.[4]

The SmithKline Beecham (SB) company, where Rolinson and his team had pioneered the semisynthetic penicillins, was a leader in the push to sequence bacterial DNA. In principle, the challenge was straightforward: MRSA, for instance, had only 2,000 genes, of which SB believed just 200 might be essential to growth.[5] An antibiotic would be effective if it interfered with the protein produced by a single one of these, and if just 5 per cent of the 200 critical genes were targeted by antibiotics, that would mean another ten powerful antibiotic classes. The dream was compelling and, evoking wartime achievements, SB gave its own programme to create new drugs an appropriate name, 'Manhattan Micro'. The metaphor was attractive, but, across the industry, success was limited.

The significance of the huge corpus of genetic data about bacteria was unclear, and, accordingly, the consequences of interrupting a part of the bacterial metabolism proved to be unpredictable. Enormous numbers of chemicals could now be screened using robots and modern combinatorial chemistry.[6] However, converting all these data into commercial drugs was expensive and the returns uncertain. The dream itself began to fade. By 2002, companies were downgrading their commitment to the development of antibacterials as they looked to other more remunerative products.[7] Whereas the biotechnology revolution of the 1940s had generated not just penicillin but also a host of other antibiotics, the prospects of the 'new biotechnology' of the 1990s quickly producing an equivalent revoluton in the treatment of infection soon dimmed.

The experience of biotechnology did, however, make a substantial cultural contribution to science's combat with resistant bacteria. In dealing since the 1970s with the new techniques of genetic engineering, and potential fears such as over the 'escape' of dangerous mutated organisms from laboratories, leaders of the scientific community had learned sophisticated strategies for communicating with the public.[8] With statutory regulation of science at stake, the experience of genetic engineering had shown that such public engagement was not at the end of the scientific process, but at its heart. Mark Cantley, a key player in biotechnology strategy in the European Commission in the 1980s, has talked of the need to be trilingual in science, economics, and cultural understanding.[9]

The opportunities and experience of biotechnology helped to shape public attitudes. From the late 1980s, these perceptions were also shaped by the global experience of AIDS. Even though it was not directly affected by antibiotics, culturally AIDS changed the entire context of infectious diseases and expectations of their cure. Until the emergence of AIDS, the conquest of infectious disease had been symbolized by the historical gap between 'nowadays' and the distant time of the plague, but now plague was 'amongst us'. The scale of this threat and the widespread public awareness of its possible implications underpinned a transformation in the interpretation of historical experience, so that the relief which penicillin had apparently brought seemed merely to have been temporary.[10]

With hindsight, the arrival of AIDS, first in a few Western cities such as San Francisco and Paris around 1980, happened quickly and inflicted a sudden shock. At the time, however, its implications were so radical that they were hard to appreciate. Richard Krause, then Director of the US National Institute of Allergy and Infectious Diseases, would later regret his early references to AIDS as the 4H disease: 'Haitians, heroine addicts, haemophiliacs and homosexuals'.[11] By 1986, the USA and western Europe were in the grip of a new terror. British posters showing eerie tombstones echoed memories of history lessons about deadly epidemics of the distant past (Ill. 25). This new sexually transmitted infection linked risks to the health of individuals and danger to the entire community. It therefore highlighted some of the same cultural issues raised by antibiotic resistance. Susan Sontag, the American commentator, put the impact eloquently in her 1988 book *Aids and its Metaphors*:

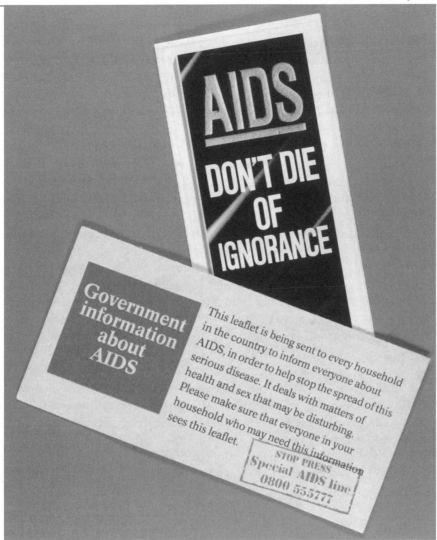

25. Emergent diseases reawaking old fears: AIDS poster 1986, Britain.
Central Office of Information.

Medicine changed mores. Illness is changing them back. Contraception and the assurance by medicine of the easy curability of sexually transmitted diseases (as of almost all infectious diseases) made it possible to regard sex as an adventure without consequences. Now AIDS obliges people to think of sex as having, possibly, the direst consequences: suicide. Or murder.[12]

Polls of popular views on sexual mores in Britain showed that attitudes against homosexuality and extra-marital sex noticeably hardened during the 1980s.[13] A majority of people asked felt that victims had only themselves to blame. Although the first treatment, AZT, was introduced in 1987, it was far from a cure. Patients' groups, influentially supported by friends of Hollywood victims, drove forward research agendas and testing protocols over the protestations of professional interests. AIDS campaigners, generally lay and often sufferers themselves, ensured that research on this still relatively exotic disease had a very high profile.

As Susan Sontag eloquently described, the incurability of AIDS had changed attitudes to the power of medicine. The so-called protease inhibitors, a second-generation treatment, were introduced in 1995. They were much more effective than AZT and would allow indefinite survival, though the patient's life was restricted. Yet they were expensive and scarcely available in developing countries, where AIDS would make a much greater impact. By 1997, when it was announced that deaths from the disease in the United States had now started to decline, 29.4 million people had been infected with the HIV virus, the precursor of AIDS, and in total 6.4 million people had already died from the illness.[14] This ongoing catastrophe would provide a vivid and immediate template for campaigners warning of the implications of a post-antibiotic age.

The experience of AIDS put other as yet little-known but potentially deadly infections in a new light. The public came to learn of other frightening syndromes, including Ebola haemorrhagic fever, dengue fever, and Lyme disease. Ebola was a virus-caused disease fortunately as hard to catch as it was gruesome to die from, ending in uncontrollable bleeding.[15] Very rare, it was generally restricted to isolated areas within Africa, but in 1989 a colony of experimental monkeys in New Jersey was wiped out and several of their keepers infected (although none fatally). Another, more common, condition was a complication of the virus-caused dengue fever already endemic in the Far East but also found in the south-eastern United States. Lyme disease was a bacterial infection borne by ticks which, though it may have been long established in the forests of New England, was only identified as a separate entity in the mid-1970s. Although quite different in their immediate cause, each of these syndromes was the result of infections hitherto restricted to forests but which now, through the expansion of human activity, had entered the human world.

At the head of the scientists urging that such challenges be taken together was Joshua Lederberg, Nobel laureate and head of the Rockefeller

University in New York from 1978 to 1990.[16] Lederberg was not alone in his scientific perceptions, but he was extraordinary in the series of activities and initiatives he put in motion to convert the single shock of AIDS into a perception of a threatening long-term process of emerging infectious diseases. He led the interpretation of spreading antibiotic-resistant bacteria as an aspect of the threat of 'emerging infections'.

With a charismatic personality, a wide reputation, and a central situation in New York city, Lederberg would become the first port of call for a veritable column of journalists, broadcasters, and writers. The writer and physician Frank Ryan, who met him at the time, described him as 'white-haired, heavy-set, speaks with a deep Brooklyn-tinged accent, and a Rabelaisian wit peppers the parry-and-thrust of his conversation'.[17] His institutional authority enabled him to build and support an impressive team at the university. As the Rockefeller Institute, the university had been the pre-war centre of the vision of a scientific medicine solving the world's ills. There, Lederberg's mentor René Dubos had discovered gramicidin, the first modern antibiotic, and later wrote his first book warning of the inadequacies of a medical approach to infection, his study of TB entitled *The White Plague*.[18]

In the light of AIDS, Lederberg was moved to revive his long-standing concern with the ecology of disease organisms. During the autumn of 1987, he presented a paper on pandemics at a New York symposium on plagues.[19] Soon his thoughts were clarified by a meeting with Steven Morse, an assistant professor at Rockefeller University, during a campus reception. In Morse he found a kindred spirit.[20] Weeks later he was giving a paper at a conference on science and humankind in Paris at a symposium of Nobel laureates organized by President Mitterrand and American writer Elie Wiesel. Lederberg's paper, later published in the *Journal of the American Medical Association*, began 'The ravaging epidemic of acquired immunodeficiency syndrome has shocked the world. It is still not comprehended widely that it is a natural, almost predictable, phenomenon.'[21] Lederberg therefore focused on the evolution of microbes, whose implications would relate to a wide variety of infectious agents and reflect on the control even of antibiotic-resistant bacteria.

With Lederberg's support, in 1988 Morse organized a conference at the Rockefeller University on 'Emerging Viruses', covering such conditions as AIDS and Ebola.[22] Again, the heart of the discussion was the flexibility of natural organisms to mutate and evolve in response to changing environments. In his keynote address, Lederberg included the evolution of bacteria and emergent antibiotic resistance within the category he now termed 'emergent diseases'.[23] Although the meeting itself was still concerned just with viruses, bacteria joined them in the next stage of the discussion organized by Lederberg. A major conference, held at the Institute of Medicine of the US Academy of Sciences in 1992, under the title 'Emerging Infections: Microbial Threats to Health in the United States', was 'official' and had long-term consequences.[24] It put infectious disease and antibiotic resistance back on the professional and legislative map. The management of expectations for such antibiotics as penicillin was now becoming a public issue.

The Institute of Medicine's 1992 conference took as its focus the emerging and incurable diseases caused by viruses, though it included a treatment of resistant bacteria. The emphasis was therefore on cause and prevention rather than cure. The long-term factors identified were largely human. These included the degradation of public health during the time when it had seemed medicines could cure what society could no longer prevent, the increasing international movement of people and goods, economic development, and uses of land that increasingly brought people into hitherto-forested territories, technologies such as air conditioning, which increased the chances of infection, the rapid growth in human population, and, only sixthly, the ability of microbes to evolve.[25] Once again, after sixty years, the focus of measures to control infection was on human behaviour rather than on the improved technology of bacterial destruction.

Effects rippled out from the Institute of Medicine's report, as if a stone had been hurled into the public-health pool. At one level the report had major effects upon US medical policies. The Centers for Disease Control (CDC) began to formulate a plan to revitalize infectious disease management. In January 1995, for instance, the organization established a new journal, *Emerging Infectious Diseases*. It also became a major resource for other papers, such as a warning written for Congress under the title 'Emerging and reemerging threats to public health'.[26] A year later, thirty-five medical journals around the world in an unprecedented act of solidarity simultaneously published theme issues dealing with the problems of emerging and re-emerging diseases. In 1996, CDC also established a National Antimicrobial Resistance Monitoring Service (NARMS) to monitor the spread of such germs as resistant salmonella within its new emerging infections programme.

The Institute of Medicine report also informed worried writers and journalists, who could bring home the threat of untreatable illness to the general public. The first and perhaps the most important was Laurie Garrett, a distinguished science journalist and erstwhile student of Joshua Lederberg (though she had abandoned her immunology doctoral studies for a career in journalism). During the late 1980s she had been increasingly devoting her efforts to depicting the AIDS crisis. She then broadened her concerns and published an essay on the topic of what might be coming next.[27] Her major 1994 book *The Coming Plague* gave flesh to the bones of the Institute of Medicine report and, through its detailed descriptions of crises across the world, vividly described an ominous present.[28] Ironically, in a review quoted on the book's back cover, her work was compared to that of a good war correspondent.[29] When, half a century earlier, the attempt to control disease had also been compared to war, that had been a guarantee of success, but now Garrett, closely connected with the scientific community, was warning of imminent defeat.

The authoritative tone of *The Coming Plague* was complemented by the more popular *The Hot Zone*, by journalist Richard Preston. As exciting as a thriller, it was nonetheless a factual account of the series of real events in 1989 when the Ebola virus, normally restricted to African jungles, infected a colony of primates in suburban New Jersey.[30] Repeatedly this book used the phrase 'species-threatening event' and, without necessarily endorsing the concept that Ebola had doomed humanity, Preston left the reader in no doubt of the threat. The success of *The Hot Zone* was indicated by the more than forty reviews of the book and six reviews of the audio version listed in one index.[31] Even this only served to whet the public's appetite for more frights. Frank Ryan's *Virus X*, published in 1996, began its acknowledgements with an expression of the author's debt to Joshua Lederberg and Steven Morse.[32] Emanating principally from the USA, these volumes had worldwide circulation and were translated into many languages. Within five years of the first discussions of 'emerging diseases' at the Rockefeller University, they were telling global audiences that, unless we managed microbes better, catastrophe would follow.

This message spread as the ideas in these books rapidly transferred to other media. Preston's book read like the script of a movie. Indeed a Hollywood studio bought the film rights to it. Another studio, Warner Brothers, also made a film, *Outbreak,* about an African virus that threatened the USA.[33] Unlike *The Hot Zone* project, which foundered at the time, this film, featuring such stars as Dustin Hoffman, Kevin Spacey, and Donald Sutherland, reached cinemas in 1995 and was a hit.[34] The UPN TV series *The Burning Zone* followed too on the success of *The Hot Zone*. Screening in the USA in 1996/7 and in Germany (RTL) in 1998, it combined fear of exotic diseases with suspicion of the powerful.[35]

Even organizations in fields remote from medicine felt they needed to take part in a growing public discussion. So, the authoritative *Economist* magazine pointed out to its international business readership in 1995 that, while Ebola had attracted a lot of attention, sleeping sickness could be 'just as deadly' and its spread across 'large parts of Zaire is virtually unchecked'.[36] That disease had not received equivalent attention and the magazine concluded that 'The chance that a plague from Kinshasa will bring the world to its knees may be small this time. But if the world fails to pay attention, next time could be worse.' At a more popular level, computer games, such as the enduring *Resident Evil* launched in 1996, drew on the theme of frightening viruses with bizarre powers.[37] And the word 'virus' entered the new language of computers, to describe the destructive programs spreading through the Internet.

Anxiety about the danger of new fatal diseases also spread quickly and beyond the control of scientists wishing to warn of a measure of long-term risk. For a week in May 1994, Britain was convulsed by a media-induced terror over an haemorrhagic bacterial infection, necrotizing fasciitis. This is a rare but endemic condition, caused by a streptococcus bacterium, which has claimed the occasional victim. In the era of Ebola its meaning was, however, greater than this death rate would suggest. Newspapers gave lurid descriptions of the consequences of a flesh-eating 'virus'. The *Guardian* newspaper's science correspondent, Tim Radford, wrote in *The Lancet* of the eagerness of a few 'cheerful' scientists to scare their audiences. 'You could almost hear the saliva flowing as they talked of flesh deliquescing, and of internal organs turning to liquid.'[38] The press's response was analysed by Bernard Dixon, the British journalist who in the 1960s had given prominence to the views of E. S. Anderson,

A deadly, flesh-eating superbug, consuming human tissues at a devastating rate, had emerged in Gloucestershire and become rampant throughout the entire country. Victims were suffering and dying in a particularly revolting fashion. There was panic on the continent of Europe too, as people began to cancel plans for holidays in Britain. Confidence in medical science plummeted. Doctors were impotent to thwart an organism resistant to all known antibiotics. Worse still, scientists had no idea where the flesh eater had come from—or how much more virulent it might become in future.[39]

Dixon pointed out that key features of the story run by newspapers, 'that the deadly foe was a virus, or a bacterium insensitive to all antibiotics', were completely fabricated. Perhaps more important, however, was the new-found ease with which public insecurity about the lack of protection from antibiotics could be aroused.

As Dixon had shown, alarm about killer viruses could be transferred easily to worry about bacteria insensitive to antibiotics. In March 1994 *Newsweek*, which had once announced the coming of penicillin as the arrival of the wonder drug, now ran a cover feature entitled 'The End of Antibiotics'.[40] A year later Virgin Publishing, whose list was stronger in popular culture than medicine, published journalist Geoffrey Cannon's book *Superbug: Nature's Revenge*.[41] So widespread was the scare that scientists began to worry that the public were being panicked. After an hour-long 1996 report about 'superbugs' on *Panorama*, the British news documentary series, generally devoted to politics rather than science, a doctor and nurse complained in the *British Medical Journal*:

The programme, although mostly factually correct, created a sinister, doom laden image of superbugs on the rampage. This was achieved by the use of low lighting of interview sets, scenes of ambulance drivers wearing face masks with visors, and an unbalanced content.[42]

While the programme may have worried members of the public, as they claimed, it may also have had other effects. Dixon suggested it may have influenced Members of Parliament to support international efforts and cautioned patients who might otherwise have demanded antibiotics from their doctors.[43] Indeed, contradictory and frightening reports clearly could raise public alarm.

The British were particularly sensitive to such scares, because they were experiencing the BSE crisis, whose interpretation would make it look like a sequel to AIDS. Although it had neither a bacterial cause nor a direct penicillin connection, its emergence would reignite the debate over industrialized agricultural practice. By popularizing the concept of nature's revenge, BSE would change the terms in which such biological technologies as penicillin were considered by the public and politicians alike.

BSE, whose cause, unusually, was a protein—not even a microbe—was first encountered during the early 1980s. Its spread among cattle led later in the decade to the setting-up of a scientific committee. This recommended an end to the use of animal offal in cattle food but discounted any risk to humans, though BSE did resemble the rare human condition

Creutzfeldt-Jakob disease (CJD).[44] The situation changed in May 1995 when a human patient died of a new variant of CJD. A year later, a link between this condition and the agent infecting cattle was demonstrated. Now there seemed the chance of a new epidemic, gruesome in both its wide extent and devastating form. The European Union banned exports of British beef, reinforcing the import bans imposed by countries around the world. The British slaughtered all cattle over 30 months old and, within four years, the EU introduced a system for tracking every cow in the Union.

The most enduring legacy of the BSE crisis may still be numerous deaths in victims within whom the protein causing CJD has been hiding. However, at the time of writing, that seems unlikely.[45] By 2003, the maximum predicted casualties had been reduced from millions to 7,000 human deaths. At that time, 135 people in Britain and a few others elsewhere had died.[46] Although this was a low number compared to that from other threats, a deep suspicion of the consequences of industrialized agricultural practices had both a very short incubation and a searing effect on populations in Britain and indeed across Europe. The link between animal and human diseases was now a matter of nightly news and international politics. The unforeseen catastrophe that had followed from feeding meat to livestock kept alive popular anxiety about the unpredictable consequences of feeding antibiotics as growth promoters to chicken and pigs. Moreover, CJD was another incurable infectious disease, and its apparently inevitable progression to disability and death underlined the limitations of modern medicine.

Amid all these new threats, antibiotic-resistant bacteria were given a high profile. A 1999 British survey of professional opinion prioritized the whole range of infectious diseases according to five criteria: '1. Present burden of ill-health; 2. Social and economic impact; 3. Potential threat to health (5 to 10 years); 4. Health gain opportunity; 5. Public concern and confidence.'[47] Using this systematic approach, right at the top of the list of professional concerns, even above sexually transmitted infections such as AIDS, came antimicrobial-resistant infections. Reflecting this concern, during the 1990s an increasing number of expert panels met. By one, albeit incomplete, count, their number increased from one a year early in the 1990s to four in 1995, six in 1997, and nine in 1998. By then alarm had been aroused even among the general public. Unlike the panels of the 1960s discussed in the previous chapter, whose briefs had been reserved for animal uses of antibiotics, these committees were amplifying the concerns of scientists worried about human uses.

The process of committee recommendations building on each other reached a crescendo in 1998. In March, the Science and Technology Committee of the British House of Lords published an influential report pulling together current thinking. In the same month, the World Health Assembly, a meeting of national representatives that directs the work of the World Health Organization, defined the problem as a priority and mandated action.[48] In September, the European Commission launched an initiative. Though they involved people who were scientists, these actions were not part of the internal working of the scientific community. Rather they had successfully translated the results of vigorous debates into science-based predictions of disaster, forcing political leaders to take them into account.

Amidst this cacophony of calls for change, the 1998 House of Lords report was one of the most cited and influential. It was thorough, but also pioneering as a political engagement with antibiotic resistance. By global standards, British doctors were not large prescribers of antibiotics. Britain's hospitals had, however, among the world's worst reported rates of MRSA infections, which were proving deeply frightening to potential patients. Thus in a short Lords debate held in November 1996 on measures taken to control MRSA, the respected Irish nationalist Gerry Fitt described to it the sudden death of his wife from a hospital-acquired infection of MRSA.[49]

When the Lords' Science and Technology committee, which periodically conducts in-depth studies of key problem areas, had called for suggestions for a 1997 study, the distinguished veterinarian and retired Cambridge professor Lord Soulsby had proposed that the committee study antibiotic resistance. An old friend of Michael Swann, who had chaired the 1969 committee into the use of antibiotics in animals, he was personally irritated that Swann's recommendation of a powerful body with oversight over the whole of antibiotic use had been passed over.[50] Soulsby had also watched debates over resistance in the USA, having served as professor of parasitology at the University of Pennsylvania in Philadelphia for fifteen years. He was therefore particularly well placed to respond to international scientific and parliamentary concerns.

Soulsby had plenty of evidence to call upon. In the USA, the Institute of Medicine was organizing a forum on infectious diseases which held a workshop in May 1997. Its summary, co-edited by Joshua Lederberg, would appear at the same time as the House of Lords report.[51] The World Medical Association meeting in South Africa in October 1996 had passed a statement warning of a potential crisis caused by antibiotic resistance.[52]

These initiatives were both high profile, but they were still within the scientific community.

The House of Lords, as part of Parliament, was by contrast a political body and addressed a political agenda. Lord Fitt's descriptions of his wife's death helped persuade members to back the proposal for a study of resistance and, in November 1997, the Science and Technology Committee started to take evidence under Soulsby's chairmanship. It not only consulted British interested parties, including doctors, pharmaceutical companies, and health lobbies, but it also visited the United States, where the committee's members met Stuart Levy. From him they would import the concept of 'prudent' use of antibiotics.

The subsequent report was distinctive not in its originality but in its combination of telling anecdote from individual physicians and analyses which had been honed within the scientific community. These were now conveniently summarized, wrapped up in blue covers, and propelled into the general political arena. Better surveillance was called for, so was more research on new drugs, support for the WHO, and better education of patients and doctors. There should be better controls of prescribing to patients and use on animals and a national strategy to safeguard the effectiveness of antimicrobials. Presenting it to the House in November 1998, Lord Soulsby reiterated what had been said in the report itself and in a press conference launching it:

Our enquiry has been an alarming experience. Misuse and overuse of antibiotics are now threatening to undo all their early promises and success in curing disease. But the greatest threat is complacency, from Ministers, the medical profession, the veterinary service, the farming community, and the public at large. Our Report is a blueprint for action. It must start now, if we are not to return to the bad old days of incurable diseases before antibiotics were available.[53]

The subsequent debate expressed the variety of opinions in society as a whole. Several peers evoked the atmosphere of pre-war medicine as they promoted the hitherto overlooked value of alternative therapies ranging from hydrogen peroxide to tea-tree oil.[54] Beyond such more extreme options, there was serious anxiety about the prospects of a society without the benefits of penicillin and other antibiotics. Repeatedly, lords pointed to the need for old attitudes to cleanliness in the hospitals and new attitudes to antibiotics in the community. The arguments that had been familiar in public-health circles, but had not been part of public debates, were now put forcefully on the public agenda.

The House of Lords report affected the political debate worldwide. Discussion in Europe was a case in point. This had begun with arguments about animal uses of antibiotics started by the accession of Sweden to the European Union in 1995. A problem had arisen because the use of antibiotic growth promoters had been totally banned in Sweden for ten years. When, however, the country joined the Union, its domestic rules were set to be compulsorily superseded by the Union's more permissive legislation. The rules of accession gave Sweden until the end of 1998 to prove its case or else change its law. There were many forces pushing for Sweden to submit. For example, southern European countries with important agricultural sectors felt dependent on the use of growth promoters. Companies which supplied them also fought for their legitimate place to be recognized.

Intensive lobbying followed at both the scientific and political levels. In their book *Killers Within*, the journalists Michael Schnayerson and Mark Plotkin have shown how two Swedish and two Danish microbiologists, 'a gang of four', lobbied the European Union to ban the use of two antibiotics, avoparcin and virginiamycin, related to the back-up antibiotic vancomycin, from use as growth promoters.[55] At first, the four seemed to be unsuccessful. When the Scientific Committee on Animal Nutrition, whose job it was formally to advise the Union, met in July 1996, it concluded that there was no overwhelming scientific evidence for banning antibiotic use as growth promoters. Yet the politics was now firmly in favour of controlling such applications of what had formerly been wonder drugs. The issue of antibiotic resistance, which had hitherto been considered of domestic political concern, was now on the international agenda.

Through the year 1996, BSE and the risk of its causing CJD became major concerns of the European Union. In March, the Union banned the export of British beef. During the very week the Scientific Committee was suggesting that an antibiotic disaster was unlikely to be caused by the misuse in agriculture, the European Parliament was examining the roots of the actual BSE disaster.[56] In the wake of the panic, beef demand had collapsed in Britain, and across Europe consumption had fallen about 5 per cent, or 1 kg per head.[57] Any repetition would be disastrous. So, in December 1996, the Standing Committee on Health and Welfare, which consisted of representatives of national governments, overruling the Scientific Committee, voted to ban avoparcin and virginiamycin as growth promoters for two years.[58] Not just an administrative act, this decision could also be read as a cultural indicator. It highlighted the conflation on the public stage of intense anxieties about diverse diseases and worries about the potential of antibiotics to control bacteria.

The European Union now went further to limit the abuse of antibiotics. Within its Research and Development Directorate it set up a section to coordinate research into antibiotic resistance. Meanwhile, the Health Directorate organized an international meeting on the 'Microbial Threat' in Copenhagen in September 1998, just a few months after the publication of the House of Lords report that would colour its proceedings.[59] The Copenhagen meeting was an impressive international affair. Industrial participants were concerned that the ongoing campaign for restrictions on the use of antibiotics in agriculture and medicine would reduce their markets. On the other hand, medical participants were worried that a laissez-faire approach would no longer suffice.

A now-familiar three-part agenda was recommended by the Copenhagen meeting—establishing levels of antibiotic resistance across the continent, research on means of mitigating the processes of bacterial evolution, and education of both doctors and patients to reduce the speed of evolutionary change. Immediately the consequence was the setting-up of a Europe-wide surveillance process, EARSS. In the longer term, the way was cleared for a five-year research funding programme worth up to 100 million euros (about $100 million). A pattern of meetings was also established, with the country holding the six-monthly presidency of the European Union also holding a summit to deal with antibiotic resistance. Exactly seventy years after the discovery of penicillin, reflection on how to maintain its effectiveness had become part of the rhythm of international politics.

The new surveillance system for the first time provided comparable international data about antibiotic use. It showed that, while across Europe penicillins constituted roughly half the antibiotics prescribed, the mix of types varied considerably.[60] In France, Italy, and Spain the most powerful drugs for combating resistant microbes, combinations such as co-amoxiclav, were widely used. In Germany and Britain broad-spectrum amoxicillin was the drug of choice and much less use was made of combination drugs. By contrast, in Scandinavia, where usage as a whole was much lower, most penicillin used was the narrow-spectrum Penicillin V, active only against a few infections and requiring an accurate diagnosis of the infective agent. Cephalosporin usage per head tripled during the 1980s in the USA, and this family of drugs came to be a favourite among doctors there.[61] Only with such information could complex patterns of bacterial resistance be interpreted and professional behaviour changed.

By itself, measurement was, however, insufficient to modify the rate of bacterial evolution. National medical authorities demanded new forms of behaviour of doctors and their professional colleagues, including more circumspection in the use of drugs and better hygienic practices, such as fastidious hand cleaning.[62] New high-speed techniques for identifying infectious organisms were introduced—so that doctors would know whether, for example, a sore throat had a bacterial or a viral cause. Although not as authoritative as laboratory cultures, these tests could give a reasonably reliable result within minutes. As the French national plan 'for the preservation of the effectiveness of antibiotics' launched in 2001 put it, all the tools were already to hand, they just needed to be deployed.[63] Within individual major medical cultures, therefore, doctors' practices were also changing.

Reports and cultural changes by themselves would be ineffective unless the 'politicization' of the issue of antibiotic resistance had an impact on the allocation of resources. To justify expenditures, the economic value of preventing further illness would have to be demonstrated to governments and insurers. It was easy to evaluate the cost of the cures: the worldwide value of the antimicrobial therapeutics market in 2000 was $27 billion.[64] It was rather harder to calculate how much freedom from resistance was worth and to whom. Yet, some valuation would be required to achieve consensus on such issues as the weight to be given to the risk of increasing resistance in animal uses. Costings were also necessary to justify greater capital expenditure on hospitals—for instance, replacing multi-person wards by individual rooms—and on anti-bacterial drugs that would encourage pharmaceutical companies to prioritize further development of this class of medicines.

Historically, it had been difficult to calculate the cost of the further illness caused were control of bacteria not to be effective, or the economic benefits of curbing use. Like the supply of water, antibiotics are goods whose use indirectly affects ultimately the global community and not just individual patients.[65] Such issues were explored through a new economic model of global public goods introduced in a 1999 book by Inge Kaul, Isabelle Grunberg, and Marc Stern, three economists working for the United Nations, subtitled *International Collaboration in the 21st Century*.[66] Global public goods were identified as non-excludable—that is, people could not be excluded from using them—and 'non-rival in consumption', like sunlight, in which 'my' consumption would not in itself compete with 'your' consumption. There was widespread debate about the implications. Could 'health' or medicines, for instance, themselves be such global public goods?[67] Although critics argued that the concepts were insufficiently precise to be effective, the attention paid to this theory by economists around the world indicated the intense concern with such shared problems as resistant bacteria.

Resources could be allocated rationally through medical establishments, but politicization entailed, too, the engagement with the expectations of patients. The World Health Organization, the most globally influential body in this field, had shown some interest in antibiotic resistance since the early 1980s, when its principal concern was with surveillance of antibiotic resistance among bacteria.[68] Much greater ambition was shown at the World Health Assembly in May 1998, when a proposal for a new global antibiotic strategy was accepted.[69] The coordinator, Rosamund Williams, proposed that, with WHO support, states each put together a strategy for managing antibiotic use. Three years later, the full global strategy for containment of antimicrobial resistance was published.[70] It was a practical document, emphasizing the 'how' and the 'what' rather than 'if' or 'why'. Above all, the organization addressed the problems of poorer countries, where it was hard to get sufficient quantities of the right drug. At the top of the list of recommendations were measures for the education of the public. This would both minimize resistance and maximize the benefits of scarce medical resources.

Whereas education can be a 'top-down' process, concepts of dialogue between doctors and patients were changing. In Western countries, urgency was added by the new-found problems of managing chronic disease. Treatments for such conditions as heart disease and high blood pressure were being prescribed in large quantities and needed to be taken for long periods. Too often, patients failed to obey doctors' instructions or forgot to take their medicines, a problem that had come to be diagnosed as a failure of 'compliance'. Criticizing was easy, but finding a more effective alternative to the now failing patriarchal relationship was hard. A new word, 'concordance', emerged as part of the perceived need for doctors to share responsibility for the medical process with the patient.[71] 'Concordance' was defined as 'an agreement between a patient and a health care professional that respects the beliefs and wishes of the patient in determining whether, when and how medicines are to be taken'. The process depended on doctor and patient discussing possible treatments and agreeing on the preferred solution. Such a patient-centred approach took patients' views not as stumbling blocks to be overcome or as demands that had to be met but as arguments that had to be incorporated in the process of deciding on a treatment.

Concordance raised substantial questions for both doctors and policy makers. How, for instance, could one give proper weight to the public interest within a dialogue which gave priority to the patient's own concerns? Nonetheless, one new and practical realization of this kind of approach did quickly prove very successful. Presented with a child screaming with pain from acute otitis media, or with a sore throat, the doctor would prescribe an antibiotic but agree with the carer that it would not be used unless it was felt improvement was unacceptably slow in coming by itself.[72] Similarly, a wider range of treatments than traditionally offered was becoming available. In an era in which patients agreed on medicines with doctors, the category of alternative medicines was reframed as complementary medicine. Increasingly, such procedures as osteopathy were taught in medical schools to future professionals who in the past would have been trained to look on such treatments as unacceptable.[73] A new medical culture, beyond the post-war industrial revolution of which penicillin had been such an important part, was developing.

Around the world, numerous initiatives to manage antibiotic use, linking patients and doctors—some public and some private—sprung up at a remarkable rate. One of the first was in California where, in February 1998, the Medical Association House of Delegates (attended by health professionals from across the state) adopted a resolution identifying antibiotic resistance as a major challenge to community health. Within two years, the resolution had been turned into a programme entitled 'Alliance Working for Antibiotic Resistance Education' (AWARE). Involving medical professionals, parents, and schools, it counted 80 organizations and 200 volunteers among its supporters. Showing the complexity of the exercise to rebrand antibiotics, the 2004 press kit issued by AWARE listed a formidable range of activities:

- A successful media campaign including spots on NBC Nightly News, *48 Hours* and Public Service Announcements featuring Bill Nye 'The Science Guy' and Dick Van Dyke. Print media exposures include *LA Times*, as well as radio interviews on the internationally broadcast 'Voice of America.'

- Establishment of an antibiotic Surveillance Data system to track *Streptococcus pneumoniae* resistance in California.

- Partnerships with those who care for and teach children in California including the California PTA, the CA Resource and Referral Agency, and the CA School Nurses Organization in order to reduce infection and increase wise antibiotic use.

- Creation of a handwashing curriculum for third graders.

- The production of patient and consumer education materials.

- Development of a Clinical Practice Guideline Compendium and clinical education program.

- A National Conference to convene those working with antibiotic resistance education.

- Antibiotic Awareness Week every year in the fall with a proclamation from the California Governor announcing the importance of this topic.

- Ethnic media campaign includes the use of over ten languages statewide, and print stories in the *China Times* and the *Korean Times*.[74]

In Britain, following the House of Lords report, a major campaign was launched by the government to change public perceptions of antibiotics.[75] The posters and leaflet designed by the agency Ogilvy and Mather had a 1940s style focused on what antibiotics would not do (see Ill. 26). There was evidence that this campaign changed public perceptions somewhat and discouraged the patients from seeking antibiotic prescriptions, but not always for the right reasons. A follow-up study found that, after the 2003 burst of activity 'There was an increase to 82% of people who agreed with the statement that taking too many antibiotics weakens the body's resistance.'[76] The lay person at the end of the century was now interested in the limitations of antibiotics, though still confused between the resistance of an individual and that of bacteria shared by the community.

At the end of the twentieth century the multiplicity of public initiatives on the one hand, and, on the other, the rapid evolution of bacteria offered grounds for both utter despondency and high hopes. They aroused contrasting emotions in Stuart Levy, veteran campaigner and head of the Alliance for the Prudent Use of Antibiotics. To the 2002 edition to his *Antibiotic Paradox* (first published in 1992), he added an introduction highlighting the encouraging developments of recent years. However, his optimism was tempered by worry.[77] The following year, in a review of progress since 1992 for the US Institute of Medicine, he reflected on the frustrations of his campaign.[78] Despite the many reports on the steps necessary to control bacterial antibiotic resistance, the lack of effective action to change behaviour had made him despondent. Bacteria were becoming resistant even to such back-stop antibiotics as vancomycin, and increasing numbers of resistant strains were becoming more common. Levy's anxieties were echoed in a 2004 report by the Infectious Diseases Society of America.[79] MRSA, once largely a hospital-acquired infection,

26 *(right)*. No longer wonder drugs: Department of Health cautionary cartoon, 1999.
Central Office of Information.

27 *(below)*. The wonder drug: penicillin in a vial, made by Merck in November 1943. Science Museum inventory no. 1984–1082.
Science Museum/Science & Society Picture Library.

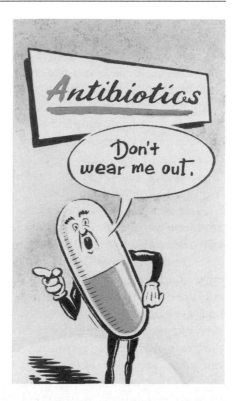

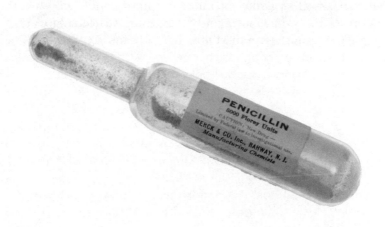

was now more widespread in the community. Sportsmen, despite their youth and fitness, seemed particularly likely to become infected, perhaps because of a lack of hygiene in the locker-room. Again, bacterial resistance was proving to be a still-worsening public problem and not merely a challenge for the professional.

On the other hand, as the twenty-first century began, doctors were changing their behaviour and patients adapting their expectations. Fewer and fewer prescriptions for antibiotics were being given: by the beginning of the century, antibiotic use in developed countries had fallen typically by a quarter since the mid-1990s.[80] So, administration to children in the USA had fallen by a third, and in a few places such as Iceland and Finland bacterial resistance was also falling.[81] Although the links between antibiotic use and bacterial resistance are complex, the public campaigns were therefore apparently already having some success.

Under the spur of AIDS and BSE, antibiotic resistance had been taken seriously, by the media and at political and professional levels. By engendering a bevy of committees and commissions, leading scientists had ensured that, internationally, the resistance of bacteria was under surveillance, medical practices were changing, and patients engaged. The problems of antibiotic resistance had not been solved, but at the beginning of the twenty-first century it was becoming clear across all the world's societies that we should no longer routinely 'trust' in antibiotics every time we experienced an infection. Increasingly, publics were becoming aware of a palette of measures for the containment of infection, including better personal hygiene, tolerance of minor conditions, and the use of vaccination as well as antibiotics. Penicillin was ceasing to be a wonder drug. There was, however, still a chance it could continue to be a really useful medicine.

Conclusion: Revolution and Tragedy

Since 1940, penicillin has evoked high hopes and profound emotions. Hearing that this book was being written, even strangers have felt spontaneously moved to share their personal experiences of penicillin. Some explained how their lives had been saved when they were young, others recalled the fiery pain of injections, and a few parents explained their worries about giving children yet more medicines. Doctors relived their guilt at prescribing penicillin unnecessarily, while their colleagues described the guilt of not prescribing it soon enough.

Such memories were intensely personal, but they were also snapshots of a much more general phenomenon. Wherever we look, the history of penicillin has been interwoven with hope, trust, relief, and triumph, but also guilt and despair. A central place has been given to such feelings and the connotations associated with penicillin in this account, by interpreting the drug through the marketing model of a 'brand' as well as the scientific model of a chemical. This approach has enabled the numerous stories of penicillin's discovery to be treated as part of the public character of the drug itself. It also helps us resolve the challenge with which this book began: the apparent contradiction between the story of triumph so often associated with the drug's introduction and the anxieties about antibiotic-resistant bacteria with which the twentieth century ended.

If the story of penicillin has resembled a tragedy, this account has suggested that its unfolding has been driven by the unrealizable ambitions that had attended the brand's early years and continued late into the twentieth century. Hopes that historical experience would be transcended through technology were shaped by the widespread determination after the Second World War, in many countries, that a better life should follow the conflict. Instead of the heavy legacy of deprivation, better lives would be made possible by improving access to goods and by drawing on technologies, above all in electronics, chemicals, and pharmaceutics, whose dramatic rise characterized the 'third industrial revolution'. In its reach across society, the depth of its impact on consumers and producers, and its cultural resonance there was a parallel with previous industrial revolutions.[1] In medicine in particular, new drugs, electronics-based technologies, and better insurance shaped the image of a transformed health-care system.

Penicillin, with its enormous industrial, medical, and cultural importance, was a totem of the revolution. The wartime triumph of its production and rapid introduction to medicine had been made known worldwide, and the success of its use led to the marked reduction across entire societies in such diseases and complaints as syphilis, rheumatic fever, pneumonia, and carbuncles. Public-health analysts may have suggested that death rates from such diseases as pneumonia merely sustained in the antibiotic era the declines established earlier in the twentieth century, but penicillin had a sudden and radical impact on the popular culture of illness. In this new world, the penicillin brand seemed the very model of the means by which post-war aspirations of a break from the suffering of pre-war days would be achieved.

The very success of modern medicine meant, however, that resources were always inadequate to meet the great expectations held for it. Whether in state insurance systems, the National Health Service in Britain, or the private US system, community physicians and hospitals were all overstretched. This has been often expressed in terms of financial resources and the growing proportion of GNP devoted to medicine. However, the problem went beyond money to the overall ecology of the medical system. The Swedish professor Gunnar Biörck, addressing the British Medical Association in July 1964, complained that demand for medicine had burst old banks, 'The crisis in medical care today', he proposed, 'is one of an increase in demand, at least temporarily, vastly in excess of the concomitant increase in supply'[2]. The consequence he saw as more technology: 'more hospitals, more group practices, less individual medicine'. In the campaign to respond to the overwhelming demand for medicine, penicillin had a key role.

Doctors under pressure found that beds in hospitals could be used more efficiently, but the greater turnover raised problems of cross-infection, which were dealt with by means of antibiotics. Meanwhile, the demand for care from patients in the community had to be dealt with faster, and, again, penicillin and other antibiotics came to the aid of the medical system. They both solved short-term technical problems and maintained the faith of ever-more demanding patients in the trustworthiness of their physicians. Emerging problems of resistance were often left to such technical solutions as the development of new penicillins: superdrugs countered superbugs.

The use of penicillin to meet the pressure of modern expectations could also be seen in agriculture. Crowded cattle feed lots made possible much greater production of meat and allowed beef to become a constant in the diet of many Western families, rather than rare luxury. However, the lots would have been crippled by infections, had these not otherwise been managed by antibiotics. Similarly, farmers could engage with confidence in intensive poultry and pig farming, curing infections before they undermined production, and manage the mastitis spread by automatic milking. The low doses of antibiotics used to enhance growth rates brought animals to slaughter faster and therefore speeded up meat production.

Thinking about the drug as a brand helps us understand how the attraction of penicillin weathered the storm over the role of expertise of the early 1960s. At a time when some chemicals, such as DDT, fell under deep suspicion, penicillin joined a long tradition of drugs that were trusted as part of patients' own 'life worlds'. In consequence, warnings about the consequences of abuse would be widely discounted. As scepticism of expertise in general grew and as doctors were increasingly strangers to their patients, they prescribed antibiotics such as penicillin to build their own reputation for trustworthiness.

While the bacterial ecosystem responded to such pressures, the development of new penicillins such as methicillin and its successors proved a remarkably effective short-term remedy for the emergence of resistant strains. By itself, of course, this approach was neither microbiologically nor economically sustainable. There has been, in consequence, a startling contradiction between, on the one hand, the triumphs of the discovery and the cures it has made possible and, on the other, the emergence of resistant strains, which had been predicted even in the 1940s. Such familiar threats as MRSA and antibiotic-resistant streptococcus emerged one by one, some spreading through hospitals, others through the community, causing infections that required more and more sophisticated antibiotic responses and occasionally outwitting all known antibiotics.

Yet, while penicillin had a chemical existence in a bacterial world as well as a social existence in the human world, nobody has, until recently, taken responsibility for the bacterial commons, or has been accountable for preserving a sustainable microbiological environment. In the absence of any 'guardian of the commons', that evolutionary process has had a sense of inevitability, and the human story has been correspondingly tragic. This does not mean that disaster will strike. By the end of the twentieth century, however, it was clear that half-century-old ambitions for humans totally to transcend infectious disease had been thwarted, and would have to be abandoned for ever.

When Aristotle explored the characteristics of drama in his book *The Poetics*, he identified reversal of fortune and the sudden awareness of the hero as defining qualities of 'complex tragedy'.[3] Both can be seen to have had their counterparts in the real-life tragedy of penicillin. While there was no single precipitating cause, the peaks of several long-running historical waves coincided in a tumultuous discontinuity during the early 1960s, and that could be seen as the period in which fortune turned. Technical solutions to the spread of resistant organisms came to be outrun by bacterial change and extravagant application. The story then came to be one of society beset by dilemmas so challenging that not only was there no immediate answer—it was even difficult to accept the gravity of the problem. The second critical moment in the complex tragedy, when the hero suddenly becomes aware of the crisis that confronts him, also had its counterpart in the history of penicillin. Since the late 1990s, there has been a serious public engagement with the challenge posed by resistance: we have yet to see the outcome of that realization.

Reformulating a global brand trusted for half a century and finding new methods of managing health care is a major challenge. Up to now the Aristotelian progress of a tragedy has been faithfully followed. Will it end with the final dramatic phase: *catastrophe*? At the beginning of the twenty-first century, the prognosis is still uncertain.

Acknowledgements

The research and writing of a book is a personal but also social activity. Librarians and archivists are the essential midwives of research. I owe a deep debt of gratitude to my colleagues in the Imperial College and Science Museum Libraries and particularly to Marika Fox, Janice Lewis, and Ben Whehelen, the interlibrary loan librarians. I am grateful too to David Short who translated material from Czech, Andrew Bud who translated Italian, and Betty Chang who translated Chinese.

Over a number of years I have been indebted for advice, support, and research materials to a number of individuals. Mark Cantley, Douglas Eveleigh, Leo Hepner, and Jeffrey Sturchio have long supported my interest in matters biotechnological. Jean-Paul Gaudillière suggested that I take an interest in the history of penicillin and has encouraged me on the quest. Joshua Lederberg has generously provided time, advice, and reminiscences for a variety of projects over many years. For conversation and wise counsel about ways into, and through, the history of antibiotics I am indebted to Harry Marks, John Parascandola, Philip Scranton, John Swann, and Tilly Tansey.

In the course of the research I was privileged to benefit from the advice of a considerable number of people who gave their time by talking about their experiences. They include Alessandro Ballio, Jessie Carter, the late I. B. Cohen, Bernard Dixon, David Felmingham, Wolfgang Forth, the late Ian Fraser, the late John Kenneth Galbraith, the late Norman Heatley, Andrew Herxheimer, Sir Gordon Hobday, Marc Lappé, Joshua Lederberg, Stuart Levy, Alan Linton, Anna Lönnroth, Richard Novick, George Rolinson, Mildred Savage, Orville Schell, Lord Soulsby, Sir Frederick Warner, the late Trevor Williams, Richard Wise, and Boyd Woodruff. For their time, forthright comments, and illumination I am most grateful.

Audiences at conferences in many countries have responded to presentations about this work and have honed my ideas. I am therefore grateful to participants at meetings organized by the American Association for the History of Medicine, British Medical Association, British Society for the History of Science, Gesellschaft Deutscher Chemiker, Medical Sciences Historical Society, Society for the History of Technology, and the Society for the Social History of Medicine, the Wellcome Trust Centre for the History of Medicine at University College London, the 'Drug Trajectories' series of workshops, and audiences at departmental seminars at the Department of History and Philosophy of Science at Cambridge University, the Department of Science and Technology Studies at University College London, and the Department of History of Medicine at the University of Wisconsin-Madison.

Several scholars have most generously shared the products of their own unpublished research. Sona Štrbànova led me to the manuscript diary of Ivan Málek, Susan Lindee provided the manuscript study of her work on Pfizer and penicillin conducted for the Brooklyn Historical Society, Gilberto Corbellini kindly gave me material he had collected on the development of the penicillin plant in Rome. Kathryn Hillier showed me drafts of her ongoing dissertation at the University of Sydney. Jackie James of the Murray Research Center at Harvard University provided the computer data generated through the Health and Personal Styles research project. John Parascandola shared several pieces of unpublished work.

I am indebted to those who have read and criticized, in part or in whole, earlier drafts of this book. They include Julian Anderson, Rima Apple, Emma Back, Tim Boon, Nicky Britten, Bernard Dixon, Douglas Eveleigh, Simon Garfield, Sir Gordon Hobday, Brian Hurwitz, Stuart Levy, Alan Linton, Anna Lönnroth, Marshall Marinker, Dianna Melrose, Peter Morris, Richard Novick, Carol Richenberg, George Rolinson, Lord Soulsby, Gordon Stewart, Harriet Strimpel, Jon Turney, Sir Frederick Warner, and Anthony White. For the errors that remain, I alone am responsible.

London's Science Museum has been a hospitable host and generous sponsor of this work. For help with photography I am indebted to the photographers of the Science Museum including David Exton and Jennie Hills. For their support I am grateful to Jon Tucker, Heather Mayfield, Tim Boon, Derek Robinson, and Tom Wright. A special debt of gratitude is due to Ela Ginalska who has been reading and criticizing innumerable drafts with a constant commitment to excellence.

Permissions

Where possible, the permission of copyright owners for using quoted extracts and photographs has been obtained. The author is grateful to those owners who gave permission for their material to be used and apologizes for any inadvertent omissions.

The following copyright owners requested that their permission be acknowledged.

The following, photograph of a box of Amoxil, is used with the permission of the GlaxoSmithKline Group of Companies.

Crown copyright material is reproduced with the permission of the Controller of HMSO and the Queen's Printer for Scotland.

Introduction

Quotation from Hayden White, *Metahistory: The Historical Imagination in Nineteenth Century Europe*, p. 9 © 1973 Hayden White. Reprinted with permission of the Johns Hopkins University Press (n. 4).

Chapter 1

Quotation from *Ghosts* by Henrik Ibsen reproduced by permission of Penguin Books Ltd. (n. 9).

Quotations from Mass Observation, 'Preliminary Report on General Attitudes to Venereal Disease', reproduced with permission of Curtis Brown Group Ltd., London, on behalf of the Trustees of the Mass-Observation Archive. Copyright © Mass Observation Archive (nn. 11 and 13).

Quotation from *Morning Post* © The Telegraph Group Ltd. 1933 (n. 15).

Excerpts from *The Sweeping Wind: A Memoir*, copyright © 1962 by Paul De Kruif and renewed 1990 by Eleanor Lappage De Kruif and Dr Henrik De Kruif, reprinted by permission of Harcourt, Inc. (n. 43).

Quotation from *Sunday Graphic* © NI Syndication (n. 55).

Quotation from the *Star Weekly*. From an article originally appearing in the *Star Weekly*, January 1939. With permission Torstar Syndication Services (n. 56).

Chapter 2

Quotation from André Maurois, *The Life of Sir Alexander Fleming*, reproduced with permission of Curtis Brown Ltd. on behalf of the Estate of André Maurois. Copyright © The Estate of André Maurois (n. 8).

Quotation from Coulthard's 'Notes' by permission of Boots Archives (n. 90).

Chapter 3

Quotation from Peter Vansittart, *In the Fifties*, reproduced by permission of John Murray Publishers (n. 80).

Chapter 4

Quotation from J. C. Hoogerheide, 'Address by the Symposium Co-Sponsor'. Copyright © 1973 J. C. Hoogerheide. Reprinted with the permission of Wiley-Liss, Inc., a subsidiary of John Wiley & Sons (n. 56).

Chapter 5

Quotation from the *American Journal of Public Health* reprinted with permission of the American Public Health Association (n. 27).

Quotation from the *Journal of Obstetrics and Gynaecology in the British Empire*, volume 67, Bryan Williams, 'Discussion', 738, 1960, reprinted with permission from the Royal College of Obstetricians and Gynaecologists (n. 34).

Quotation from Gordon T. Stewart and John P. McGovern (eds.), *Penicillin Allergy: Clinical and Immunologic Aspects*, 1970. Courtesy of Charles C. Thomas Publisher, Ltd., Springfield, Illinois (n. 51).

Chapter 7

Quotation excerpted from the Institute for Motivational Analysis, *A Psychological Study of the Doctor–Patient Relationship*, California Medical Association, May 1950. Copyright California Medical Association. Published with the permission of and by arrangement with the California Medical Association (n. 20).

Quotation from 'What we Know about Young Ears' by Louise Fox Connell, first appeared in *Parents Magazine*, March 1954. Copyright © 1954 by Louise Fox Connell, reprinted by permission of Brandt and Hochman Literary Agents, Inc. (n. 45).

Quotations from the *British Medical Journal* reprinted with permission of the BMJ Publishing Group (nn. 46 and 47).

Quotation from Stuart B. Levy, *The Antibiotic Paradox: How Miracle Drugs are Destroying the Miracle*, reproduced with kind permission of Springer Science and Business Media (n. 54).

Quotation from *The Lancet* reprinted with permission from Elsevier (*The Lancet*, 1996, 348, 1703–4) (n. 83).

Chapter 8

Quotation reprinted from *The Control of Antibiotic-Resistant Bacteria*, ed. Charles H. Stuart-Harris and David M. Harris, 196 (1982), with permission from Elsevier (n. 6).

Quotation from the *Guardian* reproduced by permission of the Guardian Media Group (n. 27).

Quotations from Medical Research Council files held at The National Archives, UK, are by permission of the Medical Research Council (nn. 59 and 61).

Quotation from Alan I. Marcus, *Cancer from Beef: Federal Food Regulation and Consumer Confidence*, p. 127, © 1994 Alan Marcus. Reprinted with the permission of Johns Hopkins University Press (n. 74).

Chapter 9

Quotation from *Emerging Infections: Biomedical Research Reports*, Richard M. Krause, 'Introduction to Emerging Infectious Diseases: Stemming the Tide', 1–22, 1998, reprinted with permission from Elsevier (n. 11).

Excerpt from *AIDS and its Metaphors* by Susan Sontag. Copyright © 1988, 1989 by Susan Sontag. Reprinted by permission of Farrar, Straus and Giroux, LLC and the Penguin Press (n. 12).

Quotation from Frank Ryan, *Virus X*, courtesy of HarperCollins Publishers © Frank Ryan (n. 17).

Quotation from Joshua Lederberg, 'Medical Science, Infectious Disease, and the Unity of Humankind', *Journal of the American Medical Association*, 260 (1988), 684–5. Copyright © 1988 American Medical Association. All rights reserved (n. 21).

Quotation from 'Disease Fights Back', © Economist Newspaper Ltd., London, 1995 (n. 36).

Quotation from Tim Radford, 'Medicine and the Media', reprinted with permission from Elsevier (*The Lancet*, 1996, 347, 1533–55) (n. 38).

Quotation from *Current Biology*, 6, Bernard Dixon, 'Killer Bug Ate my Face', 493, copyright 1996, reprinted with permission from Elsevier (n. 39).

Quotation from the *British Medical Journal* reprinted with permission of the BMJ Publishing Group (n. 42).

Quotation from *Communicable Diseases and Public Health* reproduced with permission of the Health Protection Agency, © HPA.

Conclusion

Quotation from the *British Medical Journal* reprinted with permission of the BMJ Publishing Group (n. 2).

Notes

Introduction

1. 'First A-bomb Use Called the Century's No. 1 News Story', *Christian Science Monitor*, 24 December 1999. For Fleming's place in the Great Britons poll see the National Portrait Gallery's website **www.npg.org.uk/live/greatbritop100.asp** accessed 1 December 2004.
2. See Wally Olins, *On B®and* (London: Thames and Hudson, 2003). Wally Olins, 'Branding the Nation: The Historical Context', *Brand Management*, 9 (2002), 241–8. I am very grateful to Wally Olins for his care in initiating a tyro to the world of branding. The literature on the meaning of brands is summarized by Giep Franzen and Margot Brouwman: *The Mental World of Brands: Mind, Memory and Brand Success* (Henley-on-Thames: World Advertising Research Centre, 2001).
3. Macfarlane Burnet, *The Natural History of Infectious Disease* (2nd edn. Cambridge: Cambridge University Press, 1953), p. ix.
4. Hayden White, *The Historical Imagination in Nineteenth-Century Europe* (Baltimore: Johns Hopkins University Press, 1973), 9. The literature on tragedy in literature and history was recently reviewed by Terry Eagleton in *Sweet Violence: The Idea of the Tragic* (Oxford: Blackwell, 2003).

Chapter 1

1. Barbara Lewis, born 25 August 1930, recorded for the Millennium Memory Bank, British Archive of Recorded Sound, British Library.
2. Patrick Slater, *Survey of Sickness, October 1943 to December 1945: A Report on a Series of Surveys on the State of Health of the Civilian Population between these Dates, Made for the Ministry of Health* (London: GRO, 1946), 14.
3. G. L. Armstrong, L. A. Conn, and R. W. Pinner, 'Trends in Infectious Disease Mortality in the United States during the 20th Century', *Journal of the American Medical Association*, 281 (1999), 61–6.
4. The best general introduction to this area is Nancy Tomes, *The Gospel of Germs: Men, Women, and the Microbe in American Life* (Cambridge, Mass.: Harvard University Press, 1998). Tomes distinguishes between the period of emergence

of worries about germs, 1870–90, and the era of 'The gospel triumphant', which she sees as 1890–1920.

5. Sue Ellen Hoy, *Chasing Dirt: The American Pursuit of Cleanliness* (New York: Oxford University Press, 1995).

6. Dr Robert Huchinson's lecture in Winnipeg was discussed in an editorial in the *Lancet*. See 'Health Propaganda', *The Lancet*, 220 (14 February 1931), 357; Also see J. Mackintosh, *Trends of Opinion about the Public Health 1901–51* (Oxford: Oxford University Press, 1953). On medicine and consumerism before the Second World War, see Nancy Tomes, 'Merchants of Health: Medicine and Consumer Culture in the United States, 1900–1940', *Journal of American History*, 88 (2001), 519–47.

7. This is based on studies of older people in the 1960s. See Alan Radley, *Making Sense of Illness* (London: Sage, 1994), 59; Ruthbeth Finerman and Linda A. Bennett, 'Guilt, Blame and Shame: Responsibility in Health and Sickness', *Social Science and Medicine*, 40 (1995), 1–3. See also Anne Karpf, *Doctoring the Media: The Reporting of Health and Medicine* (London: Routledge, 1988).

8. Jocelyn Cornwell, *Hard-Earned Lives: Accounts of Health and Illness from East London* (London: Tavistock, 1984), 153.

9. Henrik Ibsen, *Ghosts*, in *Ghosts and Other Plays,* trans. Peter Watts (London: Penguin, 1964), 75 and 92.

10. Joseph Earle Moore, 'Venereology in Transition', *British Journal of Venereal Diseases*, 32 (1956), 217–25 (p. 217).

11. Mass Observation, 'Preliminary Report on General Attitudes to Venereal Disease', 24 December 1942; TC 12, 'First Venereal Disease Survey, November–December 1942' 12/1/A. Mass Observation Archive, Special Collections, Sussex University.

12. Mass Observation, 'Preliminary Report', 24.

13. Ibid. 13.

14. Over the swimming pool in Iris Murdoch's novel *The Philosopher's Pupil* hung the Latin motto 'Natando virtus' (virtue through swimming).

15. Peter Lawless, 'Along the Broad Highway to Health: Bringing back Physical Well-Being to the Youth of Britain', *Morning Post*, 14 February 1933.

16. Peter Bartrip, *Themselves Writ Large: The British Medical Association 1832–1966* (London: BMJ Publishing Group, 1996), 206–10; see also Hiroyuki Onuma, 'The Development of the Physical Training and Recreation Policy in Britain 1937–1939: Mainly Concerned in the Measures of National Fitness Council', *Japanese Journal of Sports History*, 7 (1994), 1–17.

17. L. S. Amory, 'Annual Report', British Social Hygiene Council, 17 June 1936, p. 3.

18. Gladys V. Swackhamer, *Choice and Change of Doctors: A Study of the Consumer of Medical Services* (New York: Committee on Research on Medical Economics, 1939), 44.

19. Ray Sturgess, 'The Magic Bottle', *Pharmaceutical Journal*, 263 (1999), 1015–17.

20. Quotation from North Shields Library Club, **www.libraryclub.co.uk/ Memories/memory_37.html**, accessed 30 November 2004. Quoted with permission.

21. *Medical Care for the American People*, The Final Report of the Committee on the Costs of Medical Care, adopted 31 October 1932 (Chicago: University of Chicago Press, 1932), 28.

22. A. J. Clark, *Patent Medicines* (London: FACT, 1938), 36–7.

23. 'Beecham's will have Million-a-Year Press Appropriation', *World's Press News*, 14 July 1938.

24. James F. Hoge, 'An Appraisal of the New Drug and Cosmetic Legislation from the Viewpoint of the Industries', *Law and Contemporary Problems*, 6 (1939), 111–28 (see p. 112 for his figures based on the 1938 report of the FTC).

25. *Radio Pictorial* (30 June 1939), 34; Sean Street, 'Radio for Sale: Sponsored Programming in British Radio during the 1930s', **www.kent.ac.uk/sdfva/sound-journal/Street19991.html**, accessed 14 December 2004.

26. Roland Marchand, *Advertising the American Dream: Making Way for Modernity, 1920–1940* (Berkeley and Los Angeles: University of Califomia Press, 1985), 16–20.

27. H. L. Wehrbein, 'Therapy in Gonorrhea: An Historical Review', *Annals of Medical History*, 7 (1935), 492–7.

28. John Parascandola and Aaron J. Ihde, 'Edward Mellanby and the Antirachitic Factor', *Bulletin of the History of Medicine*, 51 (1977), 507–15.

29. Quotation from North Shields Library Club, **www.libraryclub.co.uk/ Memories/memory_37.html**, accessed 30 November 2004. Quoted with permission.

30. Richard D. Semba, 'Vitamin A as "Anti-Infective" Therapy, 1920–1940', *Journal of Nutrition*, 129 (1999), 783–91.

31. Stuart Reed, '300 Years of Cod Liver Oil', *Pharmaceutical Historian*, 18 (1988), 6–7; see the papers in the file entitled 'Proposed Schemes: Cod Liver Oil', MAF 34/700, National Archives, UK.

32. Seven Seas Health Care, *A History of British Cod Liver Oils: The First Fifty Years with Seven Seas* (Cambridge: Martin Books, 1984).

33. 'Report of Taking Medicines in Wartime', Mass Observation, 25 May 1943, FR 1793, Mass Observation Archive.

34. Rima Apple, 'Vitamins Win the War: Nutrition, Commerce, and Patriotism in the United States during World War II', presented at the 'Medicine, Science, and Food Policy in the 20th Century' conference, University of Aberdeen, April 1999.

35. Herman Kogan, *The Long White Line* (New York: Random House, 1963), 153.

36. E. McCollum, *History of Nutrition* (Boston: Houghton Mifflin, 1957).

37. Georg Widmann, *Das ärgerliche Leben und schreckliche Ende des viel-berüchtigten Ertzschwartzkünstlers D. Johannis Fausti . . . und einem Anhange von den Lapponischen Wahrsager-Pauken, etc.* (Nuremberg, 1681), 683. This edition had first

been published in 1674, and an earlier edition had appeared in 1599. It was reprinted, with its appendix, in Tübingen: Gedruckt für den Litterarischen Verein in Stuttgart, in 1880. On Ehrlich's own use of the terms 'magic bullets' and *Zauberkugel* see Bernhard Witkop, 'Paul Ehrlich and His Magic Bullets—Revisited', *Proceedings of the American Philosophical Society*, 143 (1999), 540–57, though this source highlights the resonance with the 'Freikugel' described in Weber's popular opera *Der Freischütz*.

38. Udo Benzenhöfer, 'Zum Paracelsusbild im Dritten Reich: Unter besonderer Berücksichtigung der Paracelsusfeier in Tübingen/Stuttgart im Jahre 1941', in Ulrich Fellmeth and Andreas Kotheder (eds.), *Paracelsus—Theophrast von Hohenheim: Naturforscher, Arzt, Theologe* (Stuttgart: Wissenschaftliche Ver-lagsgesellschaft, 1993), 63–70. E. Rentschler, 'Pabst Redesigned: Paracelsus', *Germanic Review*, 66 (1991), 16–24.

39. An illustration of this fascination was the 1936 founding in London of the Society for the History of Alchemy and Early Chemistry. See William H. Brock, '*Ambix* Celebrates its Jubilee', *Chemical Heritage*, 23 (Fall 2005), 42.

40. Ludwig Fulda, *Das Wundermittel: Komödie in drei Aufzügen* (Stuttgart: J. G. Cotta'sche Buchhandlung Nachfolger, 1920).

41. Holger Dauer, *Ludwig Fulda, Erfolgsschriftsteller: Eine mentalitätsgeschichtlich ori-entierte Interpretation populardramatischer Texte* (Tübingen: M. Niemeyer, 1998).

42. Fulda, *Das Wundermittel*, 104–5.

43. Paul De Kruif, *The Sweeping Wind* (New York: Harcourt, 1962), 6. On *Arrowsmith* see Ilana Löwy, 'Immunology and Literature in the Early Twentieth Century: *Arrowsmith* and *The Doctor's Dilemma*', *Medical History*, 32 (1988), 314–32. Also see 'Martin Arrowsmith: The Scientist as Hero', in Charles E. Rosenberg, *No Other Gods* (Baltimore: Johns Hopkins University Press, 1976), 123–32.

44. Arthur Kallet and Frederik Schlink, *100,000,000 Guinea Pigs: Dangers in Everyday Foods, Drugs and Cosmetics* (New York: Vanguard Press, 1933).

45. Clement & Johnson Ltd., *The Yadil Book: The Careful Study of this Book and the Use of Yadil Everywhere for Every Disorder will Save Hundreds of Thousands of Lives Every Year* (London: Clement & Johnson, 1922); Clement & Johnson Ltd., *Tuberculosis: The Problem Solved: Yadil Antiseptic Cures & Prevents the White Scourge* (London: Clement & Johnson, 1923).

46. Willliam J. Pope, '"Yadil" An Exposure', *Daily Mail,* 22 July 1924.

47. 'The Chemotherapy of Streptococcal Infections', *The Lancet*, 230 (6 June 1936), 1303–4.

48. 'Nationalized Doctors?', *Time* (21 June 1937), 26–30. This event was identified as the key moment in the popularization of sulphanilamide by Daniel Bovet, *Une chimie qui guérit: histoire de la découverte des sulfamides* (Paris: Payot, 1988), 212.

49. 'Conquering Streptococcus', *New York Times* (18 December 1936), 24.

50. 'New Drug Arrests Roosevelt Jr's Sinus Trouble', *Newsweek* (26 December 1936), 8.

51. Donald B. Armstrong, 'Magic Bullets', *Hygeia* (October 1938), 892.

52. Iago Galdston, *Behind the Sulfa Drugs: A Short History of Chemotherapy* (New York: Appleton-Century, 1943). See also Margaret Goldsmith, *The Road to Penicillin: A History of Chemotherapy* (London: Lindsay Drumond, 1946), 141–8.

53. Arnold Jeaves, 'Disease You Need no Longer Dread', *Everybody's*, 25 July 1938.

54. '"Miracle" Drug saves Life of W'ton Girl', *Express and Star (Wolverhampton)*, 9 September 1938: also in *Midland Counties Express*, 10 September 1938. The story was covered also by the nationally read newspapers the *Manchester Guardian* (9 September 1938) and the *Daily Mail* (10 September 1938).

55. James Harpole, 'A Surgeon's Case-Book', *Sunday Graphic*, 2 October 1938. James Harpole was the pseudonym of J. Johnston Abraham.

56. R. M. Farrington, 'Fighting Death with "693" Medical Men are Tirelessly Testing a Miracle Drug Bordering on Witch Cures of the Middle Ages, That Promises to Wipe out Pneumonia', *Star Weekly* (Toronto), 14 January 1939.

57. See the discussion and enclosures in *Congressional Record*, 83/1 (1938), 418–19.

58. The story of the attempts to get the food and drug bill through Congress was vividly told at the time by Ruth deForest Lamb, *American Chamber of Horrors* (New York: Little and Ives, 1936). For a modern history, see Charles O. Jackson, *Food and Drug Legislation in the New Deal* (Princeton: Princeton University Press, 1970).

59. Edith Summerskill, 8 July 1941, in *Parliamentary Debates* (Commons), 5th ser. 373 (1940–1), col. 77.

60. 'Pneumonia Yields to New Chemical', *New York Times*, 9 September 1939. Jill E. Cooper, 'Of Microbes and Men: A Scientific Biography of René Jules Dubos', Ph.D. thesis, Rutgers University, 1998, is a convenient introduction to Dubos.

61. 'Edward Mellanby Celebrates New Hospitals Centre at Birmingham', *Birmingham Post*, 4 July 1938.

Chapter 2

1. Charles Wilson to Beaverbrook 8 May 1929, House of Lords Records Office, Beaverbrook papers bbk/d/407. For Wilson see R. R. H. Lovell, 'Wilson, Charles McMoran, first Baron Moran (1882–1977)', *Oxford DNB* (2004).

2. Wilson to Beaverbrook, 8 May 1929, enclosure: 'What Medical Education Means to the Country', 11. For the development of St Mary's at this time and Wilson's complex ambitions for research see E. A. Heaman, *St Mary's: The History of a London Teaching Hospital* (Montreal: McGill University Press, 2003).

3. Alexander Fleming, 'On the Antibacterial Action of Cultures of a Penicillium, with Special Reference to their Use in the Isolation of *B. influenzae*', *British Journal of Experimental Pathology*, 10 (1929), 226–36. Kevin Brown, *Penicillin Man: Alexander Fleming and the Antibiotic Revolution* (Stroud: Sutton, 2004); R. Hare, *The Birth of Penicillin* (London: George Allen & Unwin, 1970).

4. Ian Fraser, 'Penicillin: Early Trials in War Casualties', *British Medical Journal*, 289 (22 December 1984), 1723–5.

5. Frederick Ridley, one of the students, moved to the Moorfield Eye Hospital to pursue an interest in ophthalmology; the other, Stuart Craddock, went to the Wellcome Research Laboratories associated with the Burroughs Wellcome pharmaceutical company. Brown, *Penicillin Man*, 92–3.

6. David Masters, *Miracle Drug: The Inner History of Penicillin* (London: Eyre and Spottiswoode, 1946), 51.

7. Brown, *Penicillin Man*, 95.

8. André Maurois, *The Life of Sir Alexander Fleming: Discoverer of Penicillin* (London: Jonathan Cape, 1959), 148. He gave MacLeod a sample of his mould, which is believed to be the Science Museum object inventory number 1997–731. The 1935 inscription seems to have been an error.

9. Nicolas Rasmussen, 'The Moral Economy of the Drug Company–Medical Scientist Collaboration in Interwar America', *Social Studies of Science*, 34 (April 2004), 161–85; John P. Swann, *Academic Scientists and the Pharmaceutical Industry* (Baltimore: Johns Hopkins University Press, 1988).

10. Jack Morrell, *Science at Oxford 1914–1939: Transforming an Arts University* (Oxford: Clarendon Press, 1997).

11. Ibid. 351.

12. Florey to H. M. Miller, 18 December 1939, Folder 457, Box 37, Series 401D, Record Group 1.1, Rockefeller Archives.

13. The finest work on Chain is the biographical memoir by his former Oxford colleague Edward Abraham, 'Chain, Ernst Boris 19 June 1906–12 August 1979', *Biographical Memoirs of the Royal Society*, 29 (1983), 43–92.

14. 'A Chemical Study of the Phenomenon of Bacterial Antagonism', Chain papers, B107, Wellcome Library for the History and Understanding of Medicine.

15. Miller to Florey, 11 December 1939; Warren Weaver to H. M. Miller, 30 November 1939, folder 457, Rockefeller archives.

16. Weaver to Miller, 30 November 1939.

17. Miller to Florey, 11 December 1939, folder 457, Rockefeller Archives.

18. For Warren Weaver see Robert E. Kohler, *Partners in Science: Foundations and Natural Scientists, 1900–1945* (Chicago: University of Chicago Press, 1991) and Lily Kay, *The Molecular Vision of Life: Caltech, the Rockefeller Foundation, and the Rise of the New Biology* (Oxford: Oxford University Press, 1993).

19. This comparison was attributed to John Smith of Pfizer in Samuel Mines, *Pfizer: An Informal History* (New York: Pfizer, 1978), 73.

20. The mice were held by Josep Trueta, a refugee Spanish surgeon who had been in charge of one of the main Barcelona hospitals, was a pioneer of blood transfusion during the Spanish civil war, and was a specialist in treating wounds in danger of infection. In January 1939, when Catalonia fell to Franco, he had fled to England. Joseph Trueta, *Trueta: Surgeon on War*

and Peace: The Memoirs of Joseph Trueta, trans. Meli and Michael Strubell (London: Gollancz, 1980), 149–51. Trueta shared with Chain an interest in snake poison, but his intense interest in wound infection was born out of wartime problems Chain had not hitherto experienced himself.

21. Chain, Chain papers, B67, p. 9, Wellcome Library for the History and Understanding of Medicine. Ronald W. Clark, *The Life of Ernst Chain: Penicillin and Beyond* (London: Weidenfeld and Nicolson, 1985) discusses evidence of penicillin's non-protein nature such as the fact it could pass through cellophane.

22. Heatley's detailed designs are preserved in his notes held in the archives of the Wellcome Library for the History and Understanding of Medicine, see files GC/48 C2 and C3.

23. Eric Lax, *The Mould in Dr Florey's Coat* (New York: Henry Holt, 2004), 118–43 describes the Chain relationship with Heatley and Florey at this time drawing on the Heatley manuscripts at the Wellcome Library.

24. The replica has the Science Museum inventory number 1986–1116. It was constructed for the Chemical Industry gallery opened in 1986 and taken off display in 2004 when that gallery was demounted.

25. This event is described in detail by many books on the history of penicillin, recently by Lax, *The Mould in Dr Florey's Coat*, 144–55.

26. Interview with Muriel Burge by Max Blythe conducted August 2000, Medical Sciences Video Archive, MSVA 192, Oxford Brookes University.

27. Dishes growing the mould typically took 7–10 days to produce broth yielding approximately 2,000 units each. To support a patient needing 100,000 units a day, about 50 dishes a day would have to be harvested from a total stock of 500. See also Gwyn Macfarlane, *Howard Florey: The Making of a Great Scientist* (Oxford: Oxford University Press, 1979), 324–5 which gives very comparable figures of 500 litres per week to support a patient.

28. Lennard Bickel, *Rise up to Life: A Biography of Howard Walter Florey who Gave Penicillin to the World* (London: Angus and Robertson, 1972), 121–4.

29. Notebook C7, 18 February 1941, E. P. Abraham papers, NCUAS, University of Bath. At the time of writing these papers were due to be deposited at the Bodleian Library, University of Oxford.

30. E. P. Abraham, E. Chain, H. W. Florey, M. E. Florey, N. G. Heatley, M. A. Jennings, and A. G. Sanders, 'Historical Introduction', in H. W. Florey, E. Chain, N. G. Heatley, M. A. Jennings, A. G. Sanders, E. P. Abraham, and M. E. Florey (eds.), *Antibiotics*, vol. ii (Oxford: Oxford University Press, 1949), 631–71 (see pp. 647–9).

31. 'Interviews: WW Visit in England April 14, 1941: Dr. H. W. Florey, of Oxford University', Folder 481, Box 37 Series 401D, Rockefeller Archives.

32. Ibid.

33. 'Grant-In Aid: New York RA-NS 4128 June 19 1941', Folder 481, Rockefeller Archives.

34. Frank Blair Hanson to Thomas Parran, 25 June 1941, Folder 481, Rockefeller Archives.

35. Clark, *The Life of Ernst Chain*, 68.

36. Gladys L. Hobby, *Penicillin: Meeting the Challenge* (New Haven: Yale University Press, 1985), 73–5.

37. Percy Wells, 'Some Aspects of the Early History of Penicillin in the United States', *Journal of the Washington Academy of Sciences*, 65 (1975), 96–101.

38. P. A. Wells to O. E. May, 10 July 1941; Charles Thom to O. E. May, 10 July 1941, Box 1, Folder 1, RG97, US National Archives.

39. Wells, 'Some Aspects of the Early History of Penicillin in the United States'.

40. 'Kenneth Bryan Raper', Autobiographical Memoir dated July 1986, National Academy of Sciences Deceased Members Record Group, National Academy of Sciences Archives.

41. Robert Bud, *The Uses of Life* (Cambridge: Cambridge University Press, 1994), 45–50.

42. A. F. Kamp, J. W. M. La Riviere, and W. Verhoeven (eds.), *Albert Jan Kluyver: His Life and Work, Biographical Memoranda, Selected Papers, Bibliography and Addenda* (Amsterdam: North-Holland Publishing Company, 1959).

43. A. L. Bacharach and B. A. Hern, 'Chemistry and Manufacture of Penicillin', in Alexander Fleming (ed.), *Penicillin* (London: Butterworth, 1946), 24–45 (on p. 33).

44. Peter Neushul, 'Science, Government and the Mass Production of Penicillin', *Journal of the History of Medicine and Allied Sciences*, 48 (1993), 371–95 tells the story of the Color Laboratory work. Their work is described in P. A. Wells, D. F. J. Lynch, H. T. Herrick, and O. E. May, 'Translating Mold Fermentation Research to Pilot Plant Operation', *Chemical and Metallurgical Engineering*, 44 (April 1937), 188–90. Percy Wells was later director of the Eastern Regional Research Laboratory, David Lynch became head of the Southern Regional Research Laboratory, and Orville May headed the Northern Regional Research Laboratory.

45. See the illustration of the Color Laboratory deep fermenter on p. 188 of Wells et al., 'Translating Mold Fermentation Research to Pilot Plant Operation'.

46. Wells, 'Some Aspects of the Early History of Penicillin in the United States'.

47. Heatley, private communication, 31 May 1996.

48. Abraham et al., 'Historical Introduction', 650.

49. The complex sequence of the penicillin patents and assignments is recorded in detail by Gladys Hobby in a page-long footnote. See Hobby, *Penicillin*, 284–5.

50. Kenneth B. Raper, 'The Penicillin Saga Remembered', *ASM News*, 44 (1978), 645–53. The technician who found this melon was memorialized as 'Moldy Mary' though apparently she did not buy the melon herself.

51. Kenneth B. Raper, 'Research in the Development of Penicillin', in E. C. Andrus et al. (eds.), *Science in World War II: Advances in Military Medicine* (Boston: Little, Brown, 1948), ii. 729.

52. P. A. Wells to A. J. Moyer, 9 August 1943, American Institute for the History of Pharmacy Archives, University of Wisconsin.

53. Masters, *Miracle Drug*, 111.

54. Boyd Woodruff, personal communication, 31 May 1996.

55. Florey to John Fulton, 9 October 1941, copies in Abraham Archive. Original in the Yale University Library, Fulton Archive MS 1236.

56. R. C. von Borstel and Charles M. Steinberg, 'Alexander Hollaender: Myth and Mensch', *Genetics*, 143 (1996), 1051–6; Raper, 'Memoir', 11. On the background of studies of mutagenesis and radiation see M. Susan Lindee, *American Science and the Survivors at Hiroshima* (Chicago: University of Chicago Press, 1999), 61–3.

57. Hollaender to Demerec, 11 January 1942, Demerec papers, American Philosophical Society.

58. Demerec to W. M. Gilbert, 24 March 1944, Demerec papers.

59. Lily E. Kay, 'Selling Pure Science in Wartime: The Biochemical Genetics of G. W. Beadle', *Journal of the History of Biology*, 22 (1989), 73–101.

60. Demerec to Vannevar Bush, 21 April 1944, Demerec papers.

61. Interview with Robert H. Burris, University of Wisconsin-Madison Archives, Oral History Project, Madison 1983.

62. D. Perlman, 'How Penicillin Research Came to the University of Wisconsin', *Mortar and Quill*, 15/1 (1978–9), 5–8.

63. M. P. Backus and J. F. Stauffer, 'Fundamental Studies on Variability in *Penicillium notatum* with Special Emphasis on Penicillium Production', Botany Dept, General subject files L–S, series 7/5/3, Box 2, University of Wisconsin, Madison, Archives.

64. M. P. Backus, J. F. Stauffer, and M. J. Johnson, 'Penicillin Yields from New Mold Strains', *Journal of the American Chemical Society*, 68 (1946), 152–3; M. P. Backus and J. F. Stauffer, 'The Production and Selection of a Family of Strains in *Penicillium chrysogenum*', *Mycologia*, 47 (1955), 429–63.

65. Florey to Fulton, 7 December 1943, Yale University Archives.

66. The extensive correspondence with Florey about the summary volume *Antibiotics* is included in file B52 in the Chain papers at the Wellcome Library for the History and Understanding of Medicine.

67. Lorraine Daston, 'The Moral Economy of Science', *Osiris*, 2nd ser. 10 (1995), 1 26; Robert Kohler, *Lords of the Fly: Drosophila Genetics and the Experimental Life* (Chicago: Chicago University Press, 1994); W. Patrick McCray, 'Large Telescopes and the Moral Economy of Recent Science', *Social Studies of Science*, 30 (2000), 685–711.

68. Michael Aaron Dennis, 'A Change of State: The Political Cultures of Technical Practice at the MIT Instrumentation Laboratory and the Johns Hopkins University Applied Physics Laboratory, 1930–1945', doctoral dissertation, Johns Hopkins University, 1991. Michael Aaron Dennis, 'Accounting for Research: New Histories of Corporate Laboratories and the Social History of American Science', *Social Studies of Science*, 17 (1987), 479–518.

69. Steve Shapin, 'Who is the Industrial Scientist? Commentary from Academic Sociology and from the Shop-Floor in the United States, ca. 1900–ca. 1970', in Karl Grandin, Nina Wormbs, Anders Lundgren, and Sven Widmalm (eds.), *The Science–Industry Nexus: History, Policy, Implications*, Nobel Symposium 123 (New York: Science History Publications, 2005), 337–63.

70. The shifting relationship between chemistry's role as an academic subject and its place in industry is mapped in Arnold Thackray, Jeffrey L. Sturchio, P. Thomas Carroll, and Robert Bud, *Chemistry in America, 1876–1976* (Dordrecht: Reidel, 1984). For the 1941 survey see figure 5.1–9, p. 121.

71. Kenneth Raper to Chester S. Keefer, 3 July 1947, Box 2 Liaison Folder, RG227, US National Archives.

72. Raper to Norman Heatley, 15 January 1948, Box 2 Liaison Folder.

73. The meeting is graphically described in Masters, *Miracle Drug*, 135–37.

74. MRC retained however responsibility for the more long-term chemical and academic work on penicillin.

75. Raymond G. Rettew, *A Quiet Man from Chester County* (West Chester, Pa.: Chester County Historical Society, 1975), 25–9.

76. Robert Coghill to A. N. Richards, 3 May 1943, listed Parke Davis and Takamine Laboratories as working on a bran-based fermentation, Box 1, Folder 2, RG 97, US National Archives.

77. Hobby, *Penicillin*, 183.

78. Interview between Weber and Mines, n.d., p. 10, Pfizer archives.

79. Florey to J. F. Fulton, August 1944, Fulton Archive MS 1236, Yale University.

80. Mines, *Pfizer*, 88.

81. Vannevar Bush, 'The Case for Biological Engineering', in Karl Compton (ed.), *Scientists Face the World of 1942* (New Brunswick, NJ: Rutgers University Press, 1942), 33–45. For the context see Bud, *The Uses of Life*, 86–7.

82. The detailed story of the use of the word biotechnology and its application to this journal is told in Bud, *The Uses of Life*.

83. Jeffrey Sturchio (ed.), *Values and Visions: A Merck Century* (Rahway, NJ.: Merck, 1991).

84. Production had increased from 21 billion units in 1943 to almost 7,000 billion units in 1945. See R. D. Coghill and R. S. Koch, 'Penicillin: A Wartime Accomplishment', *Chemical and Engineering News*, 23 (1945), 2310.

85. US Federal Trade Commission, *Economic Report on Antibiotics Manufacture* (Washington, DC: US Government Printing Office, 1958), 51–4.

86. J. P. Swann, 'The Search for Synthetic Penicillin during World War 2', *British Journal for the History of Science*, 16 (1983), 154–88.

87. Bacharach and Hern, 'Chemistry and Manufacture of Penicillin', 33.

88. Jonathan Liebenau, 'The British Success with Penicillin', *Social Studies of Science*, 17 (1987), 69–86.

89. On Boots see Simon Phillips, 'Jesse Boot and the Rise of Boots the Chemists *The Pharmaceutical Journal* 296 (2002), 925–28.

90. 'Notes on the History of the Bacteriological Laboratories and Other Departments of Boots Pure Drug Co. Ltd with Special Reference to the Research and Fine Chemical Departments. Reminiscences of Retail and Army (1915–1919) Experiences by C E Coulthard', 47, Boots Archives, Nottingham.

91. C. E. Coulthard, R. Michaelis, W. F. Short, G. Sykes, G. E. H. Skrimshire, A. F. B. Standfast, J. H. Birkinshaw, and H. Raistrick, 'Notatin and Anti-bacterial Glucose-aerohydrogenase from *Penicillium notatum* Westling and Penicillium resticulosum sp. Nov.', *Biochemical Journal*, 39 (1945), 24–36; Coulthard, 'Notes', 482.

92. 'Improvements Relating to Bactericidal Substances', British Patent Specification 552,619, application dated 14 October 1941, accepted 16 April 1943.

93. Boris Sokoloff, *Penicillin: A Dramatic Story* (London: George Allen and Unwin, 1946), 50–2 describes work in the USA which led to this material being described as Penicillin B. See also D. Keilin and E. F. Hartree, 'Properties of Glucose Oxidase (Notatin)', *Biochemical Journal*, 42 (1948), 221–9.

94. Trevor Williams, *Howard Florey: Penicillin and After* (Oxford: Oxford University Press, 1984), 157–58. For I.C.I. investment in Penicillin see Liebenau, 'The British Success with Penicillin', 78. For the tour of the USA see Hobby, *Penicillin*, 134–36.

95. Kane interview, 21 and 41, Pfizer archives, New York.

96. J. Ward, 'Memorandum', 22 September 1942, Kemball Bishop papers, Pfizer Ltd.

97. The production figures for Clevedon come from 10th general penicillin committee, 11 May 1944, Kemball Bishop papers, File 6, Pfizer UK. For information on the use of gin bottles I am grateful to G. T. Stewart who was trained at Clevedon.

98. L. Anderson to Mr Coulthard, n.d., in Coulthard, 'Notes', 95–7.

99. Report of the Penicillin Conference, 21 July 1943.

100. Sir Frederick Warner, personal communication.

101. See Hobby, *Penicillin*, 136–40.

102. *Bridging a Gap: The Story of Boots Achievement in the Wartime Production of Penicillin* (Nottingham: Boots, 1946), 18.

103. L. Miall, 'Note', n.d., Kemball Bishop papers.

104. Hobby, *Penicillin,* 130; Edgar Jones, *The Business of Medicine: The Extraordinary History of Glaxo, a Baby Food Producer, Which Became One of the World's Most Successful Pharmaceutical Companies* (London: Profile, 2001), 71.

105. Jones, *The Business of Medicine,* 69.

106. Brown, *Penicillin Man,* 135.

107. Hobby, *Penicillin,* 131; Sir Austin Bide, private communication. Sir Austin, later Chairman of Glaxo, had been deputed to find a site for the new factory.

108. Hobby, *Penicillin,* 130: Glaxo produced 2.6 billion units 1943; Pfizer produced 6.8 billion units that year. The 2.5% figure was given in Masters, *Miracle Drug,* 179.

109. E. W. Pates, 'A Visit to Barnard Castle', *Glaxo Staff Bulletin,* 96 (April 1946), 6.

110. For the investment in the Speke plant see J. R. Harman, 'Penicillin', 24 January 1947, 'Penicillin: Question of Patent Right in Connection with Scheme for Pooling Research', AVIA 22/1591, National Archives, UK. Harman estimated that £1.1 million had already been spent and another £258,000 still needed to be spent for economic operation.

111. Distillers' lack of experience caused anxieties about its competence even when it was first asked to run the plant. S. Warebak to M. Roe, 13 November 1946, 'Penicillin Bill', MH 80/42, National Archives, UK. On Commercial Solvents' production see US Federal Trade Commission, *Economic Report on Antibiotics Manufacture,* 331. It was subsequently sold to Eli Lilly who still manufacture on the site.

112. E. Lester Smith, 'British Penicillin Production', *Transactions of the Society of Chemical Industry,* 65 (1946), 308–13. He compares British monthly production in mid-1946 of 260,000 MU with US production of 800,000 MU.

113. Swann, 'The Search for Synthetic Penicillin during World War 2'. John C. Sheehan, *The Enchanted Ring: The Untold Story of Penicillin* (Cambridge, Mass.: MIT Press, 1982), 4.

114. 'Committee for Co-ordinating Departmental Policy Connection with Patented and Unpatented Inventions', 12th Meeting, 2 December 1944, 'Penicillin: Question of Patent Rights in Connection with Scheme for Pooling Research', AVIA 22/1591, National Archives, UK.

115. Albert Elder, 'The Role of the Government in the Penicillin Program', in Albert Elder (ed.), *The History of Penicillin Production,* Symposium Series No. 100, *Chemical Engineering Progress,* 66 (1970), 3–11, see p. 4.

116. The hypothesis that Penicillin (F) stood for Penicillin (Florey) is proposed by Sydney Selwyn, 'The Role of Beta-lactam Agents in Antibiotic Policies and Strategy' in Sydney Selwyn (ed.), *The Beta-lactam Antibiotics: Penicillin and Cephalosporins in Perspective,* (London: Hodder and Stoughton, 1980), 299–318. This is substantiated by the use of the phrase Penicillin (Florey) in the title of a report by Major R. J. V. Pulvertaft in March 1943 entitled 'Report from the Middle East Forces to the War Office of an Investigation

on the action of Penicillin (Florey) on War Wounds', in 'Penicillin Clinical Trials Committee'.

117. Georgina Ferry, *Dorothy Hodgkin: A Life* (London: Granta, 1998).

118. H. J. C. Herrald, MRC to Dorothy Crowfoot (Hodgkin), 4 November 1946, b351 ms eng.c.5599, Hodgkin papers, Bodleian Library, Oxford University.

119. Private communication, Sir Frederick Warner.

120. Raper, 'Research in the Development of Penicillin'.

121. This refers to the work of O. Behrens and his team. See E. J. Kahn Jr., *All in a Century: The First Hundred Years of Eli Lilly and Company* (Indianapolis: Eli Lilly, 1976), 137–8.

122. This calculation is based on the fact that penicillin was bought by the US government at $20 for 100,000 units. Since penicillin had roughly 1,600 units to the mg, a gram cost $320 or roughly $9,000 an ounce at a time when gold cost $35 an ounce!

123. Allan J. Greene and Andrew J. Schmitz, 'Meeting the Objective', in Elder (ed.), *The History of Penicillin Production*, 80–97.

Chapter 3

1. *Penicillin: Its Properties, Uses and Preparations* (London: Pharmaceutical Press, 1946), 83.

2. Ibid. 84.

3. David P. Adams, *The Greatest Good to the Greatest Number: Penicillin Rationing on the American Home Front, 1940–1945* (New York: Peter Lang, 1991), 134–42.

4. C. S. Davidson, 'The Cocoanut Grove Disaster: Maxwell Finland', *Journal of Infectious Diseases*, 125 (March 1972), Suppl.: 58–73. See Peter Neushul, 'Fighting Research: Army Participation in the Clinical Testing and Mass Production of Penicillin during the Second World War', in Roger Cooter, Mark Harrison, and Steve Sturdy (eds.), *War, Medicine and Modernity* (Stroud: Sutton, 1998), 203–24.

5. 'Penicillin', *Time* (8 February 1943), 41.

6. In my treatment of the early clinical work on penicillin I follow the work of Lennard Bickel, *Rise up to Life* (London: Argus and Robertson, 1972).

7. Ibid. 204; the early advertisement showing a soldier rescued by penicillin (Ill. 9) was evoked in a 1995 report: Office of Technology Assessment, *Impacts of Antibiotic-Resistant Bacteria: 'Thanks to Penicillin, He will Come Home!'*, Publication OTA-H-6297 (Washington, DC: Office of Technology Assessment, 1995).

8. Champ Lyons, 'Penicillin Therapy of Surgical Infections in the US Army' *Journal of the American Medical Association*, 123 (1943), 1007–18.

9. Champ Lyons to B. M. Carter, Box 20 ff20, RG 97, US National Archives.

10. J. H. Burn, 'Penicillin', 31 May 1943, submitted by E. Mellanby to Penicillin Clinical Trials Committee, 9 June 1943, 'Penicillin Clinical Trials Committee', FD1/6870, National Archives, UK.

11. Sir Ian Fraser, *Blood, Sweat and Cheers* (London: BMJ, 1989), 45.
12. A. E. Porritt and G. A. G. Mitchell, 'Penicillin and Sulphonamides in Prophylaxis', in *Penicillin Therapy and Control in 21 Army Group* (London: Published under the Direction of the Director of Medical Services, 21 Army Group, May 1945), 17.
13. Porritt and Mitchell, 'Factors Influencing the Occurrence of Infection in War Wounds', ibid. 21.
14. Mark Harrison, *Medicine & Victory: British Military Medicine in the Second World War* (Oxford: Oxford University Press, 2004).
15. F. H. K. Green and Gordon Covell, *Medical Research: Medical History of the Second World War* (London: HMSO, 1953), 64.
16. Harrison, *Medicine & Victory*, 88–91.
17. Ibid. 91.
18. 'Penicillin Administration in Wartime Surgery', in *Statistical Report on the Health of the Army 1943–45* (London: HMSO, 1948), 281–8.
19. Ibid. 281 and 288.
20. H. G. Mayne, 'The Army Medical Services', in Franklin Mellor (ed.), *Casualties and Medical Statistics: History of the Second World War United Kingdom Medical Services* (London: HMSO, 1972), 444–5.
21. Ernest Bulmer, 'Penicillin in Medicine', in *Penicillin Therapy and Control in 21 Army Group*, 219.
22. Gordon Stewart, *The Penicillin Group of Drugs* (Amsterdam: Elsevier, 1965), 175.
23. John Parascandola, 'John Mahoney and the Introduction of Penicillin to Treat Syphilis', *Pharmacy in History*, 43 (2001), 1–56.
24. Gladys L. Hobby, *Penicillin; Meeting the Challenge* (New Haven: Yale University Press, 1985), 155–6.
25. Albert Elder, 'The Role of the Government in the Penicillin Program', in Albert Elder (ed.), *The History of Penicillin Production*, Chemical Engineering Progress Symposium Series No. 100, *Chemical Engineering Progress*, 66 (1970), 4.
26. J. Howie, 'Gonorrhoea: A Question of Tactics', *British Medical Journal*, 2 (22 December 1979), 1631–2.
27. G. T. Stewart, 'Toxicity of the Penicillins', *Postgraduate Medical Journal*, 40 (1964), Suppl.: 160–9.
28. Florey to Mellanby, 15 February 1943; Mellanby to Florey, 23 February 1943, 'Penicillin Clinical Trials Committee', FD1/6870, National Archives, UK.
29. 'Requests for Penicillin', Florey papers, HF/1/3/2/10, at the Royal Society. The two quoted are contained in letters, Barbara Lingwood to Florey, 14 April 1943; Dr S. C. Dyke to Florey, 30 April 1943, to which Florey replied on 6 May 1943.
30. The death of Anne Miller and a subsequent article in *Yale Medicine* stimulated a fascinating correspondence from several then junior doctors who had attended her. John Curtis, 'Fulton, Penicillin and Chance', *Yale Medicine*, 34 (Fall 1999–Winter 2000) and available on the web at **http://info.med. yale.edu/external/pubs/ym_fw9900/capsule.html**, accessed 1 December

2004; Charles M. Grossman, 'The First Use of Penicillin', *Yale Medicine*, 34 (Spring 2000), 3; Thomas S. Sappington,'The Early Days of Antibiotics', *Yale Medicine*, 34 (Summer 2000), 2.

31. Maria Riva, *Marlene Dietrich* (London: Bloomsbury, 1994), 586.
32. Adams, *The Greatest Good to the Greatest Number*.
33. Burn, 'Penicillin'.
34. Paul De Kruif, *The Sweeping Wind* (New York: Harcourt, 1962), 208.
35. Bickel, *Rise up to Life*, 205–7. For the introduction of penicillin into US army surgery see Elliot C. Cutler, 'The Chief Consultant in Surgery', in B. Noland Carter (ed.), *Activities of Surgical Consultants* (Washington, DC: Office of the Surgeon General, Dept. of the Army, 1962–4), 19–358 (see pp. 133–46).
36. 'Report of a Meeting Held at the Ministry of Health on May 5th 1944 to Consider the Principles on which Supplies of Penicillin should be Distributed when it Becomes Available to Civilians, and the Machinery of Distribution', minutes of the 10th general meeting of the Penicillin Committee, Kemball Bishop papers, Pfizer Ltd.
37. Dr Walter Ehrlich interviewed for the Brooklyn Historical Society. I am indebted to Susan Lindee of the University of Pennsylvania for kindly letting me use her manuscript research on the history of penicillin, 'Technology for a Miracle: Pfizer Inc.'s Production of Penicillin in Brooklyn, 1941–1945', a report to the Brooklyn Historical Society, Brooklyn, NY, 1990, which quoted the interview, and to Dr Ehrlich for his support.
38. Mrs Jessie Carter, London. From an interview conducted with the Science Museum in September 2002.
39. The work of Bodenham is reported by Bickel who was able to talk to him about his work on Procaine. See Bickel, *Rise up to Life*, 163–5.
40. G. W. S. Andrews and J. Miller, *Penicillin and Other Antibiotics* (London: Todd, 1949), 100; W. Howard Hughes, 'Methods of Administration', in Alexander Fleming (ed.), *Penicillin: Its Practical Application* (London: Butterworth, 1946), 93–104 (see p. 102).
41. Herman Kogan, *The Long White Line* (New York: Random House, 1963), 216.
42. George Bankoff, *The Conquest of Disease* (London: Macdonald, 1946), 176.
43. 'Penicillium', *The Times*, 27 August 1942.
44. 'Penicillin', *The Times*, 31 August 1942.
45. Gwyn Macfarlane, *Alexander Fleming: The Man and the Myth* (London: Chatto and Windus, 1984), 256.
46. '20th Century Seer', *Time* (15 May 1944), 61–8. The *Time* story and the response in Britain are covered by Kevin Brown, *Penicillin Man* (Stroud: Sutton, 2004), 140–1.
47. Chain to Tizard, 17 July 1945, Chain papers, Wellcome Library for the History and Understanding of Medicine.
48. Moran to Prime Minister, 8 March 1944, 'Penicillin', Prem 4/88/7, National Archives, UK.

49. This argument was first put by Macfarlane, *Alexander Fleming*, 256–7. Beaverbrook's extended discussion of his asthma is included in his correspondence with Charles Wilson, BBK/D/407, House of Lords Records Office.

50. A. J. P. Taylor, *Beaverbrook* (London: Hamish Hamilton, 1992).

51. The correspondence between Beaverbrook and Moran is preserved in the Beaverbrook papers, BBK c/232, House of Lords Records Office.

52. 'We Will Remember Them', *Royal British Legion Journal*, 57/8 (August 1977).

53. See Robert Bud, 'Penicillin and the New Elizabethans', *British Journal for the History of Science*, 31 (1998), 305–33.

54. Florey to Mellanby, 19 June 1944, Florey papers, HF 36.4.107, Royal Society. The reply came within a few days: Mellanby to Florey, 30 June 1944, Florey papers, HF 36.4.106, Royal Society.

55. Alice Nicholls, 'Lord Nuffield's Gift of an Iron Lung to any Hospital or Institution in the Empire, November 1938: An Appropriate Gift for the Colonies?', MA dissertation, Birkbeck College, University of London, 2000.

56. Taylor, *Beaverbrook*, 423.

57. Lindee, 'Technology for a Miracle', 179–80.

58. A. N. Richards to A. Baird Hastings, 8 January 1945, Richards papers, Box 24 FF17, University of Pennsylvania.

59. Labor FSA Appropriations Hearings 1947, House, 79th Congress, 2nd session, p. 180.

60. Vannevar Bush, *Science: The Endless Frontier: A Report to the President* (Washington DC: United States Government Printing Office, 1945).

61. Isaiah Berlin, *The Hedgehog and the Fox: An Essay on Tolstoy's View of History* (New York: Bantam, 1957; first published 1953). On the back of this US edition the publisher's blurb highlighted this book's contribution to the debate about whether man was a free agent of his own life or a mere victim of larger forces.

62. I. Bernard Cohen, *Science, Servant of Man* (Boston: Little Brown, 1948), 20–32. See also Cohen's letter to Florey, 20 July 1948, Florey papers, HF37.1.39, Royal Society. Professor Cohen was distressed by a review by Waldemar Kaempffert, 'On Great Discoveries and What Precedes Them', *New York Times*, 22 August 1948. Private communication from the late Professor Cohen to Robert Bud.

63. Robert Bud, 'Strategy in American Cancer Research after World War 2: A Case Study', *Social Studies of Science*, 8 (1978), 425–59.

64. See for instance 'Penicillin and Modern Research', *The Lancet*, 1 (14 January 1950), 76–7.

65. 'Penicillin: Notes on the Question of Mr Gormley's Visit to U.S.A.', 'Penicillin', Prem 4/88/7, National Archives, UK.

66. '"Penicillin Won't be Ready for Second Front"—M.P.', *Daily Mirror*, 14 February 1944.

67. Memo by Churchill, 14 February 1944, 'Penicillin', Prem 4/88/7.

68. D. Kelly, telegram dated 28 June 1944; Gerald Meade, telegram 3 July 1944; Sir Gerald Meade to Sir Anthony Eden, 6 July 1944, FO 371/38213, National

Archives, UK. On the sense of being robbed, the evolution of protest, and its meaning see Bud, 'Penicillin and the New Elizabethans'.

69. Wyatt C. Wells, *Antitrust and the Making of the Postwar World* (New York: Columbia University Press, 2002), 99–107.

70. See Bud, 'Penicillin and the New Elizabethans' for this and for a broader discussion of the propaganda value of innovation.

71. Ibid. Brown, *Penicillin Man*, 141.

72. Kay Mander, private communication. See also a film made by Adele Carroll, *One Continuous Take: Kay Mander's Life In Film* (2001). I am grateful to Adele Carroll for sight of this film.

73. Galvin Wright to Florey, 26 May 1944, Florey papers, 35.11.18, Royal Society.

74. See Brown, *Penicillin Man*, 193–94.

75. The text of this letter from Hugh-Jones to Conant is reproduced in John T. Connor to Vannevar Bush, 28 October 1952, Container 27, Bush papers, Library of Congress.

76. Connor to Bush, 28 October 1952, p. 9, Container 27, Bush papers.

77. R. P. T. Davenport-Hines and Judy Slinn, *Glaxo: A History to 1962* (Cambridge: Cambridge University Press, 1992), 246 and 372.

78. '£5 million to Stop Foreigners Filching our Ideas', *Daily Herald*, 14 April 1948.

79. 'The 1946 Campaign: This is the Policy and Purpose of the *Daily Express*', *Daily Express*, 1 January 1946.

80. Colleagues and I have explored the concept of defiant modernism in more detail in Robert Bud, Simon Niziol, Tim Boon, and Andrew Nahum, *Inventing the Modern World* (London: Dorling Kindersley, 2000).

81. Peter Vansittart, *In the Fifties* (London: John Murray, 1995), 98.

82. *Daily Telegraph*, 19 March 1955.

83. Brenda Heagney, *Half a Century of Penicillin: An Australian Perspective* (Canberra: The Royal Australasian College of Physicians, 1991), 8.

Chapter 4

1. Appendix to 'Control of Epidemics, Report of the Medical Commission to Germany and Austria', GEN93, in 'Control of Epidemics', CAB 78/38 pt2, National Archives, UK.

2. See Milton Wainwright, 'Hitler's Penicillin', *Perspectives in Biology and Medicine*, 47 (2004), 189–98.

3. E. H. G. Lutz, *Penicillin: Die Geschichte eines Heilmittels und seines Entdeckers Alexander Fleming* (Bad Worishofen: Kindler, 1954). The author describes this event as happening in the aftermath of the battle of the Kasserine Pass but before the fall of Tunis, probably April 1943 when it would have been very unlikely that penicillin would have been available in the way described.

4. Joseph Garrity, 'Soldiers without Weapons', *Eighth Army News*, 8 June 1945. Harrison points also to the correspondence between Porritt and Tomlinson, 4

September 1944, RAMC 406/3/7, CMAC, Wellcome Library for the History and Public Understanding of Medicine. Mark Harrison, *Medicine & Victory: British Military Medicine in the Second World War* (Oxford: Oxford University Press, 2004), 255.

5. Málek in Czechoslovakia would be a pioneer of continuous fermentation, while Bernhauer was later professor at the University of Stuttgart where he trained the leaders of German biotechnology in the 1970s. See Robert Bud, *The Uses of Life: A History of Biotechnology* (Cambridge: Cambridge University Press, 1994), 150.

6. The authoritative description of German wartime work in this area is Wolfgang Forth, Dietmar Gericke, and Reinhard Klimmek, *Men & Fungi: Penicillin Research and Production in World War II Germany* (Munich: W. Zuckschwerdt, 2000); translation of *Von Menschen und Pilzen* (1997). Where no other source is given, this is the basis for the treatment here. I am grateful to Professor Forth for his guidance. Also Gilbert Shama and Jonathan Reinarz, 'Allied Intelligence Reports on Wartime German Penicillin Research and Production', *Historical Studies in the Physical and Biological Sciences*, 32 (2002), 347–67.

7. The Zeiss work is reported in Horst Heinecke (ed.), *Dokumente zu den Anfängen der Penicillin-Forschung in Deutschland* (Erfurt: Akademie Gemeinnütziger Wissenschaften zu Erfurt, 2001).

8. David Irving (ed.), *The Secret Diaries of Hitler's Doctor*, revised and abridged by Susanna Scott-Gall (London: Grafton, 1990); E. Wondrák, 'Die Pharmaindustrie von Hitlers Leibarzt Dr. T. Morell während des Zweiten Weltkrieges in Olmütz: Gab es ein Olmützer Penicillin?', *Acta Universitatis Palackianae Olumuciensis, Facultas Rerum Naturalium 112, Chemica*, 32 (1993), 127–37. See also Milton Wainwright, 'Hitler's Penicillin', *Perpectives in Biology and Medicine*, 47 (2004), 189–98. Paul Weindling, *Epidemics and Genocide in Eastern Europe 1890–1945* (Oxford: Oxford University Press, 1999), 379 describes how Morell turned to penicillin after his insecticide Russla was rejected in favour of DDT.

9. R. Brunner, 'In Memoriam: Konrad Bernhauer', *Mitteilungen der Versuchsstation für das Gärungsgewerbe in Wien*, 2 (1976), 22.

10. Konrad Bernhauer, *Gärungschemisches Praktikum* (Berlin: Julius Springer, 1936).

11. For Bernhauer's wartime political activity, see Alena Mišková and Petr Svobodny, 'Hermann Hubert Knaus, 1892–1970', in Monika Gettler and Alena Mišková (eds.), *Prager Professoren 1938–1948* (Essen: Klartext, 2001), 437.

12. Forth, Gericke, and Klimmek, *Men & Fungi*, 38.

13. Joseph Koenig, *Die Penicillin-V Story: Eine Erfindung aus Tirol als Segen für die Welt* (Innsbruck: Haymon Verlag, 1984), 15.

14. Ivan Málek, 'Penicillin in Czechoslovakia', Manuscript Memoir from: Ivan Málek, Personal Papers, Archives of the Academy of Sciences of the Czech Republic. I am very grateful to Professor Sona Strbanova who provided this to me and to David Short who translated it from the Czech. For the wartime and post-war history of Czech penicillin see also the memoirs of another Fragner

chemist Josef Koštiř, 'O "Českem" Penicilinu', *Chemické Listy*, 84 (1990), 827–42. I am grateful to my colleague Jiri Staraček for his interpretation of this text for me.

15. The linkage of post-war to wartime work is emphasized by Koštiř, 'O "Českem" Penicilinu'. See also the Royal Society obituary of Wiesner: W. G. Schneider and Z. Valenta, 'Karel František Wiesner', *Biographical Memoirs of the Royal Society*, 37 (1991), 463–90. This also describes the exciting first use of BF510 and cites the work on its separation that was published.

16. I am grateful for conversations with Andrew Nahum for this perception.

17. Melanie Burns and Piet W. M. van Dijck, 'The Development of the Penicillin Production Process in Delft, the Netherlands, during World War II under Nazi Occupation', *Advances in Applied Microbiology*, 51 (2002), 185–200. Melanie Burns, J. W. Bennett, and Piet W. M. van Dijck, 'Code Name Bacinol', *ASM News*, 69 (2003), 25–31. I am grateful to Professor Ernst Homburg for bringing the work of Melanie Burns to my notice and to Melanie Burns for copies of her papers.

18. Delft would maintain its importance in the penicillin story. In 1995, Gist-Brocades, the local pharmaceutical company, would be the world's largest producer of the drug. H. J. M. Van Nistelrooij, J. Krijgsman, E. de Vroom, and C. Oldendof, 'Penicillin Update—Industrial', in Richard I. Mateles (ed.), *Penicillin: A Paradigm for Biotechnology* (Chicago: Candida, 1998), 85–91.

19. The immediate post-war development of penicillin production in France has been described in detail by Jean-Paul Gaudillière, *Inventer la biomédecine: la France, l'Amérique et la production des savoirs du vivant (1945–1965)* (Paris: La Découverte, 2002), 36–68 and in J. P. Gaudillière and B. Gausemeier, 'Molding National Research Systems: The Introduction of Penicillin to Germany and France', *Osiris*, 20 (2005), 180–202. Also see Université de Paris, 'Exposition de la pénicilline décembre 1945–janvier 1946', Paris: Palais de la Découverte, Archives of the Palais de la Découverte. Also Viviane Quirke, 'Experiments in Collaboration: The Changing Relationship between Scientists and Pharmaceutical Companies in Britain and in France, 1935–1965'. D.Phil. thesis, Oxford University, 1999.

20. Joseph Needham, 'Science in South-West China', *Nature*, 152 (3 July 1943), 9–10; (10 July 1943), 36–7.

21. Ibid. 36.

22. Niu Yahua, ['The Manufacture of Penicillin in China in 1940s'], *Zhonghua yi shi za zhi*, 31 (2001), 184–8. I am grateful to Betty Chang for her help in translating this article.

23. On Chinese production: F. F. Tang to Dr P. Z. King, 22 July 1944. In this letter Tang says his team was producing 250,000–500,000 Oxford units every 24–48 hours, Box 24, ABMAC records. For information on US penicillin supplies see 'Preliminary Report of the Central Penicillin Control Committee with Special Reference to the Activities of the Subcommittee for Civilians', Received 25

January 1945, Box 24, ABMAC records, Columbia University Rare Book and Manuscript Library.

24. 'Minutes of Conference on the Production of Penicillin Held at the Office of the American Bureau for Medical Aid to China', 6 March 1944, Box 24, ABMAC records.

25. Ibid.

26. Z. Yermolieva, T. Kaplun, and M. Levitov, 'Penicillin Crustosin', *American Review of Soviet Medicine*, 2 (February 1945), 247–50.

27. A. Baird Hastings and Michael B. Shimkin, 'Medical Research Mission to the Soviet Union: Part II', *Science*, 103 (24 May 1946), 637–44. The experience of visiting the Soviet Union was described by Michael Shimkin in 'Roads to OZ. I: A Personal Account of Some USSR Medical Exchanges and Contacts 1942–1962', *Perspectives in Biology and Medicine*, 22 (1979), 565–86.

28. Harold Truman, *Year of Decisions 1945* (London: Hodder and Stoughton, 1955), 403–6.

29. United Nations Relief and Rehabilitation Administration (UNRRA) Committee on Supplies, CS(46)3, 16 January 1946, United Nations Archives.

30. 'The Famine Threatening Half the World', 16 April 1946, NARA 200–170, US National Archives. This was a broadcast discussion between Fiorella LaGuardia of UNRRA, Clive Anderson, Secretary of Agriculture, Harry Truman, and Herbert Hoover.

31. 'Report of Official Working Party', 18 September 1945, p. 8. Control of Epidemics. Meeting 1–6, Papers 1–8, CAB 78/38, National Archives, UK.

32. 'Memorandum by the Secretary of State', Gen 93 (ministerial) in appendix to 'Control of Epidemics', CAB 78/38 pt. 2, National Archives, UK.

33. 'Report of Winter Emergency Health and Hygiene Committee. 8 Corps District, November 1945', 'Preparations for Winter Epidemic', vol. i, FO 1013/1955, National Archives, UK.

34. 'Report of Official Working Party', p. 5, Control of Epidemics, CAB 78/38.

35. Committee on Priorities, Minutes of the Third Session of the Interim Commission Held in Geneva from 31 March to 12 April 1947 (United Nations, World Health Organization Interim Commission, August 1947), annex 24, p. 137.

36. Patricia Meehan, *A Strange Enemy People: Germans under the British 1945–50* (London: Peter Owen, 2001).

37. Maria Hohn, *GIs and Frauleins: The German American Encounter in 1950s West Germany* (Chapel Hill: University of North Carolina Press, 2002).

38. Michaela Freund, 'Women, Venereal Disease and the Control of Female Sexuality in Post-War Hamburg', in Roger Davidson and Lesley A. Hall (eds.), *Sex, Sin and Suffering: Venereal Disease and European Society since 1870* (London: Routledge, 2001), 205–19; John Willoughby, 'The Sexual Behavior of American GIs during the Early Years of the Occupation of Germany', *Journal of Military History*, 62 (1998), 155–74.

39. Dr A. H. Bensch to Colonel Donelly, Headquarters Military Government, Düsseldorf, 10 October 1945, 'Control of Venereal Disease', FO 1013/1929, National Archives, UK.

40. Control Commission for Germany, 'Penicillin Imported to Fight VD', 29 June 1946, in 'Prevalence of Venereal Disease in Germany 1946', FO 371/5578, National Archives, UK.

41. Minute dated 12 February 1948, MH 136/73, National Archives, UK.

42. 'Racket in Fake Drug Smashed in Germany', *New York Times*, 21 April 1946.

43. Taylor to Secretary of State, 21 December 1944, in Myron C. Taylor, Nov.–Dec. 1944 i471, Box 53, Diplomatic Correspondence with the Vatican, Franklin D. Roosevelt Presidential Library and Museum. See also John Lamberton Harper, *America and the Reconstruction of Italy, 1945–1948* (Cambridge: Cambridge University Press, 1986).

44. United Nations Relief and Rehabilitation Administration, Report of the Director General to the Council for the Period 1 January 1946 to 31 March 1946, Washington, DC, 1946; George C. Herring Jr., *Aid to Russia 1941–1946: Strategy, Diplomacy and the Origins of the Cold War* (New York: Columbia University Press, 1973), 244 explains the balancing between the Soviet republics and Italy.

45. Peter Stursberg, *Lester Pearson and the American Dilemma* (Toronto: Doubleday Canada, 1980); Robert D. Defries, *The First Forty Years 1914–1955: Connaught Medical Research Laboratories* (Toronto: University of Toronto Press, 1968), 192–3.

46. Karel Sommer, *UNRRA a Československo* (Opava: Slezský ústav AV ČR, 1993). See Eris Holland, 'Penicillin Plant Project: Medical and Sanitation Supplies Divison', 29 July 1947, UNRRA Records, S-0527–0448 PAG 4.13.0.5.3.1 UNRRA file: 'Supply Penicillin'. Each plant cost about $240,000 and was intended to produce 40 billion units per month of penicillin. This compared to Canadian production at the end of 1945 of 20 billion units a month (Hobby, *Penicillin*, 211) but US production of 700 million units per month by then.

47. Dr M. K. Fügnerová, 'Health Services and the Two Year Plan', *Czechoslovakia* (January 1947), 48.

48. Walter Ullmann Malek, *The United States in Prague, 1945–1948* (Boulder, Colo.: East European Quarterly, distributed by Columbia University Press, 1978), 39 for US support of Czechs.

49. The debates are preserved in a surviving British government file, 'Control of Exports to Eastern Europe: "Podbielniak Penicillin extractors", 1950', FO 371/87185, National Archives, UK.

50. 'Report on the Penicillin Conference held at the Ministry of Health in Prague on June 16th to June 19th 1947'. The meeting was led by Mr Hendershott of the Merck company. This report is contained in the archives of the Istituto Superiore di Sanita in Rome and I am very grateful for the help of Gilberto Corbellini in obtaining it.

51. The developments are summarized in an English document entitled 'Memorandum' addressed to Dr F. Abbott Ingalls, Attaché at the US Embassy, dated 18 June 1948, Istituto Superiorie di Sanita.

52. 'My Activities at the Istituto Superiore di Sanita. A Brief Survey', Chain papers, EBC/C13, Box 12, Wellcome Library for the History and Understanding of Medicine.

53. Giuseppe Gualandi, 'Il Centro Internazionale di Chimica Microbiologica ed il suo capo E. B. Chain', in 'Le origini del Laboratorio di Fisica', in *Domenico Marotta nel 25° anniversario della morte: rendiconti Accademia Nazionale delle Scienze detta dei XL 23* (1999), 211–13.

54. Chain, 'My Activities at the Isituto Superiore di Sanita'.

55. Gualandi, 'Il Centro Internazionale di Chimica Microbiologica ed il suo capo E. B. Chain', I am grateful to Andrew Bud for the translation of this passage from Italian.

56. J. C. Hoogerheide, 'Address by the Symposium Co-sponsor', *Biotechnology and Bioengineering Symposium*, 4i (1973), p. vii. On the development of fermenter design in Rome see for instance: E. B. Chain, S. Paladino, F. Ugolini, D. S. Callow, and J. van der Sluis, 'A Laboratory Fermenter for Vortex and Sparger Aeration', *Rendiconti Istitututo Superiore di Sanita* (English edn.), 17 (1954), 61–86 and a sequence of similar papers. A 300l fermenter to the team's design was built for Beecham and was used for the research on semisynthetic penicillins and later given to the Science Museum, inventory number 1984–477 (See Ill. 17).

57. R. Falini, 'Biochemical Engineering in the Production of Fungal Metabolites', in D. A. Hems (ed.), *Biologically Active Substances: Exploration and Exploitation* (Chichester: John Wiley, 1977), 33–48.

58. N. Tyabjim, 'Gaining Technical Know-how in an Unequal World: Penicillin Manufacture in Nehru's India', *Technology and Culture*, 45 (2004), 331–49.

59. Koenig, *Die Penicillin-V Story*.

60. Penicillin V is normally known as phenoxymethyl penicillin in contrast to the benzyl penicillin which had been the standard 'penicillin G'.

61. Forth, Gerice, and Klimmek, *Men & Fungi*, 60.

62. Ibid 53–5.

63. Gaudillière and Gausemeier, 'Molding Natural Research Systems'. Wilhelm Girstenbrey, 'Der Aufstieg der Gruenenthal gmbh mit dem ''Wundermittel'' Penicillin', *die Waage*, 22 (1983), 126–32. Also see Helmüth Böttcher, *Wunderdrogen: Die abenteurliche Geschichte der Heilpilze* (Cologne: Kiepenheuer & Witsch, 1959), 298–307. This section is not included in the English translation of the book.

64. Michael Cooper, *Prices and Profits in the Pharmaceutical Industry* (Oxford: Pergamon, 1966), 128.

65. Yukimasa Yagisawa, 'Early History of Antibiotics in Japan', in John Parascandola (ed.), *The History of Antibiotics: A Symposium* (Madison: American Institute for the History of Pharmacy, 1980), 69–90. See also Hazime Mizoguchi, 'Penicillin Production and the Reconstruction of the Pharmaceutical Industry', in Shigeru Nakayama (ed.), *A Social History of Science and Technology in Contemporary Japan*, 2 vols. (Melbourne: Transpacific Press, 2005) ii. 541–51.

66. Thomas B. Turner, 'Japan and Korea', in *Civil Affairs/Military Government Public Health Activities*, vol. viii of Ebbe Curtiss Hoff (ed.), *Preventive Medicine in World War II* (Washington, DC: Office of the Surgeon General, Dept. of the Army, 1976), 659–707 (p. 680).

67. Boyd Woodruff, 'The Legacy of Jackson W. Foster', American Society of Microbiology, 1 June 1999; Jackson W. Foster, 'Three Days Symposium on Penicillin Production', separate issues of *Journal of Penicillin*, 1 (March 1947). The printing of this symposium conference is recalled by Yagisawa, 'Early History of Antibiotics in Japan', 86.

68. Jackson Foster, 'Preface', *Journal of Antibiotics*, 1 (1947), 1.

69. Boyd Woodruf, personal communication.

70. Kinichiro Sawao and Sakaguchi Murao, 'A Preliminary Report on a New Enzyme, "Penicillin-amidase"', *Journal of Agricultural Chemical Society* (Japan), 23 (1950), 411.

71. J. W. Foster, 'A View of Microbiological Science in Japan', *Applied Microbiology*, 9 (1961), 434–51.

72. Report of the Interim Commission to the First World Health Assembly 38, 'Venereal Diseases', *Official Records of the World Health Organization*, 9 (1948). Also see *Official Records of the World Health Organization*, 12, Supplementary Report of the Interim Commission to the First World Health Assembly, World Health Organization, Palais des Nations, Geneva, December 1948.

Chapter 5

1. G. L. Armstrong, L. A. Conn, and R. W. Pinner, 'Trends in Infectious Disease Mortality in the United States during the 20th Century', *Journal of the American Medical Association*, 281 (1999), 61–6.

2. Harold Coy, *The Americans: A Story about People Democracy, Free Schools, Ice Cream, Airplanes, Social Security, Penicillin, Atomic Energy and All the Things that Make our Nation Great* (Boston: Little Brown, 1958)

3. A detailed discussion of the concept of the post-war concepts of an industrial revolution is provided by Ernst Homburg in 'De "Tweede Industriële Revolutie": een problematisch historisch concept', *Theoretische Geschiedenis*,

13 (1986), 367–85. For discussions about the use of the concept of a third industrial revolution, I am indebted to Jean-François Auger, Andrew Russell, and Ernst Homburg.

4. For Bernal's most developed articulation of the concept which he had first deployed in his *Science in History* (London: Watts, 1954), see his lecture: John Desmond Bernal, 'Britain's Part in the New Scientific Industrial Revolution' (University of Newcastle-upon-Tyne: Newcastle-upon-Tyne, 1965). This vision had political ramifications too as it was famously deployed by prime ministerial candidate Harold Wilson at the Labour Party conference in 1963.

5. See for instance Alfred Chandler, *Shaping the Industrial Century: The Remarkable Story of the Evolution of the Modern Chemical and Pharmaceutical Industries* (Cambridge, Mass.: Harvard University Press, 2005). On the enthusiasm for 'wonder drugs', see Alan Yoshioka, 'Streptomycin in Postwar Britain: A Cultural History of a Miracle Drug', in M. Gijswijt-Hofstra, G. M. Van Heteren, and E. M. Tansey (eds.), *Biographies of Remedies: Drugs, Medicines and Contraceptives in Dutch and Anglo-American Healing Cultures* (Amsterdam: Rodopi, 2002), 203–27.

6. US Federal Trade Commission, *Economic Report on Antibiotics Manufacture* (Washington, DC: US Government Printing Office, 1958), 67.

7. R. H. Liss and F. R. Batchelor, 'Economic Evaluations of Antibiotic Use and Resistance: A Perspective Report of Task Force 6', *Reviews of Infectious Diseases*, 9 (1987), S297–S312.

8. For Britain see P. G. Davey, R. P. Bax, J. Newey, D. Reeves, D. Rutherford, R. Slack, R. E. Warren, B. Watt, and J. Wilson, 'Growth in the Use of Antibiotics in the Community in England and Scotland in 1980–93', *British Medical Journal*, 312 (9 March 1996), 613. For the USA see Anita G. Carrie and George G. Zhanel, 'Antibacterial Use in Community Practice: Assessing Quantity, Indications and Appropriateness, and Relationship to the Development of Antibacterial Resistance', *Drugs*, 57 (1999), 871–81.

9. This term has been used by Peter Temin, *Taking your Medicine: Drug Regulation in the United States* (Cambridge, Mass.: Harvard University Press, 1980).

10. Herman Goossens, Matus Ferech, Robert Vander Stichele, Monique Elseviers, and the ESAC Project Group, 'Outpatient Antibiotic Use in Europe and Association with Resistance', *The Lancet*, 365 (12 February 2005), 579–87.

11. Seymour E. Harris, *The Economics of American Medicine* (New York: Macmillan, 1964), 171. On the technological revolution in medicine there is of course an enormous literature. See for instance Stanley Joel Reiser, *Medicine and the Reign of Technology* (Cambridge: Cambridge University Press, 1978), 196–22; Stuart Blume, *Insight and Industry: The Dynamics of Technological Change in Medicine* (Cambridge, Mass.: MIT Press, 1992); Ghislaine Lawrence (ed.), *Technologies of Modern Medicine: Proceedings of a Seminar Held at the Science Museum, London, March 1993* (London: Science Museum, 1994); James Le Fanu, *The Rise and Fall of Modern Medicine* (London: Little, Brown, 1999); David Rothman, *Beginnings Count: The Technological Imperative in American Health Care* (Oxford:

Oxford University Press, 1997); Jennifer Stanton (ed.), *Innovations in Health and Medicine: Diffusion and Resistance in the Twentieth Century* (London: Routledge, 2002).

12. David Armstrong, 'Decline of the Hospital: Reconstructing Institutional Dangers', *Sociology of Health and Illness*, 20 (1998), 445–57. The precise growth had been 85% from 263,000 beds in 1938 to 488,000 in 1960.

13. Louise K. Martell, 'Maternity Care during the Post-World War II Baby Boom', *Western Journal of Nursing Research*, 21 (1999), 387–404 (quotation on p. 394).

14. Carl Walter, 'The Personal Factor in Hospital Hygiene', in *Prevention of Hospital Infection* (London: Royal Society of Health, 1963), 37–46.

15. S. D. Elek and P. C. Fleming, 'A New Technique for the Control of Hospital Cross-Infection: Experience with BRL. 1241 in a Maternity Unit', *The Lancet*, 2 (10 September 1960), 569–72; J. Jacobs, T. J. Livsey, and B. J. Stephens, 'Methicillin Spray and Staphylococcal Carriage in a Neonatal Unit', *Journal of Obstetrics and Gynaecology in the British Commonwealth*, 71 (1964), 543–55.

16. This famous description of pneumonia was given by William Osler, *The Principles and Practice of Medicine* (4th edn. New York: Appleton, 1901), 26.

17. C. C. Dauer, 'A Demographic Analysis of Recent Changes in Mortality, Morbidity, and Age Group Distribution in our Population', in Iago Galdston (ed.), *The Impact of the Antibiotics on Medicine and Society*, Monograph 2, Institute of Social and Historical Medicine, New York Academy of Medicine (New York: International Universities Press, 1958), 98–120.

18. Benedict F. Massell, *Rheumatic Fever and Streptococcal Infection: Unravelling the Mysteries of a Dread Disease* (Cambridge, Mass.: Harvard University Press, 1997), 265–75.

19. Joseph Earle Moore, 'Venereology in Transition', *British Journal of Venereal Diseases*, 32 (1956), 217–25.

20. Annet Mooij, *Out of Otherness: Characters and Narrators in the Dutch Venereal Disease Debates 1850–1990*, trans. from the Dutch by Beverley Jackson (Amsterdam: Rodopi, 1998), 179.

21. Moore, 'Venereology in Transition'.

22. W. P. D. Logan, *General Practitioners' Records: An Analysis of the Clinical Records of Eight Practices during the Period April 1951 to March 1952*, GRO Studies on Medical and Population Subjects 7 (London: HMSO, 1953).

23. T. McKeown, *The Role of Medicine: Dream, Mirage or Nemesis?* (London: Nuffield Provincial Hospitals Trust, 1976), 97. See also John B. McKinlay and Sonja M. McKinlay, 'The Questionable Contribution of Medical Measures to the Decline of Mortality in the United States in the Twentieth Century', *Health and Society*, 55 (1977), 405–28. McKeown accepts that his figures aggregate a variety of separately caused conditions, both viral and bacterial, under the

heading 'pneumonia'. On the other hand see the fresh analysis by Scott F. Dowell, Benjamin A. Kupronis, Elizabeth R. Zell, and David K. Shay, 'Mortality from Pneumonia in Children in the United States, 1939 through 1996', *New England Journal of Medicine*, 342 (2000), 1399–407. This attributes a sharp fall in childhood pneumonia deaths during the 1940s to penicillin.

24. The results of the *Economic Report on Antibiotics Manufacture* were further digested by John Parascandola, 'The Introduction of Antibiotics into Therapeutics', in Yosio Kawakita, Shizu Sakai, and Yasuo Otsuka (eds.), *History of Therapy: Proceeding of the 10th Internation Symposium on the Comparative History of Medicine—East and West, September 8–September 15, 1985* (Ishiyaku: Euroamerica, 1990), 261–81.

25. For Britain see W. Logan and E. Brook, *The Survey of Sickness 1943–1952*, Studies of Medical and Population Subjects 12 (London: HMSO, 1957). The shifts in use of doctors is described by David Morrell, 'As I Recall', *British Medical Journal*, 317 (1998), 40–5. More broadly see Paul Starr, *The Social Transformation of American Medicine* (New York: Basic Books, 1982); Ellen M. Immergut, *Health Politics: Interests and Institutions in Western Europe* (Cambridge: Cambridge University Press, 1992).

26. Ritchie Calder, *Medicine and Man: The History of the Art and Science of Healing* (London: George Allen and Unwin, 1958), 204.

27. J. M. Andrews and A. D. Langmuir, 'The Philosophy of Disease Eradication', *American Journal of Public Health*, 53 (1963), 1–6. They were not alone; see T. A. Cockburn, *The Evolution and Eradication of Infectious Diseases* (Baltimore: Johns Hopkins University Press, 1963); Socrates Litsios, 'René J. Dubos and Fred L. Soper: Their Contrasting Views on Vector and Disease Eradication', *Perspectives in Biology and Medicine*, 41 (1997), 138–49; F. L. Soper, 'Rehabilitation of the Eradication Concept in Prevention of Communicable Diseases', *Public Health Reports*, 80 (1965), 855–69.

28. C. J. Hackett, 'Yaws', in E. Sabben-Clare, D. J. Bradley, and K. Kirkwood (eds.), *Health in Tropical Africa during the Colonial Period: Based on the Proceedings of a Symposium Held at New College Oxford 21–23 March 1977* (Oxford: Oxford University Press, 1980), 62–92.

29. Marc H. Dawson, 'The Social History of Africa in the Future', *African Studies Review*, 30 (1987), 83–91.

30. Theodor Rosebury, *Microbes and Morals: The Strange History of Venereal Disease* (London: Secker and Warburg, 1971), 267; T. Guthe and J. L. de Vries, 'Surveillance Reports: Epidemiological/Serological Evaluation of Tropical Yaws Following Mass Penicillin Campaigns', World Health Organization, GES/SR/662 WHO/VDT/66.336.

31. The consequences would be complex, for early yaws infections protected against syphilis, which is an even worse disease, and a future generation would grow up without the syphilis immunity. Dawson, 'The Social History of Africa in the Future'.

32. Newell Stewart, 'Pharmaceutical Concatenations', Maine Pharmaceutical Association Convention, 12–14 Sept. 1959.

33. L. P. Garrod, 'The Waning Power of Penicillin', *British Medical Journal*, 2 (1947), 874.

34. Bryan Williams, 'Discussion', *Journal of Obstetrics and Gynaecology in the British Empire*, 67 (1960), 738.

35. R. H. Moser, *Diseases of Medical Progress* (Springfield, Ill.: Charles Thomas, 1959), 8. Attention to Moser's work was drawn by James C. Whorton, '"Antibiotic Abandon": The Resurgence of Therapeutic Rationalism', in John Parascandola (ed.), *The History of Antibiotics: A Symposium* (Madison: American Institute of the History of Pharmacy, 1980), 125–36.

36. Malcolm Muggeridge, 'London Diary', *New Statesman* (3 August 1962), 139–40.

37. Michael Winstanley in 'Medicine Bill', *Parliamentary Debates* (Commons), 5th ser. 758 (1967–8), col. 1633. On the talismanic appeal of drugs see also Yoshioka, 'Streptomycin in Postwar Britain: A Cultural History of a Miracle Drug'.

38. Talcott Parsons, *The Social System* (London: Routledge and Kegan Paul, 1951).

39. Claudine Herzlich and Janine Pierret, *Illness and Self in Society*, trans. Elborg Forster (Baltimore: Johns Hopkins University Press, 1987), 38–48.

40. Alan Radley, *Making Sense of Illness* (London: Sage, 1994), 59; Ruthbeth Finerman and Linda A. Bennett, 'Guilt, Blame and Shame: Responsibility in Health and Sickness', *Social Science and Medicine*, 40 (1995), 1–3; Dorothy Nelkin and Sander Gilman, 'Placing Blame for Devastating Disease', *Social Research*, 55 (1988), 361–78; Mildred Blaxter, 'Whose Fault is It? People's Own Conceptions of the Reasons for Health Inequalities', *Social Science and Medicine*, 10 (1997), 747–56; Mildred Blaxter, 'Why do Victims Blame Themselves', in Alan Radley (ed.), *Worlds of Illness: Biographical and Cultural Perspectives on the Worlds of Illness* (London: Routledge, 1993), 124–42 (p. 129); R. Pill and N. C. H. Stott, 'Concepts of Illness Causation and Responsibility: Some Preliminary Data from a Sample of Working Class Mothers', *Social Science and Medicine*, 16 (1982), 43–52; eid., 'Preventive Procedures and Practices among Working-Class Women: New Data and Fresh Insights', *Social Science and Medicine*, 21 (1985), 975–93; Margot Jefferys, J. H. Brotherton, and Ann Cartwright, 'Consumption of Medicines on a Working-Class Housing Estate', *British Journal of Preventive and Social Medicine*, 14 (1960), 64–76; R. Williams, *A Protestant Legacy: Attitudes to Death and Illness among Older Aberdonians* (Oxford: Clarendon Press, 1990).

41. This research used the Health and Personal Styles 1989 data set (made accessible in 1997, original paper records and electronic data file). These data were collected and donated by Dr Margie Lachman and Dr Jackie James and are made available through the archive of the Henry A. Murray Research

Center of the Radcliffe Institute for Advanced Study, Harvard University, Cambridge, Mass. (Producer and Distributor). The study was based upon questionnaires issued to 150 men and women accessed through a variety of economically diverse treatment centres operated by a health membership organization in the greater Boston area.

42. These results are based on my own reanalysis of the original data.

43. C. G. Helman, '"Feed a Cold, Starve a Fever": Folk Models of Infection in an English Suburban Community, and their Relation to Medical Treatment', *Culture, Medicine and Psychiatry*, 2 (1978), 107–37.

44. Sue Ellen Hoy, *Chasing Dirt: The American Pursuit of Cleanliness* (New York: Oxford University Press, 1995), 179.

45. See Simon Garfield, *Our Hidden Lives: The Remarkable Diaries of Post-War Britain* (London: Ebury, 2005).

46. H. Walker to Sir Austin Strutt, 23 September 1953, HO 302/10, National Archives, UK; See also C. S. Nicol, 'Venereal Diseases: Moral Standards and Public Opinion', *British Journal of Venereal Diseases*, 39 (1963), 169–70. Richard Davenport-Hines, *Sex, Death and Punishment: Attitudes to Sex and Sexuality in Britain since the Renaissance* (London: Collins, 1990).

47. See Mary Lines, 'From Wonder Drug to Potential Killer: Penicillin Allergies, 1941 to 1960', M.Sc. thesis, London Centre for the History of Science, Technology and Medicine, University of London, 1999.

48. *Federal Food, Drug and Cosmetic Act: Hearings before the Committee on Interstate and Foreign Commerce, House of Representatives*, 82nd Congress, 1st session, on HR 3298, A Bill to Amend Section sec503(b) of the Federal Food, Drug and Cosmetic Act (Washington, DC: US Government Printing Office, 1951).

49. George L. Waldbott, 'Anaphylactic Death from Penicillin', *Journal of the American Medical Association*, 139 (1949), 526–7; Henry Welch, 'Antibiotics 1943–1955: Their Development and Role in Present-Day Society', in Galdston (ed.), *The Impact of the Antibiotics on Medicine and Society*, 70–87 (see pp. 79–80).

50. O. Idsøe and T. Guthe, 'Penicillin Side Reactions and Fatalities', presented at the 5th International Congress of Chemotherapy, Vienna, 26 June to 1 July 1967, WHO paper WHO/VDT/67.340.

51. Gordon T. Stewart, Brian T. Butcher, and John P. McGovern, 'Penicillin Allergy: The Nature of the Problem', in Gordon T. Stewart and John P. McGovern (eds.), *Penicillin Allergy: Clinical and Immunologic Aspects* (Springfield, Ill.: Charles C. Thomas, 1970), 176–91 (p. 189).

52. Toby Helm, 'Tragic Allergy to Light Drives Kohl Wife to Suicide', *Daily Telegraph*, 6 July 2001.

53. On Taiwan see Arthur Kleinmann, *Patients and Healers in the Context of Culture* (Berkeley and Los Angeles: University of California Press, 1980), 287–8, where he describes the searing effect on Taiwanese doctors of the experience of allergic reactions and for the response Y. J. Chou, W. C. Yip, N. Huang, Y. P. Sun, and H. J. Chang, 'Impact of Separating Drug Prescribing and Dispensing on Provider

Behaviour: Taiwan's Experience', *Health Policy and Planning*, A. 18 (2003), 316–29. For Japan, R. Fujii, 'Changes in Antibiotic Consumption in Japan during the Past 40 Years', *Japanese Journal of Antibiotics*, 37 (1984), 2261–70. He shows declining use in the mid–1950s in response to allergic reactions.

54. Details of the prices and profits of penicillin are presented in detail in US Federal Trade Commission, *Economic Report on Antibiotics Manufacture*. In 1950 one major company made net profits on its antibiotic operations equivalent to 101% of its assets (p. 215).

55. Bristol-Myers Company, General Executive Committee Meeting of Operating Heads dated 25 May 1953, p. 1, CX 958, 7211-1-2-1 box 201, RG122, US National Archives.

56. Cross-examination of Mr John Tuohy, General Manager of Squibb, Tr 2956–57, 7211-2-5 Box 219, RG122; for the Pfizer opinion see 'Statement by John McKean, President of Charles Pfizer & Co.', quoted in US Senate, Subcommittee on Antitrust and Monopoly, *Report of the Study on Administered Prices in the Drug Industry*, 87th Congress, 1st session, 1961, pp. 81–8.

57. On the work of Waksman and the Waksman school see the personal account of one of its distinguished members (and discoverer of neomycin) Hubert Lechevalier, 'The Search for Antibiotics at Rutgers University', in John Parascandola (ed.), *The History of Antibiotics: A Symposium* (Madison: American Institute for the History of Pharmacy, 1980), 113–24. The role of Waksman himself in the discovery of streptomycin was highly contested. See William Kingston, 'Streptomycin, Schatz v. Waksman, and the Balance of Credit for Discovery', *Journal of the History of Medicine and Allied Sciences*, 59 (2004), 441–62.

58. Waksman defined an antibiotic as 'inhibiting the growth or the metabolic activities of bacteria and other micro-organisms by a chemical substance of microbial origin'. See Selman Waksman, 'What is an Antibiotic or Antibiotic Substance?', *Mycologia*, 39 (1947), 565–9.

59. Peter Costello, 'The Tetracycline Conspiracy: Structure, Conduct and Performance in the Drug Industry', *Antitrust Law and Economics Review*, 1 (1968), 13–44; E. J. Kahn Jr., *All in a Century: The First Hundred Years of Eli Lilly and Company* (Indianapolis: Eli Lilly, 1976), 133.

60. The history of chloramphenicol has been studied in detail by Thomas Maeder, *Adverse Reactions* (New York: William Morrow, 1994). See also Wesley W. Spink, *Infectious Diseases: Prevention and Treatment in the Nineteenth and Twentieth Centuries* (London: W. M. Dawson, 1978), 116–21; Henry Welch and Felix Marti-Ibanez, *The Antibiotic Saga* (New York: Medical Encyclopedia, 1960).

61. Mildred Savage, *In Vivo* (London: Longmans, 1965; first published 1964). Marvin Johnson wrote to Ernest Weber of Pfizer commending the accuracy with which the book captured the atmosphere of the early days of antibiotics. Johnson to Weber, 2 July 1964, Johnson papers, University of Wisconsin, Madison.

62. The history of Terramycin development is told by Samuel Mines, *Pfizer: An Informal History* (New York: Pfizer, 1978), 110–21.

63. Costello, 'The Tetracycline Conspiracy: Structure, Conduct and Performance in the Drug Industry'. See also Peter Temia, *Taking your Medicine: Drug Regulation in the United States* (Cambridge, Mass.: Harvard University Press, 1980), 70–2.

64. The story is recounted by Richard E. McFadyen, 'The FDA's Regulation and Control of Antibiotics in the 1950s: The Henry Welch Scandal, Felix Marti-Ibanez, and Charles Pfizer & Co.', *History of Medicine*, 53 (1979), 159–69. However McFadyen did not have the benefit of the interviews with FDA staff conducted subsequently. Moreover, he saw this merely as an account of corruption without reflecting on the unexpectedness of Welch's income. This account benefits from the interview with Dr Lloyd C. Miller by Fred L. Lofsvold, 27 January 1981, FDA Oral History Project, History of Medicine Division, NLM, pp. 30–4. He also does not seem to have had access to the original correspondence now in the 44 FRC 17, US National Archives. However nearly all the correspondence was published by the Committee in an entire volume of reproduced letters, US Senate, *Administered Prices. Hearings before Subcommitee on Antitrust and Monopoly*, 86th Congress, 2nd session, pt. 23. On his partner Felix Ibanez see H. A. Bogdan, 'Felix Marti Ibanez—Iberian Daedalus: The Man behind the Essays', *Journal of the Royal Society of Medicine*, 86 (1993), 593–6.

65. Lloyd C. Miller, interview.

66. Louis Lasagna, *The Doctor's Dilemmas* (New York: Harper, 1962), 131. Turnover had increased from $149 million to $1,677 million.

67. Milton Moskowitz, 'Wonder Profits in Wonder Drugs', *The Nation*, 184 (1957), 357.

68. Newell Stewart, 'Pharmaceutical Concatenations', Maine Pharmaceutical Association Convention, 12–14 Sept. 1959.

69. Jeffrey Sturchio (ed.), *Values and Visions: A Merck Century* (Rahway, NJ: Merck, 1991), 185.

70. Du Pont sales are given in David Hounshell and John K. Smith, *Science and Corporate Strategy: Du Pont R & D, 1902–1980* (Cambridge: Cambridge University Press, 1988), 602. On Merck see Sturchio, *Values and Visions*, 185. In 1998 Du Pont sales were $24.7 billion, see *Du Pont Annual Report* (1998), 2; the sales of Merck that year were 26.8 billion, 1998 *Annual Report*, 3.

71. Julius J. Mastro, 'The Pharmaceutical Manufacturers' Association. The Ethical Drug Industry and the 1962 Drug Amendments: A Case Study of Congressional Action and Interest Group Reaction', Ph.D. thesis, New York University, 1965, p. 72.

72. US Federal Trade Commission, *Economic Report on Antibiotics Manufacture*, 139.

73. C. K. Piercy to H. Wendt, Cyanamid File Copy, 1–25 RACX 755 11942, US FTC Docket No. 7211, Box 248, RG122, US National Archives.

74. *Emergency Ward 10 Girls Annual* (London: Purnell, 1963), 60.

75. 'Trends in the Supply and Demand of Medical Care', Study Paper No. 5, US Congress Joint Economic Committee, 10 November 1959 (Washington, DC: US Government Printing Office, 1959), cited by Daniel M. Fox, *Health Policies,*

Health Politics: The British and American Experience 1911–1965 (Princeton: Princeton University Press, 1986), 199–200.

76. Herman Miles Somers and Anne Ramsay Somers, *Doctors, Patients, and Health Insurance: The Organization and Financing of Medical Care* (Washington, DC: Brookings Institution, 1961), table A–9, p. 545.
77. Costs of prescriptions and the ensuing crisis are described by Charles Webster, *The Problems of Health Care: The National Health Service before 1957*, vol. i of *The National Health Services since the War* (London: HMSO, 1988), 223.
78. See Robert Bud, 'Antibiotics, Big Business and Consumers', *Technology and Culture*, 46 (2005), 329–49.
79. Question put by Rand Dixon, United States Congress, Senate Committee on the Judiciary. Subcommittee on Antitrust and Monopoly, *Administered Prices in the Drug Industry (Antibiotics)*, pt. 24, p. 13671.
80. William S. Comanor, 'The Political Economy of the Pharmaceutical Industry', *Journal of Economic Literature*, 24 (1986), 1178–217.
81. Richard E. MacFadyen, 'Thalidomide in America: A Brush with Tragedy', *Clio Medica*, 11(1976), 79–93.
82. On the history of thalidomide see Beate Kirk, *Der Contergan-Fall: Eine unvermeidbare Arzneimittelkatastrophe* (Stuttgart: Wissenschafts-Verlag, 1999).
83. MacFadyen, 'Thalidomide in America: A Brush with Tragedy'.
84. Mrs Stella Lief, 'Chairman's Address', Annual Meeting of the National Antivaccination League, *Vaccination Observer* (July–September 1963), 26–7.
85. 'Joyce Butler', obituary in *The Times*, 8 January 1992.
86. Joyce Butler, Parliamentary Sessions, 30 October 1962–24 October 1963.
87. Carol Moberg and Zanvil Cohn, 'René Jules Dubos', *Scientific American* (May 1991), 58–65. C. L. Moberg, 'René Dubos: A Harbinger of Microbial Resistance to Antibiotics', *Microbial Drug Resistance*, 2 (1996), 287–97.
88. René Dubos, interview with Saul Benison, 1955–6, transcript, Columbia University Oral History Research Office, New York, 10 volumes combining interview transcript with offprints, viii. 564 led to René Dubos, 'The Philosopher's Search for Health', *Transactions of the Association of American Physicians*, 66 (1953), 31–41.
89. René Dubos, *Mirage of Health: Utopias, Progress, and Biological Change* (New York: Harper & Row, 1959), 161–2.
90. This phrase was coined by Dubos as an adviser to the 1972 United Nations Conference on the Human Environment. R. A. Eblen and W. Eblen, *The Encyclopedia of the Environment* (Boston: Houghton Mifflin, 1994), 702.

Chapter 6

1. E. A. North and R. Christie, 'Observations on the Sensitivity of Staphylococci to Penicillin', *Medical Journal of Australia*, 2 (1945), 44–6.

2. Craig H. Steffen, 'Penicillins and Staphylococci: A Historical Interaction', *Perspectives in Biology and Medicine*, 35 (1991–2), 596–608; Donald I. McGraw, 'The Golden Staph: Medicine's Response to the Challenge of the Resistant Staphylococci in the Mid-Twentieth Century', *Dynamis*, 4 (1984), 219–37.

3. L. P. Garrod, 'Mary Barber 3 April 1911–11 September 1965', *Journal of Pathology and Bacteriology*, 92 (1966), 603–10; Mary Barber, 'Staphylococcal Infection Due to Antibiotic-Resistant Strains', *British Medical Journal*, 2 (1947), 863–5 and a long sequence of further works.

4. Mary Barber, 'The Incidence of Penicillin Sensitive Variant Colonies in Penicillinase Producing Strains of *Staphylococcus aureus*', *Journal of General Microbiology*, 3 (1949), 274.

5. Richard Harris, *The Real Voice* (New York: Macmillan, 1964), 18–19.

6. R. T. Ravenholt and G. D. La Veck, 'Staphylococcal Disease: An Obstetric, Pediatric and Community Problem', *American Journal of Public Health*, 46 (1956), 1287–96.

7. M. Finland, W. J. Jones Jr., and M. W. Barnes, 'Occurrence of Serious Bacterial Infections since Introduction of Antibacterial Agents', *Journal of the American Medical Association*, 170 (1959), 2188–97.

8. See for example Robert Williams, 'Hospital Infection', in Philips S. Brachman and Theodore C. Eickhoff (eds.), *Proceedings of the International Conference on Nosocomial Infections, Center for Disease Control, August 3–6 1970* (Chicago: American Hospital Association, 1971), 1–10.

9. Ravenholt and La Veck, 'Staphylococcal Disease: An Obstetric, Pediatric and Community Problem'.

10. Mary Barber, 'Drug-Resistant Staphylococcal Infection', *Journal of Obstetrics and Gynaecology in the British Empire*, 67 (1960), 727–32.

11. Phyllis M. Rountree, 'History of Staphylococcal Infection in Australia', *Medical Journal of Australia*, 2 (1978), 543–6. Rountree described her career in a 1991 oral history conducted by Kerry Gordon, Victoria Barker (ed.), 'Phyllis Margaret Rountree', University Interviews Project, University of New South Wales Archive.

12. R. E. O. Williams, 'Investigations of Hospital-Acquired Staphylococcal Disease and its Control in Great Britain', *Proceedings of the National Conference on Hospital-Acquired Staphylococcal Disease, Sponsored by US PHS and NAS Atlanta Georgia* (Washington, DC: US DHEW, CDC, 1958), 11–29.

13. Jonathan S. Nguyen-Van-Tam and Alan W. Hampson, 'The Epidemiology and Clinical Impact of Pandemic Influenza', *Vaccine*, 21 (2003), 1762–8.

14. N. C. Oswald, R. A. Shooter, and M. P. Curwen, 'Pneumonia Complicating Asian Influenza', *British Medical Journal*, 2 (29 November 1958), 1305–11; 'Deaths from Asian Influenza, 1957: A Report by the Public Health Laboratory Service Based on Records from Hospital and Public Health Laboratories', *British Medical Journal*, 1 (19 April 1958), 915–18; Walsh McDermott, 'The Problem of Staphylococcal Infection', *British Medical Journal*, 2 (13 October 1956), 837–40.

15. Ministry of Health, *The Influenza Epidemic in England and Wales 1957–1958*, Reports on Public Health and Medical Subjects No. 100 (London: HMSO, 1960); C. C. Dauer and R. E. Scrfling, 'Mortality from Influenza, 1957–1958 and 1959–1960', *American Review of Respiratory Diseases*, 83 (1961), 15–28.

16. Oswald, Shooter, and Curwen, 'Pneumonia Complicating Asian Influenza'.

17. 'Influenzal Pneumonia', *British Medical Journal*, 2 (29 November 1958), 1342–3.

18. Barbara Rosencrantz, 'Coverage of Antibiotic Resistance in the Popular Literature 1950 to 1994', appendix to Office of Technology Assessment, *Impacts of Antibiotic-Resistant Bacteria: 'Thanks to Penicillin, He will Come Home!'*, Publication OTA-H-6297 (Washington, DC: Office of Technology Assessment; 1995).

19. Stanley Schneierson, 'Hazards of Antibiotics', *Consumer Reports* (April 1953), 162–4.

20. The events were summarized by Richard I. Wise, Elizabeth A. Ossman, and Dwight R. Littlefield, 'Personal Reflections on Nosocomial Infections and the Development of Hospital Surveillance', *Reviews of Infectious Diseases*, 11 (1989), 1005–19.

21. Standing Medical Advisory Committee, Central Health Services Council, *Staphylococcal Infections in Hospitals: Report of the Subcommittee* (London: HMSO, 1959), 1.

22. Eleazar Lipsky, *The Scientists* (London: Longman Green, 1959), 265.

23. Sir George Godber, 'Opening Address', in *Prevention of Hospital Infection: The Personal Factor. Report of a Conference Held in London on 19 June 1963* (London: Royal Society of Health, 1963), 1–3. There is considerable evidence that many ordinary clinicians were indeed unaware of the scale of the problem. See Steffen, 'Penicillins and Staphylococci'.

24. Toine Pieters, *Interferon: The Science and Selling of a Miracle Drug* (London: Routledge, 2004).

25. G. E. W. Wolstenholme and Cecilia M. O'Connor (eds.), *The CIBA Foundation Symposium on Drug Resistance in Micro-organisms: Mechanisms of Development* (London: J. & A. Churchill, 1957).

26. Sir Charles Harington, 'Opening Remarks', ibid. 3.

27. E. B. Chain, 'Penicillinase Resistant Penicillins and the Problern of the Penicillin Resistant Staphylococci', in A. V. S. De Reuck and Margaret P. Cameron (eds.), *Resistance of Bacteria to the Penicillins: In Honour of Sir Charles Harington*, Ciba Foundation Study Group 13 (London: J. & A. Churchill, 1962), 3–18 (p. 5).

28. J. Sheehan, 'Discussion', ibid. 24.

29. E. P. Abraham and P. B. Loder, 'History of Cephalosporin C', in E. H. Flynn (ed.), *Cephalosporins and Penicillins: Chemistry and Biology* (New York, Academic Press, 1972), 3–11; E. P. Abraham, 'Some Aspects of the History of the Penicillins and Cephalosporins', Invitational ONR Lecture, *Journal of Industrial Microbiology and Biotechnology*, 22 (1999), 275–87.

30. Brotzu's journal was entitled *The Works of the Institute of Hygiene of Cagliari*.
31. While there had been attempts to modify penicillin before, begun at the Northern Regional Research Laboratory in Peoria, the Peoria team, which focused on the hydroxyl group of Penicillin X, took a less fruitful direction than their European colleagues and were not successful in developing new therapeutic compounds. R. D. Coghill, F. H. Stodola, and J. L. Wachtel, 'Chemical Modifications of Natural Penicillins', in Hans T. Clarke, John R. Johnson, and Sir Robert Robinson (eds.), *The Chemistry of Penicillin* (Princeton: Princeton University Press, 1949), 680–7.
32. I am grateful to Professor Ballio for discussing this with me.
33. For background work on para-aminobenzyl penicillin see Glebb A. Brewer and Marvin J. Johnson, 'Activity and Properties of Para-aminobenzyl Penicillin', *Applied Microbiology*, 1 (1953), 163–6.
34. H. G. Lazell, *From Pills to Penicillin: The Beecham Story—a Personal Account* (London: Heinemann, 1975), 62.
35. Lazell, ibid. 140–4 reproduces the minutes of a 1955 meeting which set Beecham on the path to penicillin.
36. These experiments are described by F. P. Doyle, 'Some Contributions to Chemotherapy', *Särtryck ur Farmaceutisk Revy*, 62 (1963), 443–63.
37. Doyle, ibid. 451 provides the detailed figures of their experiments.
38. The notebook describing these experiments has been donated to the Science Museum where it is kept as accession number 1996–309. J. H. Nayler, 'Early Discoveries in the Penicillin Series', *Trends in the Biochemical Sciences*, 16 (1991), 195–7 and Doyle, 'Some Contributions to Chemotherapy'. Doyle explains that the material added was sodium carbonate and a solution of phenylacetyl chloride in acetone.
39. A. Ballio, E. B. Chain, D. I. Dentice, F. Accadia, G. N. Rolinson, and F. R. Batchelor, 'Penicillin Derivatives of p-aminobenzylpenicillin', *Nature*, 183 (17 January 1959), 180–1. 6-APA has the chemical name 6 amino penicillanic acid.
40. Kinichiro Sawao and Sakaguchi Murao, 'A Preliminary Report on a New Enzyme, "Penicillin-amidase" ', *Journal of Agricultural Chemical Society* (Japan), 23 (1950), 411; K. Kato, 'Occurrence of Penicillin-Nucleus in Culture Broths', *Journal of Antibiotics*, 6 (1953), 130–6; K. Kato, 'Further Notes on Penicillin-Nucleus', *Journal of Antibiotics*, 6 (1953), 184–5. See Sydney Selwyn, *The Beta-lactam Antibiotics: Penicillins and Cephalosporins in Perspective* (London: Hodder and Stoughton, 1980).
41. Lazell, *From Pills to Penicillin*, 149.
42. The story of Sheehan is told in his *Enchanted Ring: The Untold Story of Penicillin* (Cambridge, Mass.: MIT Press, 1982).
43. Lazell, *From Pills to Penicillin*, 166. The first product, phenethicillin, had the chemical name phenoxyethyl penicillin. See David Wilson *Penicillin in Perspective* (London: Faber & Faber, 1976), 266–68.

44. For criticism of the Beecham approach see 'A New Penicillin', *British Medical Journal*, 2 (7 November 1959), 940.

45. Chapman Pincher, 'The Big Penicillin Robbery', *Daily Express*, 6 November 1959.

46. Steffen,'Penicillins and Staphylococci'; McGraw, 'The Golden Staph'

47. See E. M. Tansey and L. R. Reynolds (eds.), *Post-Penicillin Antibiotics, from Acceptance to Resistance?*, Wellcome Witnesses to Twentieth Century Medicine 6 (London: Wellcome Institute for the History of Medicine, 2000), 31.

48. I am grateful to George Rolinson for the account of the testing of methicillin. The drug was initially marketed by Beecham as Celbenin after the initials of the subsidiary which made it, C. L. Bencard.

49. Tansey and Reynolds (eds.), *Post-Penicillin Antibiotics*, 30 and 34.

50. William L. Laurence, 'Drug for Staph: Widespread Germ Succumbs to a New Synthetic Penicillin', *New York Times* (12 March 1961), section 4.

51. H. Koprowski, 'Future of Infectious and Malignant Diseases', in Gordon Wolstenholme (ed.), *Man and his Future* (London: Ciba Foundation, 1963), 196–216.

52. Mary Barber, ' "Celbenin"-Resistant Staphylococci', *British Medical Journal*, 2 (24 September 1960), 939; Patricia Jevons wrote of her findings in ' "Celbenin"-Resistant Staphylococci', *British Medical Journal*, 1 (14 January 1961), 124–5.

53. G. T. Stewart, ' "Celbenin"-Resistant Staphylococci', *British Medical Journal*, 2 (8 October 1960), 1085.

54. Ernest Earl, *Queen Mary's Hospital for Children* (Knebworth: Able, 1996). The atmosphere in such institutions was summarized by the campaigner and former worker at Queen Mary's Maureen Oswin in her *The Empty Hours: A Study of the Week-End Life of Handicapped Children in Institutions* (Harmondsworth: Penguin, 1973).

55. G. T. Stewart and R. J. Rolt, 'Evolution of Natural Resistance to the Newer Penicillins', *British Medical Journal*, 1 (2 February 1963), 308–11.

56. K. Riewerts Eriksen and Ingrid Eriksen, 'Resistance to Newer Penicillins', *British Medical Journal*, 1 (16 March 1963), 746.

57. 'Future of Methicillin', *British Medical Journal*, 1 (2 February 1963), 280–2.

58. F. F. Barrett, R. F. McGehee, and M. Finland, 'Methicillin-Resistant *Staphylococcus aureus* at Boston City Hospital', *New England Journal of Medicine*, 279 (1968), 441–8.

59. M. C. Enright, D. A. Robinson, G. Randle, E. J. Feil, H. Grundmann, and B. G. Spratt, 'The Evolutionary History of Methicillin-Resistant *Staphylococcus aureus* (MRSA)', *Proceedings of the National Academy of Science*, 99 (2002), 7687–92.

60. Stuart Mudd, 'Staphylococcic Infections in the Hospital and Community', *Journal of the American Medical Association*, 166 (1956), 1177–8.

61. Elizabeth Temkin, 'Rooming-in: Redesigning Hospitals and Motherhood in Cold War America', *Bulletin of the History of Medicine*, 76 (2002), 271–98.

62. See Williams, 'Hospital Infection'.

63. Lazell, *From Pills to Penicillin*, 169.

64. Stuart B. Levy, 'Survey of a Conference: Turista or not Turista', in Stuart B. Levy, Royston B. Clowes, and Ellen L. Koenig (eds.), *International Plasmid Conference on Molecular Biology, Pathogenicity and Ecology of Bacterial Plasmids* (New York: Plenum Press, 1981), 676–7.

65. Marc Lappé, *Germs that Won't Die: Medical Consequences of the Misuse of Antibiotics* (Garden City, NY: Anchor Press, 1982), 131.

66. H. Lundbeck, U. Plazsikowski, and L. Silverstolpe, 'The Swedish Salmonella Outbreak of 1953', *Journal of Applied Bacteriology*, 18 (1955), 535–48.

67. George N. Rolinson, 'Forty Years of β-lactam Research', *Journal of Antimicrobial Chemotherapy*, 41 (1998), 589–603.

68. Lipsky, *The Scientists*.

69. Richard Wise, 'β-Lactamase Inhibitors', *Journal of Antimicrobial Chemotherapy*, 9 (1982), Supp. B: 31–40.

70. G. N. Rolinson, 'Evolution of β-Lactamase Inhibitors', *Review of Infectious Diseases*, 13 (1991), Supp.: 727–32.

71. 'Doctors Get the "Superbug" Drug', *Daily Mail*, 17 September 1981.

72. See Rolinson, 'Evolution of β-Lactamase Inhibitors'.

73. Keith Klugman, 'Pneumococcal Resistance to Antibiotics', *Clinical Microbiology Reviews*, 3 (1990), 171–96.

74. Vincent A. Fischetti, 'The Streptococcus and the Host: Present and Future Challenges', *Advances in Experimental Medicine and Biology*, 418 (1997), 15–20.

75. Charles F. Gilks, 'HIV and Pneumococcal Infection in Africa: Clinical, Epidemiological and Preventative Aspects', *Transactions of the Royal Society of Tropical Medicine and Hygiene*, 91 (1997), 627–31.

76. 'Acute Respiratory Infections: The Forgotten Pandemic. Communiqué from the International Conference on Acute Respiratory Infections, Held in Canberra, Australia, 7–10 July 1997', *International Journal of Tuberculosis and Lung Diseases*, 2 (1998), 2–4.

77. Stephen Berman, 'Otitis Media in Developing Countries', *Pediatrics*, 96 (1995), 126–31.

78. J. W. Kislak, L. M. B. Razavi, A. K. Daly, and M. Finland, 'Susceptibility of Pneumococci to Nine Antibiotics', *American Journal of Medical Science*, 250 (1965), 261–8.

79. D. Hansman and M. M. Bullen, 'A Resistant Pneumococcus', *The Lancet*, 2 (29 July 1967), 264–5.

80. D. Hansman, 'Type Distribution and Antibiotic Sensitivity of Pneumococci from Carriers in Kiriwina, Trobriand Islands (New Guinea)', *Medical Journal of Australia*, 14 (1972), 771–3.

81. Hendrik J. Koornhof, Avril Wasas, and Keith Klugman, 'Antimicrobial Resistance in *Streptococcus pneumoniae*: A South African Perspective', *Clinical Infectious Diseases*, 15 (1992), 84–94.

82. Robert Austrian, 'Confronting Drug-Resistant Pneumococci', *Annals of Internal Medicine*, 121 (1994), 807–9.

83. Fernando Baquero, 'Pneumococcal Resistance to β-lactam Antibiotics: A Global Geographic Overview', *Microbial Drug Resistance*, 1 (1995), 115–20.

84. J. Casal, A. Fenol, M. D. Vicioso, and R. Munoz, 'Increase in Resistance to Penicillin in Pneumococci in Spain', *The Lancet*, 1 (1 April 1989), 735.

85. Raquel Sá-Leão, Sigurdur E. Vilhelmsson, Hermınia de Lencastre, Karl G. Kristinsson, and Alexander Tomasz, 'Diversity of Penicillin-Nonsusceptible Streptococcus pneumoniae Circulating in Iceland after the Introduction of Penicillin-Resistant Clone Spain 6B-2', *Journal of Infectious Diseases*, 186 (2002), 966–75.

86. D. Felmingham and J. Washington, 'Trends in the Antimicrobial Susceptibility of Bacterial Respiratory Tract Pathogens: Findings of the Alexander Project 1992–1996', *Journal of Chemotherapy*, 11 (1999), Suppl. 1: 5–21.

87. Baquero, 'Pneumococcal Resistance to β-lactam Antibiotics: A Global Geographic Overview'.

88. Klugman, 'Pneumococcal Resistance to Antibiotics'.

89. Lazell, *From Pills to Penicillin*, 169.

90. W. L. Hewitt, 'Penicillin: Historical Impact on Infection Control', *Annals of the New York Academy of Sciences*, 145 (1967), 212–15. On the subsequent growth to 1971 see H. E. Simmons and Paul D. Stolley, 'This is Medical Progress? Trends and Consequences of Antibiotic Use in the United States', *Journal of the American Medical Association*, 227 (1974), 1023–8.

91. For US patterns of antibiotic use 1980–92, see Linda F. McCaig and James M. Hughes, 'Trends in Antimicrobial Drug Prescribing among Office-Based Physicians in the United States', *Journal of the American Medical Association*, 273 (1995), 214–19. This shows that in 1992 the penicillins, including amoxicillin and ampicillin, still constituted about 40% of outpatient antibacterial prescriptions, and for 1992–2000 see Linda F. McCaig, Richard E. Besser, and James M. Hughes, 'Antimicrobial Drug Prescription in Ambulatory Care Settings, United States, 1992–2000', *Emerging Infectious Diseases*, 9 (2003), 432–7.

Chapter 7

1. Milan Čižman, 'The Use and Resistance to Antibiotics in the Community', *International Journal of Antimicrobial Agents*, 21 (2003), 297–307; see also James Trostle, 'Inappropriate Distribution of Medicines by Professionals in Developing Countries', *Social Science and Medicine*, 42 (1996), 1117–20. Thus penicillin and other antibiotics were being widely used to treat the common cold although this is a syndrome caused by a virus unaffected by penicillin. In the USA, the two Harvard physicians reported in 2000 that, of the 51 million visits for 'colds', upper respiratory tract infections, and bronchitis in

the United States in a single year, one-half to two-thirds culminated in an antibiotic prescription.

2. Brian Balogh, 'Reorganising the Organisational Synthesis: Federal–Professional Relations in Modern America', *Studies in American Political Development*, 5 (1991), 119–70.

3. 'Future Control of Penicillin', 3 October 1946, in 'Penicillin Bill', MH 80/42, National Archives, UK.

4. Alexander Fleming to P. Panton, 5 October 1946, 'Penicillin Bill', MH 80/42.

5. Aneurin Bevan, speaking to the 2nd reading of the Penicillin Bill, 9 June 1947, *Parliamentary Debates* (Commons), 5th ser. 438 (1946–7), cols. 821–3.

6. On the Hinchliffe Inquiry and the question of forcing doctors to change prescribing habits see Charles Webster, *Government and Health Care: The National Health Service 1958–1979, vol. ii of The Health Services since the War* (London: The Stationery Office, 1996), 141–8.

7. In discussing the dilemmas of population control, Hardin drew a parallel with the problem of the medieval peasants who shared use of the common land. They each suffered from the progressive deterioration of the land due to overexploitation whereas any one peasant benefited from grazing his cattle as much as possible. Hardin himself suggested that his model fitted the problem of freeloading in domains other than population, for instance pollution. Here again, he suggested, there was the problem of balancing individual rights to produce against the costs to society. Garrett Hardin, 'The Tragedy of the Commons', *Science*, 162 (13 December 1968), 1243–8.

8. Robert D. Putnam, *Bowling Alone: The Collapse and Revival of American Community* (New York; Simon and Schuster, 2000).

9. Seymour Martin Lipset and William Schneider, *The Confidence Gap: Business, Labor and Government in the Public Mind* (New York: Free Press, 1982), 48–9.

10. Ibid. See also Bernice A. Pescosolido, Stephen A. Tuch, and Jack A. Martin, 'The Profession of Medicine and the Public: Examining Americans' Changing Confidence in Physician Authority from the Beginning of the "Health Care Crisis" to the Era of Health Care Reform', *Journal of Health and Social Behavior*, 42 (2001), 1–16.

11. For a review of long-term decline in trust in British politicians see John Curtice and Roger Jowell, 'Trust in the Political System', in Roger Jowell, John Curtice, Alison Park, Lindsay Brook, Katarina Thomson, and Caroline Bryson (eds.), *British Social Attitudes: The 14th Report* (Aldershot: Ashgate, 1997), 89–109; Gerry McKie, 'Patterns of Social Trust in Western Europe and their Genesis', in Karen Cook (ed.), *Trust in Society* (New York: Russell Sage, 2001), 245–82. See also Onora O'Neill, *A Question of Trust* (Cambridge: Cambridge University Press, 2002).

12. Lucy Gilson, 'Trust and the Development of Health Care as a Social Institution', *Social Science and Medicine*, 56 (2003), 1453–68. See also B. Misztal, *Trust in Modern Societies* (Cambridge: Polity Press, 1996). David Mechanic, 'Changing

Medical Organization and the Erosion of Trust, *Milbank Quarterly*, 74 (1996), 171–89.

13. E. L. Koos, *The Health of Regionsville* (New York: Columbia University Press, 1954). I am grateful to Professor S. J. Kunitz of the University of Rochester for the information about Regionsville.

14. Ibid. 54.

15. Charles P. Loomis and J. Allan Beegle, *Rural Social Systems: A Textbook in Rural Sociology and Anthropology* (New York: Prentice Hall, 1950), 712.

16. On the Institute of Community Studies see Jennifer Platt, *Social Research in Bethnal Green* (London: Macmillan, 1971); On the USA see Samuel W. Bloom, *The Word as Scalpel: A History of Medical Sociology* (Oxford: Oxford University Press, 2002); Howard E. Freeman and Leo G. Reeder, 'Medical Sociology: A Review of the Literature', *American Sociological Review*, 22 (1957), 73–81. See also Dorothy Porter (ed.), *Social Medicine and Medical Sociology in the Twentieth Century* (Amsterdam: Rodopi, 1997) and Eliot Freidson, 'The Development of Design by Accident', in R. H. Elling and M. Sokoloska (eds.), *Medical Sociologists at Work* (New Brunswick, NJ: Transaction Books, 1978), 115–32.

17. See for instance J. T. Young, 'Illness Behaviour: A Selective Review and Synthesis', *Sociology of Health and Illness*, 26 (2004), 1–31.

18. Vance Packard, *The Hidden Persuaders* (London: Longman, 1960; first published 1957), 32–4; Ernest Dichter, *Getting Motivated by Ernest Dichter: The Secret Behind Individual Motivations by the Man Who was not Afraid to Ask 'Why?'* (New York: Pergamon Press, 1979).

19. Packard, *The Hidden Persuaders*, 33.

20. Institute for Motivational Analysis, *A Psychological Study of the Doctor–Patient Relationship*, Submitted to California Medical Association (Sacramento: California Medical Association, May 1950), 6.

21. Ibid. 11.

22. Selig Greenberg, 'The Decline of the Healing Art', in Marion Sanders (ed.), *The Crisis in American Medicine* (New York: Harpers, 1960), 20–9.

23. O. L. Peterson, L. P. Andrews, R. S. Spain, and B. G. Greenberg, 'An Analytical Study of North Carolina General Practice', *Journal of Medical Education*, 31 (1956), 1–165 (quotation is from p. 40).

24. 'Doctors See a Split Personality', *Business Week* (22 February 1958), 160–70.

25. Victor Steiger and A. Victor Hansen, 'A Definition of Comprehensive Medicine', *Journal of Health and Human Behavior*, 2 (1961), 82–6.

26. J. Collings, 'General Practice in England Today', *The Lancet*, 1 (25 March 1950), 555–85.

27. Social Surveys (Gallup Poll) Ltd., 'Report on the National Health Service Medical Service: Report Prepared on Behalf of the "The Daily Telegraph"', in *A Review of the Medical Services in Great Britain* (Porritt Report) (London: Social Assay, on behalf of the Medical Services Review Committee, 1963), appendix 3, see table 6, p. 214.

28. Elizabeth Bott, *Family and Social Network* (2nd edn. London: Tavistock, 1971), 14.

29. Mildred Blaxter, *Mothers and Daughters: A Three Generation Study of Health Attitudes and Behaviour* (London: Heinemann, 1982).

30. 'A National Health Service', Mass Observation Report 3140, July 1949, p. 28. Mass Observation Archive, University of Sussex.

31. Institute for Motivational Analysis, *A Research Study on Pharmaceutical Advertising* (New York: Pharmaceutical Advertising Club, 1955), 25.

32. J. S. Coleman, E. Katz, and H. Menzel, *Medical Innovation: A Diffusion Study* (Indianapolis: Bobbs-Merrill, 1966), 12.

33. M. H. Pappworth, 'Human Guinea Pigs: A Warning', *Twentieth Century* (Autumn 1962), 66–75; M. H. Pappworth, *Human Guinea Pigs* (London: Routledge, 1967).

34. In November 1962 a letter was written to a British Sunday newspaper, the *Sunday Times*, complaining about news of an experiment of a new drug on twenty-one pregnant women, and this led directly to the formation of the Association. See Helen Hodgson, 'A Patients' Group', *Sunday Times*, 25 November 1962. Also 'The Voice of the Patient', *Daily Telegraph*, 3 October 1963. See also *The Times,* 17 June 1963. Harold Carr, 'The Patients Association', *Hospital and Health Management*, 4 (1963), 287–8. For the USA see Murray Wax, 'On Public Dissatisfaction with the Medical Profession: Personal Observations', *Journal of Health and Human Behavior*, 3 (1962), 152–6.

35. In the debates over the fluoridation of water one can see frequent references to the threat of human experimentation. See the memorandum from the National Pure Water Association in CAB 124/1641, National Archives, UK.

36. For the raising of numerous such concerns to the Ministry of Health in Britain in 1962 and 1963, see MH 148/177, National Archives, UK.

37. Kenneth J. Arrow, 'Uncertainty and the Welfare Economics of Medical Care', *American Economic Review*, 53 (1963), 941–73.

38. See W. Tousijn, 'Medical Dominance in Italy: A Partial Decline', *Social Science and Medicine*, 55 (2002), 733–41; W. Tousijn, 'Medical Professionalisation in Italy: A Comparative Perspective', in I. Hellberg, M. Saks, and C. Benoit, (eds.), *Professional Identities in Transition: Cross-Cultural Dimensions* (Sodertalje: Almqvist & Wiksell, 1999). For East Africa see John Illiffe, *East African Doctors: A History of the Modern Profession* (Cambridge: Cambridge University Press, 1978). On the USA see J. D. McKinlay and L. D. Marceau, 'The End of the Golden Age of Doctoring', *International Journal of Health Services*, 32 (2002), 379–416. See also F. Hafferty and J. McKinlay (eds.), *The Changing Character of the Medical Profession: An International Comparison* (New York: Oxford University Press, 1993); Renée Fox, 'The Medicalization and Demedicalization of American Society', in J. Knowles (ed.), *Doing Better and Feeling Worse* (New York: W. W, Norton, 1977), 9–22.

39. For the USA, B. Lavin, M. Haug, L. L. Balgrave, and N. Breslau, 'Change in Student Physicians' Views on Authority Relations with Patients', *Journal of Health and Social Behavior*, 28 (1987), 258–72. The proportion cited was 64%. See also Mark Schlesinger, 'A Loss of Faith: The Sources of Reduced Political Legitimacy for the American Medical Profession', *Milbank Quarterly*, 80 (2002), 185–235.

40. For the USA see Knowles (ed.), *Doing Better and Feeling Worse*. For the UK see Peter Taylor-Goody, 'Attachment to the Welfare State', in Roger Jowell, Lindsay Brook, Bridget Taylor, and Gillian Prior (eds.), *British Social Attitudes: The 8th Report* (Aldershot: Dartmouth Publishing, 1991), 23–42.

41. For an introduction to this large literature see Simon J. Williams and Michael Calnan, 'The "Limits" of Medicialization? Modern Medicine and the Lay Populace in "Late" Modernity', *Social Science and Medicine*, 42 (1996), 1609–20.

42. Among sociologists of medicine there is an ongoing debate about whether trust in doctors has been enduringly problematic in the post-war years or has declined. For the analysis here it is important only to show how questionable it has indeed been. See Fiona Stevenson and Graham Scambler, 'The Relationship between Medicine and the Public: The Challenge of Concordance', *Health*, 9 (2005), 5–21; David Armstrong, 'The Myth of Concordance: Response to Stevenson and Scambler', *Health*, 9 (2005), 23–7.

43. Marshall Marinker, 'The Doctor and his Patient: An Inaugural Lecture' (Leicester: Leicester University Press, 1975), 16.

44. Jack Feldman, 'What Americans Think about their Medical Care', in American Statistical Association, *Proceedings of the Social Statistics Section 1958* (Washington, DC: American Statistical Association, 1959), 102–5. Another study giving rather similar results was reported by M. F. Cahal, What the Public Thinks of the Family Doctor: Folklore and Facts', *GP* 25 (1962), 146–57.

45. Louise Fox Connell, 'What We Now Know about Young Ears', *Parents Magazine*, 29 (March 1954), 40–1.

46. Christopher C. Butler, Stephen Rollnick, Roisin Pill, Frances Maggs-Rapport, and Nigel Stott, 'Understanding the Culture of Prescribing: Qualitatative Study of General Practitioners' and Patients' Perceptions of Antibiotics for Sore Throats', *British Medical Journal*, 317 (5 September 1998), 637–42.

47. Len Ratoff, 'Antibiotics are Seen as Having Magical Powers', *bmj.com*, 9 September 1998. See **http://bmj.bmjjournals.com/cgi/eletters/317/7159/637#734**, accessed 1 December 2004.

48. R. Mangione-Smith, E. A. McGlynn, M. N. Elliott, L. McDonald, C. E. Franz, and R. L. Kravitz, 'Parent Expectations for Antibiotics, Physician–Parent Communication, and Satisfaction', *Archives of Pediatrics and Adolescent Medicine*, 155 (2001), 800–6.

49. J. G. Scott, D. Cohen, B. DiCicco-Bloom, A. J. Orzano, C. R. Jaen, and B. F. Crabtree, 'Antibiotic Use in Acute Respiratory Infections and the Ways Patients

Pressure Physicians for a Prescription', *Family Practice*, 50 (2001), 853–8; T. Stivers, 'Participating in Decisions about Treatment: Overt Parent Pressure for Antibiotic Medication in Pediatric Encounters', *Social Science and Medicine*, 54 (2002), 1111–30.

50. *Antibiotic Resistance Survey: Report of Findings*, Conducted for the Royal Pharmaceutical Society by Business Diagnostics, September/October 1999, p. 9. On the cycle of prescription for colds and belief that antibiotics would be active see D. Chandler and A. E. Dugdale, 'What do Patients Know about Antibiotics?', *The Lancet*, 2 (21 August 1976), 422.

51. G. Mazzaglia, A. P. Caputi, A. Rossi, G. Bettoncelli, G. Stefanini, G. Ventriglia, R. Nardi, O. Brignoli, and C. Cricelli, 'Pharmacoepidemiology and Prescription: Exploring Patient- and Doctor-Related Variables Associated with Antibiotic Prescribing for Respiratory Infections in Primary Care', *European Journal of Clinical Pharmacology*, 59 (2003), 651–7.

52. Nicola Britten, 'Lay Views of Medicines and their Influence on Prescribing: A Study in General Practice', Ph.D. thesis, London University, 1996. She is however sceptical of the blaming of patients. See Nicky Britten, 'Patients' Demands for Prescriptions in Primary Care: Patients Cannot Take All the Blame for Overprescribing', *British Medical Journal*, 310 (29 April 1995), 1084–5.

53. Britten, 'Lay Views of Medicines and their Influence on Prescribing: A Study in General Practice'.

54. Stuart B. Levy, *The Antibiotic Paradox: How Miracle Drugs are Destroying the Miracle* (New York: Plenum Press, 1992), 50.

55. Jerry Avorn and Daniel H. Solomon, 'Cultural and Economic Factors That (Mis)Shape Antibiotic Use: The Nonpharmacologic Basis of Therapeutics', *Annals of Internal Medicine*, 133 (2000), 128–35.

56. 'Resistance to Antibiotics: Select Committee Report', *Parliamentary Debates* (Lords), 16 November 1998, 5th ser. 594 (1997–8), cols. 1048–9.

57. P. Auinger, B. Lamphear, H. J. Kalkwarf, and M. E. Mansour, 'Trends in Otitis Media among Children in the United States', *Pediatrics*, 112 (2003), 514–20.

58. L. F. McCaig and J. M. Hughes, 'Trends in Antimicrobial Drug Prescribing among Office-Based Physicians in the United States', *Journal of the American Medical Association*, 273 (1995), 214–19.

59. F. L. van Buchem, J. H. Dunk, and M. A. van't Hof, 'Therapy of Acute Otitis Media: Myringotomy, Antibiotics or Neither', *The Lancet*, 2 (24 October 1981), 883–7; N. Mygind, K. L. Meistrup-Larsen, J. Thomsen, V. F. Thomsen, K. Josefsson, and H. Sorenson, 'Penicillin in Acute Otitis Media: A Double-Blind Placebo-Controlled Trial', *Clinical Otolaryngology*, 6 (1981), 5–13.

60. R. A. Damoiseaux, R. A. deMelker, M. J. Ausems, and F. A. van Belen, 'Reasons for Non-Guideline-Based Antibiotic Prescriptions for Acute Otitis Media in the Netherlands', *Family Practice*, 16 (1999), 50–3.

61. Robert Bell, *Impure Science: Fraud, Compromise and Political Influence in Scientific Research* (New York: Wiley, 1992), 144–82.

62. N. F. Col and R. W. O'Connor, 'Estimating Worldwide Current Antibiotic Usage: Report of Task Force 1', *Reviews of Infectious Diseases*, 9 (1987), Suppl. 3: S232–43.

63. On a comparison between French and German uses see Stephan Harbarth, Werner Albrich, and Christian Brun-Buisson, 'Outpatient Antibiotic Use and Prevalence of Antibiotic-Resistant Pneumococci in France and Germany: A Sociocultural Perspective', *Emerging Infectious Diseases*, 8 (2002), 1460–7.

64. There was some evidence that the differences began to reduce some-what thereafter, Massimo Fillipini, Giuliano Masiero, and Karine Moschetti, 'Regional Differences in Outpatient Antibiotic Consumption in Switzer-land', Department of Management and Information Technology Working Paper n.2/EM—2004, University of Bergamo. Published on the web at **www.unibg.it/dati/bacheca/432/12080.pdf.**

65. Otto Cars and Sigvard Mölstad, 'Variation in Antibiotic Use in the European Union', *The Lancet*, 357 (9 June 2001), 1851–3.

66. Fernando Baquero, Gregorio Baquero-Artigao, Rafael Canton, and Cesar Garcia-Rey, 'Antibiotic Consumption and Resistance Selection in *Streptococcus pneumoniae*', *Journal of Antimicrobial Chemotherapy*, 50 (2002), Suppl. S2: 27–37.

67. A. Orero, J. Gonzalez, and J. Prieto, 'Antibiotics in Spanish Households: Medi-cal and Socioeconomic Implications', *Medicina Clinica*, 109 (1997), 782–5. For a very similar finding in a study of Russian cabinets see L. S. Stratchounski, I. V. Andreeva, S. A. Ratchina, D. V. Galkin, N. A. Petrotchenkova, A. A. Demion, V. B. Kuzin, S. T. Kusnetsova, R. Y. Likhatcheva, S. V. Nedogoda, E. A. Orten-berg, A. S. Belikov, and J. A. Toropova, 'The Inventory of Antibiotics in Russian Home Medicine Cabinets', *Clinical Infectious Diseases*, 15 (2003), 498–505.

68. Baquero et al., 'Antibiotic Consumption and Resistance Selection in *Streptococcus pneumoniae*'.

69. McKie, 'Patterns of Social Trust in Western Europe and their Genesis', 245–82.

70. Reginald Deschepper, Robert H. Vander Stichele, and Flora M. Haaijer-Ruskamp, 'Cross-Cultural Differences in Lay Attitudes and Utilisation of Antibiotics in a Belgian and a Dutch City', *Patient Education and Counselling*, 48 (2002), 161–9.

71. These terms are derived from the work of Habermas for whose impact on the study of health see Graham Scambler (ed.), *Habermas, Critical Theory and Health* (London: Routledge, 2001) and in the history of medicine see Steve Sturdy (ed.), *Medicine, Health and the Public Sphere in Britain, 1600–2000* (London: Routledge, 2002); these works discuss the ideas introduced in Jürgen Habermas, *The Theory of Communicative Action* i. *Reason and Rationalization of Society*, trans. Thomas McCarthy (London: Heinemann, 1984).

72. A. Branthwaite and J. C. Pechère, 'Pan-European Survey of Patients' Attitudes to Antibiotic and Antibiotic Use', *Journal of International Medical Research*, 24 (1996), 229–38; Jean Claude Pechère, 'Patients' Interviews and Misuse of Antibiotics', *Clinical Infectious Diseases*, 33 (2001), Suppl. 3: S170–3.

73. C. J. Hackett, 'Yaws', in E. Sabben-Clare, D. J. Bradley, and K. Kirkwood (eds.), *Health in Tropical Africa during the Colonial Period: Based on the Proceedings of a Symposium Held at New College Oxford 21–23 March 1977* (Oxford: Oxford University Press, 1980), 62–92.

74. S. R. Whyte, 'Penicillin, Battery Acid and Sacrifice: Cures and Causes in Nyole Medicine', *Social Science and Medicine*, 16 (1982), 2055–64.

75. For a summary of the detailed evidence from the 1990s see Melinda Pavin,Tafgat Nurgozhin, Grace Hafner, Farruh Yusufy, and Richard Laing, 'Prescribing Practices of Rural Primary Health Care Physicians in Uzbekistan', *Tropical Medicine and International Health*, 8 (2003), 182–90.

76. Dianna Melrose, *Bitter Pills: Medicine and the Third World Poor* (Oxford: Oxfam, Public Affairs Unit, 1983), 110–12.

77. Ibid. 23.

78. David Morley, *Paediatric Priorities in the Developing World* (London: Butterworth, 1973), 4.

79. E. E. Obaseiki-Ebor, J. O. Akerele, and P. O. Ebea, 'A Survey of Antibiotic Outpatient Self-Medication', *Journal of Antimicrobial Chemotherapy* (1987), 759–63.

80. J. Calva and R. Bojalil, 'Antibiotic Use in a Periurban Community in Mexico: A Household and Drugstore Survey', *Social Science and Medicine*, 42 (1996), 1121–8.

81. Caroline H. Bledsoe and Monica F. Goubaud, 'The Reinterpretation and Distribution of Western Pharmaceuticals: An Example from the Mende of Sierra Leone', in Sjaak Van Der Geest and Susan Reynolds Whyte (eds.), *The Context of Medicines in Developing Countries* (Dordrecht: Kluwer, 1988), 253–76.

82. Melrose, *Bitter Pills*, 114.

83. J. P. Loefler, 'Microbes, Chemotherapy, Evolution, and Folly', *The Lancet*, 348 (21 December 1996), 1703–4.

84. C. E. Taylor, 'The Doctor's Role in Rural Health Care', *International Journal of Health Services*, 6 (1976), 219–30.

85. Ozzie G. Simmons, 'Popular and Modern Medicine in Mestizo Communities of Coastal Peru and Chile', *Journal of American Folklore*, 68 (1955), 57–71.

86. Richard and Eva Blum, *Health and Healing in Rural Greece* (San Jose, Calif: Stanford University Press, 1965), 86.

87. R. Burghart, 'Penicillin: An Ancient Ayurvedic Medicine', in Van Der Geest and Whyte (eds.), *The Context of Medicines in Developing Countries*, 289–98.

88. Anne Ferguson, 'Commercial Pharmaceutical Medicine and Medicalization: A Case Study from El Salvador', in Van Der Geest and Whyte (eds.), *The Context of Medicine in Developing Countries: Studies in Pharmaceutical Anthropology*, 19–46.

89. Glen Williams, 'WHO: The Days of the Mass Campaigns', *World Health Forum*, 9 (1988), 7–23.

90. Division of Strengthening of Health Services, WHO, *Strengthening of Health Services: WHO's Response to the Changing Needs of Countries* (Geneva: Division

of Strengthening of Health Services, WHO, 1994). This manuscript history is accessible through the WHO library at xx.(31221.2).

91. Ibid. 22.

92. Andrew Chetley, *A Healthy Business: World Health and the Pharmaceutical Industry* (London: Zed Books, 1990).

93. David A. Tejada de Rivero, 'Alma-Ata Revisited', *Perspectives in Health Magazine*, 8/2 (2003). Available on the web at **www.paho.org/English/DD/ PIN/Number17_article1_4.htm**, accessed 7 March 2004.

94. Chetley, *A Healthy Business*, 85–90.

95. Stephen J. Fabricant and Norbert Hirschhorn, 'Deranged Distribution, Perverse Prescription, Unprotected Use: The Irrationality of Pharmaceuticals in the Developing World', *Health Policy and Planning*, 2 (1987), 204–13. See also the document which emerged, 'Pharmaceutical Distribution, Prescription and Use', WHO/Conrad/WP/2.3, in the WHO library, Geneva.

96. Chetley, *A Healthy Business*, 133–45.

97. Management Sciences for Health, *Interventions and Strategies to Improve the Use of Antimicrobials in Developing Countries* (Geneva: WHO, 2001).

98. D. Greenwood, 'Resistance to Antimicrobial Agents: A Personal View', *Journal of Medical Microbiology*, 47 (1998), 751–5.

Chapter 8

1. US Federal Trade Commission, *Economic Report on Antibiotics Manufacture* (Washington, DC: US Government Printing Office, 1958), 81.

2. Alan Linton, 'The Role of Meat in the Spread to Man of Pathogenic and Antibiotic-Resistant Bacteria', *Meat Hygienist*, 25 (February/March 1980), 22–7.

3. A. Fleisch, 'Antibiotika in Nahrungsmitteln', *Schweize Ärztezeitung*, 49 (1959), 722. This paper is cited and abstracted by J. C. Somogyi, 'Antibiotics in Agriculture and Human Health', in J. C. Somogyi and A. C. François (eds.), *Antibiotics in Agriculture: Proceedings of the 5th Symposium of the Group of European Nutritionists in Jouy-en-Josas April 25–27 1966* (Basel: Karger, 1968), 204–6.

4. Kevin Woodward, *Antibiotics: The Resistance Issue* (London: PJB Publications, 1999), 61.

5. 'Use of Antibiotics and Antibiotic Residues in the Feeding of Livestock', Note of an Informal Meeting Held at the Council's Offices on Friday 12 October 1951, ARC 853/51, National Archives, UK.

6. L. M. Crawford, comment on A. Linton, 'The Swann Report and its Impact', in Charles H. Stuart-Harris and David M. Harris (eds.), *The Control of Antibiotic-Resistant Bacteria* (New York: Academic Press, 1982), 196.

7. **http://xroads.virginia.edu/~1930s/DISPLAY/39wf/bordenextim.htm**, accessed 20 November 2004.

8. www.elsie.com/about_elsie/press/cowhistorian.htm, accessed 25 March 2001. Dean Muellerleile, 'On the Moove...The Evolution of America's First Cow', *Milk Route*, 152 (May 1993). Available on **http://home. twcny.rr.com/dgillett/tmr1/tmr4.html**, accessed 18 November 2004. Mark Williams, 'Elsie the Cow Changed Industry's Image: Ad Age Ranks Icon among Century's Best', *Cincinnati Enquirer*, 23 October 1999.

9. René Dubos, interview with Saul Benison, 1955–6, transcript, Columbia University Oral History Research Office, iii. 450–1. The cattle treated are listed in R. B. Little, R. J. Dubos, R. D. Hotchkiss, C. W. Bean, and W. T. Miller, 'The Use of Gramicidin and Other Agents for the Elimination of the Chronic Form of Bovine Mastitis', *American Journal of Veterinary Research*, 11 (1941), 305–12.

10. **www.elmers.com/funFacts/index.asp**, accessed 18 November 2004.

11. National Academy of Sciences, *The Effects on Human Health of Subtherapeutic Use of Antimicrobials in Animal Feeds* (Washington, DC: Office of Publications, 1980), 341.

12. **http://www.mcdonalds.ca/pdfs/history_final.pdf**, accessed 18 November 2004.

13. National Academy of Sciences, *The Effects on Human Health of Subtherapeutic Use of Antimicrobials*, 341. On antibiotics and hogs see Mark R. Finlay, 'Hogs, Antibiotics, and the Industrial Environment of Postwar Agriculture', in Susan R. Schrepfer and Philip Scranton (eds.), *Industrializing Organisms: Introducing Evolutionary History* (London: Routledge, 2004), 237–60.

14. Ruth Harrison, *Animal Machines: The New Factory Farming Industry* (London: Vincent Stuart, 1964), 62.

15. E. S. Anderson, 'Drug Resistance in *Salmonella typhimurium* and its Implications', *British Medical Journal*, 2 (10 August 1968), 333–9.

16. Finlay, 'Hogs, Antibiotics, and the Industrial Environments of Postwar Agriculture'; K. L. Robinson, 'Use of Antibiotics in Feeds: The Value of Antibiotics for Growth of Pigs', in Malcolm Woodbine (ed.), *Antibiotics in Agriculture: Proceedings of the University of Nottingham Ninth Easter School in Agricultural Science, 1962* (London: Butterworths, 1962), 285–302; Damon Catron, 'Recent Development in Swine Nutrition', *Veterinary Medicine*, 44 (May 1949), 215–20.

17. John Maddox, 'Obituary: Thomas Hughes Jukes (1906–99)', *Nature*, 402 (2 December 1999), 478.

18. 'Antibiotics in the Barnyard', *Fortune* (March 1952), 118–40.

19. 'Livestock and Meat Production in the United States: An Overview', figure 7, 'Per capita Consumption of Meat and Seafood in the United States by Commodity, 1909–2000', **www.usda.gov/gipsa/pubs/01assessment/section2.pdf**, accessed 20 December 2004.

20. 'Major Trends in U.S. Food Supply, 1909–99', *Food Review*, 23 (2000), 9–15 (see figure 6, p. 11).

21. 'Countries by Commodity', Major Food and Agricultural Commodities and Producers, Statistics Division, Food and Agriculture Organization, published on the web at: **www.fao.org/es/ess/top/commodity.jsp?lang=EN&commodity=1094&CommodityList=1094&year=1961&yearLyst=1961**, accessed 1 December 2004.

22. See also Orville Schell, *Modern Meat: Antibiotics, Hormones and the Pharmaceutical Farm* (New York: Random House, 1984); Catron, 'Recent Development in Swine Nutrition'.

23. Robert Bud, *The Uses of Life: A History of Biotechnology* (Cambridge: Cambridge University Press, 1994), 32.

24. S. J. Edwards, 'Antibiotics in the Treatment of Mastitis', in *Antibiotics in Agriculture: Proceedings of the University of Nottingham Ninth Easter School in Agricultural Science, 1962*, 43–57.

25. H. R. Vickers, L. Bagratuni, and Suzanne Alexander, 'Dermatitis Caused by Penicillin in Milk', *The Lancet*, 1 (15 February 1958), 351–2.

26. WHO Expert Committee on the Public Health Aspect of the Use of Antibiotics in Food and Feedstuffs, *The Public Health Aspects of the Use of Antibiotics in Food and Feedstuffs: Report of an Expert Committee*, meeting held in Geneva 11–17 December 1962 (Geneva: World Health Organization, 1963).

27. Michael Winstanley, 'Cow Punch: Antibiotics in Milk through Treatment of Cows', *The Guardian*, 25 June 1963.

28. Ralph H. Lutts, 'Chemical Fallout: Rachel Carson's Silent Spring, Radioactive Fallout and the Environmental Movement', *Environmental Review*, 9 (1985), 214–25; Robert Divine, *Blowing on the Wind: The Nuclear Test Ban Debate, 1954–1960* (New York: Oxford University Press, 1978), 262–80.

29. Peter George, *Dr Strangelove, or, How I Learned to Stop Worrying and Love the Bomb* (London: Transworld, 1963), 586.

30. A. J. D. Winnifrith, 25 July 1962, MAF 251/369, National Archives, UK.

31. A. J. D. Winnifrith, 2 November 1962, MAF 251/369, National Archives, UK.

32. H. Mol, *Antibiotics and Milk* (Rotterdam: A. A. Balkema, 1975); see also **www.cdfa.ca.gov/ahfss/mdfc/pdfs/M-I-04-4_DelvoScanReader_-FINAL.pdf**, accessed 1 December 2004.

33. National Research Council, *The Use of Drugs in Food Animals* (Washington, DC: National Academy Press, 1999), 14. This was based on a review of the 'agricola' and 'biosis' databases.

34. Ruth Harrison, *Animal Machines: The New Factory Farming Industry* (London: Vincent Stuart, 1964).

35. William Yates to Christopher Soames, 29 March 1961, MAF 113/565, National Archives, UK.

36. R. B. A. Carnaghan, 'Antibiotics in Poultry Feeding', ARC paper 522/60, FD1/8226, National Archives, UK.

37. Lord Netherthorpe (chair), *Report of the Joint Committee on Antibiotics in Animal Feeding to the Agricultural Research Council and the Medical Research Council* (London: HMSO, 1962).

38. T. Watanabe, 'Infectious Drug Resistance', *Scientific American*, 217 (1967), 19–28; Thomas Brock, *The Emergence of Bacterial Genetics* (Cold Spring Harbor, NY: Cold Spring Harbor Laboratory Press, 1990).

39. E. M. Tansey and L. M. Reynolds (eds.), *Post-Penicillin Antibiotics: From Acceptance to Resistance?* Wellcome Witnesses to Twentieth Century Medicine 6 (London: Wellcome Institute for the History of Medicine, 2000), 45.

40. Naomi Datta, 'Transmissible Drug Resistance in an Epidemic Strain of *Salmonella typhimurium*', *Journal of Hygiene*, 60 (1962), 301–10.

41. E. S. Anderson and M. J. Lewis, 'Drug Resistance and its Transfer in *Salmonella typhimurium*', *Nature*, 206 (8 May 1965), 579–83.

42. Anderson with Betty Hobbs had been responsible for tracing the origin of the typhoid bacilli that caused the 1964 Aberdeen typhoid epidemic. See David F. Smith and H. Lesley Diack with T. Hugh Pennington and Elizabeth M. Russell, *Food Poisoning, Policy, and Politics: Corned Beef and Typhoid in Britain in the 1960s* (Woodbridge: Boydell Press, 2005).

43. E. S. Anderson, 'Origin of Transferable Drug-Resistance Factors in the Enterobacteriaceae', *British Medical Journal*, 2 (27 November 1965), 1289–91; E. S. Anderson, 'Influence of the Delta Transfer Factor on the Phage Sensitivity of Salmonellae', *Nature*, 212 (19 November 1966), 795–9; E. S. Anderson, 'Possible Importance of Transfer Factors in Bacterial Evolution', *Nature*, 209 (5 February 1966), 637–8. See also his 'The Ecology of Transferable Drug Resistance in the Enterobacteria', *Annual Review of Microbiology*, 22 (1968), 131–80, which was recognized as a citation classic by *Science Citation Index* in 1986 by which time it had been cited in over 315 publications. For an interpretation of the significance of this work of Anderson, see S. Falkow, *Infectious Multiple Drug Resistance* (London: Pion, 1975), 87–97.

44. H. Williams Smith and Sheila Halls, 'Observations on Infective Drug Resistance in Britain', *British Medical Journal*, 1 (29 January 1966), 266–9.

45. Arthur Koestler, *The Sleepwalkers: A History of Man's Changing Vision of the Universe* (London: Hutchinson, 1959).

46. Agricultural Research Council and Medical Research Council, 'Joint Committee on Antibiotics and Animal Feeding: Second Report of the Scientific Subcommittee', MAF287/450, National Archives, UK. The subcommittee first met on 22 June 1965 and reported to a meeting of the Netherthorpe Committee as a whole on 6 April. See minute by W. D. McCrae, 18 January 1967, summarizing what the author saw as an almost incomprehensibly complex series of manoeuvrings.

47. The links between the foot and mouth catastrophe and regulation of antibiotics were explained by P. W. Daykin, 'Antibiotic Usage in Veterinary Practice

before Swann', in Donald V. Jolly, David J. S. Miller, David B. Ross, and Peter D. Simm (eds.), *Ten Years on from Swann* (London: The Association of Veterinarians in Industries, 1981), 27–36. On the outbreak itself see Abigail Woods, *A Manufactured Plague: The History of Foot and Mouth Disease in Britain* (London: Earthscan, 2004), 108–30.

48. Anthony Tucker, 'Anti-antibiotics', *The Guardian*, 30 January 1967; Anthony Tucker, 'Issues Raised by the Inquiry into the Farm Use of Antibiotics', *The Guardian*, 13 July 1968. Several leaders on antibiotic use appeared in the newspaper: 'Pharmaceutical Euphoria', *The Guardian*, 21 October 1967; 'A Drug-Taking Culture', *The Guardian*, 14 November 1967; 'The Dangers of Misusing Antibiotics', *The Guardian*, 3 February 1968.

49. Bernard Dixon, private communication.

50. Bernard Dixon, 'Antibiotics on the Farm: Major Threat to Human Health', *New Scientist* (5 October 1967), 33–5.

51. C. A. Green and E. G. Brewis, 'An Enquiry into the Outbreak of E. Coli 0128 Gastro-Enteritis in Infants under One Year Old in Tees-side', MH/60/788, National Archives, UK.

52. 'The Men who Fought It', *Evening Gazette* (Middlesbrough), 7 March 1968.

53. 'The Diary of a Tragedy', *Evening Gazette*, 7 March 1968.

54. Green and Brewis, 'An Enquiry into the Outbreak of E. Coli 0128 Gastro-Enteritis in Infants under One Year Old in Tees-side', 18. There was a television investigation in the BBC1 programme *Twenty-Four Hours* broadcast on 21 December 1967. Unfortunately the transcript of this seems now to be lost. I am grateful to the archives of the BBC for looking into this for me.

55. 'The Diary of a Tragedy', *Evening Gazette*.

56. Green and Brewis, 'An Enquiry into the Outbreak of E. Coli 0128 Gastro-Enteritis in Infants under One Year Old in Tees-side'.

57. 'Gastro-Enteritis on Tees-side', *Parliamentary Debates* (Commons), 5th ser. 762 (1967–8), cols. 1619–30, held on 11 April 1968.

58. A. T. Roden to Dr Shaw, 18 January 1968, MH 160/788, National Archives, UK.

59. World Health Organization, 'Growing Antibiotic Resistance of Enteric Bacteria', Press Release, WHO/10, 26 February 1974.

60. 'Action Sought on Antibiotics after Babies' Deaths', *The Times*, 14 April 1969; 'F and M at the Min of Ag', *Daily Mirror*, 29 April 1968.

61. G. B. Blaker to T. B. Wilkinson, 17 January 1968, FD7/894, National Archives, UK.

62. W. D. McRae to Mr Parker, 'Joint ARC/MRC Report on Antibiotics: Inter-departmental Committee Meeting 13.2.68', MA 287/450, National Archives, UK.

63. 'Note of a Meeting with the Ministry of Agriculture Fisheries and Food', 21 February 1968, FD7/900, National Archives, UK.

64. W. D. Macrae to Mr Parker, 'Joint A.R.C./M.R.C. Report on Antibiotics: Interdepartmental Committee Meeting 13.2.68', 7 February 1968, MAF 287/450, National Archives, UK.

65. For objections to Anderson's membership of the Swann Committee For objections to Anderson's membership of the Swann Committee see minute by J. C. Tame, 29 April 1968, in 'Joint A.R.C./M.R.C. Report on Antibiotics', MAF 287/450, National Archives, UK. For Ministry of Health anxieties G. J. L. Avery, 2 May 1968, p. 78, in the same file.

66. EMBC, 'Filenote', 27 September 1968, FD7/1621, National Archives, UK.

67. M. M. Swann (chair), *Report of the Joint Committee on the Use of Antibiotics in Animal Husbandry and Veterinary Medicine,* 1969–70, v Cmnd. 4190 (London: HMSO, 1969).

68. Bernard Dixon, *What is Science For?* (London: Collins, 1973), 137–40.

69. James Howie, 'The Situation Then and Now', in Jolly et al. (eds.), *Ten Years on from Swann,* 3–26.

70. V. Krécmâery, L. Rosival, and T. Watanabe, *Bacterial Plasmids and Antibiotic Resistance: International Symposium on Infectious Antibiotic Resistance 1971* (Prague: Avicenum; Berlin: Springer-Verlag, 1972).

71. Anderson and Lewis, 'Drug Resistance and its Transfer in *Salmonella typhimurium'.* R. E. O. Williams, *Microbiology for the Public Service: Evolution of the Public Health Laboratory Service 1939–1980* (London: Public Health Laboratory Service, 1985), 107.

72. E. J. Threlfall, L. R. Ward, A. S. Ashley, and B. Rowe, 'Plasmid-Encoded Trimethoprim Resistance in Multiresistant Epidemic *Salmonella typhimurium* Phage Types 204 and 193 in Britain', *British Medical Journal,* 280 (17 May 1980), 1210–11.

73. A. H. Linton, 'Antibiotic Resistance: The Present Situation Reviewed', *Veterinary Record,* 100 (23 April 1977), 354–60.

74. Mark Richmond. 'Why has Swann Failed?', *British Medical Journal,* 280 (28 June 1980), 1615.

75. Jolly, Miller, Ross, and Simm (eds.), *Ten Years on from Swann.*

76. Alan Marcus, *Cancer from Beef: DES, Federal Food Regulation and Consumer Confidence* (Baltimore: Johns Hopkins University Press, 1994), 127.

77. Marc Lappé, *Germs That Won't Die* (Garden City, NY: Anchor Press, 1982), 130–3.

78. Office of Technology Assessment, *Drugs in Livestock Feed* (Washington, DC: US Office of Technology Assessment 1979), 8.

79. Schell, *Modern Meat,* 28–36 describes an interview with Professor Novick.

80. R. Novick, 'Analysis by Transduction of Mutations Affecting Penicillinase Formation in *Staphylococcus aureus', Journal of General Microbiology,* 33 (1963), 121–36.

81. Richard Novick, 'Use of BRL 1241', *The Lancet,* 2 (29 October 1960), 978.

82. Richard Novick, 'The Situation is Completely Out of Hand', *New York Times*, 3 July 1978.
83. Richard Novick, 'Antibiotics: Use in Animal Feed', *Science*, 204 (1 June 1978), 908.
84. 'Scientists Quit Panel in Dispute over Livestock', *New York Times*, 23 January 1979.
85. Thomas H. Jukes, 'Antibiotics in Feeds', *Science*, 204 (6 April 1978), 8.
86. Novick, 'Antibiotics: Use in Animal Feed'.
87. Richard P. Novick, 'Antibiotics: Wonder Drugs or Chicken Feed', *The Sciences* (July–August 1979), 14–17.
88. Thomas H. Jukes, 'Antibiotics, Resistance and Animal Growth: Another View', *The Sciences* (April 1980), 24–6.
89. Office of Technology Assessment, *Drugs in Livestock Feed*.
90. 'New Warning on Risk from Antibiotic in Animal Feed', *Nature*, 280 (5 July 1979), 4.
91. National Academy of Sciences, *The Effects on Human Health of Subtherapeutic Use of Antimicrobials in Animal Feeds* (Washington, DC: Office of Publications, 1980).
92. S. D. Holmberg, M. T. Osterholm, K. A. Senger, and M. L. Cohen, 'Drug Resistant Salmonella from Animals Fed Anti-microbials', *New England Journal of Medicine*, 311 (1984), 617–22; Stuart B. Levy, *The Antibiotic Paradox* (2nd edn. Cambridge, Mass.: Perseus, 2002), 298.
93. Ed Quillen, 'Another Perspective on Natural Beef: Sidebar', *Colorado Central Magazine*, 55 (September 1998), 32.
94. Lappé, *Germs That Won't Die*, 75–7.
95. 'Drug Resistance in Salmonellas', *The Lancet*, 1 (19 June 1982), 1391–2.
96. S. B. Levy, R. B. Clowes, and G. L. Koenig (eds.), *International Plasmid Conference on Molecular Biology, Pathogenicity, and Ecology of Bacterial Plasmids* (New York: Plenum Press, 1981).
97. Private communication, Stuart Levy, 8 December 2003.
98. 'Worldwide Abuse of Antibiotics Poses Threat: 150 Experts Say', *Washington Post*, 5 August 1981.
99. Levy, *The Antibiotic Paradox*, 304–7.
100. 'Antibiotics: Dangers of Misuse', *Washington Post*, 8 August 1981.
101. Lappé, *Germs that Won't Die*. I am grateful to Dr Lappé for the opportunity to discuss his writing of the book.
102. E. J. Threlfall, L. R. Ward, J. A. Frost, and G. A. Willshaw, 'Spread of Resistance from Food Animals to Man: The UK Experience', *Acta Veterinaria Scandinavica*, 93 (2000), Suppl.: 63–8; discussion 68–74.
103. Michael Swann, Official Opening, British Veterinary Association Centenary Congress, Reading, 22 September 1982, File H90, Swann papers, Edinburgh University, and reported *Veterinary Record*, 109 (1982), 287–8.

104. A. H. Linton, 'Has Swann Failed?', *Veterinary Record*, 108 (1981), 328–31 (p. 331).

Chapter 9

1. M. Wood, 'The Politicization of Antimicrobial Resistance', *Current Opinion in Infectious Diseases*, 11 (1998), 649–51.
2. David M. Shlaes, 'The Abandonment of Antibacterials: Why and Wherefore?', *Current Opinion in Pharmacology*, 3 (2003), 470–3; See for example D. Shlaes, D. Levy, and G. Archer, 'Antimicrobial Resistance: New Directions', *ASM News*, 57 (1991), 455–8.
3. Joshua Lederberg, *'Escherichia coli'*, in Robert Bud and Deborah Jean Warner (eds.), *Instruments of Science: An Historical Encyclopedia* (New York: Garland, 1998), 230–2.
4. 'Memorandum by the Medical Research Council', submitted to Select Committee on Science and Technology, The House of Lords, session 1997–8, *Resistance to Antibiotics and Other Microbial Agents: Evidence*, HL Paper 81-II, pp. 428–31.
5. 'Memorandum by SmithKline Beecham Pharmaceuticals', *Resistance to Antibiotics: Evidence*, 472–85.
6. D. Hughes, 'Exploiting Genomics, Genetics and Chemistry to Combat Antibiotic Resistance', *Nature Reviews Genetics*, 4 (2003), 432–41.
7. B. Spellberg, J. H. Powers, E. P. Brass, L. G. Miller, and J. E. Edwards Jr., 'Trends in Antimicrobial Drug Development: Implications for the Future', *Clinical Infectious Diseases*, 38 (2004), 1279–86.
8. Thus Richard Novick whose activities were discussed in the previous chapter and Joshua Lederberg were active in the 1973 Asilomar conference which led to a moratorium on the practice of recombinant DNA until new regulations were in place—albeit their positions at that meeting were rather different.
9. Mark Cantley, private communication.
10. Paul Roizin and Allan Brandt (eds.), *Morality and Health* (London: Routledge, 1997).
11. Richard M. Krause, 'Introduction to Emerging Infectious Diseases: Stemming the Tide', in Richard M. Krause (ed.), *Emerging Infections: Biomedical Research Reports* (New York: Academic Press, 1998), 1–22.
12. Susan Sontag, *AIDS and its Metaphors* (New York: Farrar Straus Giroux, 1989), 76.
13. Kaye Wellings and Jane Wadsworth, 'Aids and the Moral Climate', in Roger Jowell, Sharon Witherspoon and Lindsay Brook (eds.), *British Social Attitudes: The 7th Report* (London: Gower, 1990), 10–26.
14. Reuters New Media report of the United Nations launch of 'Children Living in a World with AIDS' Initiative, Brussels, 27 June 1997.

15. Aldo A. Benini and Janet Bradford-Benini, 'Ebola Virus: From Medical Emergency to Complex Disaster', *Journal of Contingencies and Crisis Management*, 4 (1996), 10–19.

16. At the same time Joshua Lederberg was also a key participant in discussion as over 'genetic engineering'. See Robert Bud, *The Uses of Life: A History & Biotechnology* (Cambridge: Cambridge University Press, 1994), 172–5.

17. Frank Ryan, *Virus X Understanding the Real Threat of the New Pandemic Plagues* (London: HarperCollins, 1996), 331.

18. René and Jean Dubos, *The White Plague: Tuberculosis, Man and Society* (Boston: Little, Brown, 1952). Also see Elizabeth Hanson, *The Rockefeller University Achievement: A Century of Science for the Benefit of Mankind, 1901–2001* (New York: Rockefeller University Press, 2001).

19. Joshua Lederberg, 'Pandemic as a Natural Evolutionary Phenomenon', in Arien Mack (ed.), *In Time of Plague: The History and Social Consequences of Lethal Epidemic Disease* (New York: New York University Press, 1991), 21–38.

20. Joshua Lederberg, private communication.

21. Joshua Lederberg, 'Medical Science, Infectious Disease, and the Unity of Humankind', *Journal of the American Medical Association*, 260 (1988), 684–5.

22. Stephen Morse (ed.), *Emerging Viruses* (New York: Oxford University Press, 1993).

23. Joshua Lederberg, 'Viruses and Humankind: Intracellular Symbiosis and Evolutionary Competition', in Morse (ed.), *Emerging Viruses*, 3–9. I am grateful to Professor Lederberg for his elucidation of these developments.

24. J. Lederberg, R. E. Shope, and S. C. Oaks (eds.), *Emerging Infections: Microbial Threats to Health in the United States* (Washington, DC: National Academy Press, 1992).

25. Larry J. Strausbaugh, 'Emerging Infectious Diseases: No End in Sight', *American Journal of Infection Control*, 26 (1998), 3–4.

26. Judith A. Johnson, *Infectious Diseases: Emerging and Reemerging Threats to Public Health in the United States* (Washington, DC: Congressional Research Service, Library of Congress, 1995).

27. Laurie Garrett authored a chapter on future threats in J. Mann, D. J. M. Taranola, and T. W. Netter (eds.), *Aids in the World: A Global Report* (Cambridge, Mass.: Harvard University Press, 1992), 825–39.

28. Laurie Garrett, *The Coming Plague: Newly Emerging Diseases in a World out of Balance* (Harmondsworth: Penguin, 1995; first published 1994).

29. David Perlman, 'Review of *The Coming Plague*', *San Francisco Chronicle*. Quoted on back of Penguin edition.

30. R. Preston, *The Hot Zone* (New York: Random House, 1994).

31. *Book Review Index* (Detroit: Gale Research Co., 1994, 1995).

32. Ryan, *Virus X*, p. ix.

33. www.amazon.com/exec/obidos/tg/detail/-/6303484328/103-5885973-7728635?v=glance&vi=reviews, accessed 1 December 2004.

34. www.movietome.com/movietome/servlet/MovieMain/movieid-2513/-Outbreak/, accessed 1 December 2004.

35. www.epguides.com/BurningZone, accessed 22 November 2004.

36. 'Disease Fights Back', *The Economist*, 335 (20 May 1995), 15.

37. *See* www.pureresidentevil.com/, accessed 1 December 2004.

38. Tim Radford, 'Medicine and the Media: Influence and Power of the Media', *The Lancet*, 347 (1996), 1533–5. Although this scare dissipated within a week, similar gruesome tales would be told across the world. In December 1994, Lucien Bouchard, the Canadian politician and future premier of Quebec, lost a leg to the condition. Michael Schnayerson and Mark Plotkin, *The Killers Within* (London: Time Warner, 2003), 195–6.

39. Bernard Dixon, 'Killer Bug Ate my Face', *Current Biology*, 6 (1996), 493.

40. Sharon Begley, 'The End of Antibiotics', *Newsweek* (28 March 1994), 47–52.

41. Geoffrey Cannon, *Superbug: Nature's Revenge: Why Antibiotics Can Breed Disease* (London: Virgin, 1995).

42. S. G. Jones and J. Howard, 'Stories about "Doomsday Killer Bugs": The Aftermath', *British Medical Journal*, 312 (17 February 1996), 441.

43. Bernard Dixon, 'Don't Blame the Messenger', *Current Biology*, 7 (1997), R2.

44. 'The Southwood Working Party, 1988–89'. Its findings were surveyed in chapter 4 of the BSE Inquiry which reported in 2000 and the analysis was mounted on the web at www.bseinquiry.gov.uk/report/volume4/chapt102.htm#888456, accessed 1 December 2004.

45. Shaoni Bhattacharya, 'Predicted Deaths from vCJD Slashed', *New Scientist Online News*, 26 February 2003. www.newscientist.com/channel/health/bse/dn3440, accessed 1 December 2004.

46. UK Department of Health, 'Definite and Probable CJD Cases in the UK May 2003', www.dh.gov.uk/assetRoot/04/07/57/88/04075788.pdf, accessed 1 December 2004.

47. P. Horby, A. Rushdy, C. Graham, and M. O'Mahoney, On Behalf of the PHLS Overview of Communicable Diseases Committee, 'PHLS Overview of Communicable Diseases 1999', *Communicable Diseases and Public Health*, 4 (2001), 8–17.

48. 'Emerging and Other Communicable Diseases: Antimicrobial Resistance', WHA51.17, Fifty-First World Health Assembly, Geneva, 11–16 May 1998.

49. Lord Fitt, 4 November 1996, *Parliamentary Debates* (Lords), 5th ser. 575 (1996–7), cols. 581–3.

50. Lord Soulsby, private communication.

51. Polly F. Harrison and Joshua Lederberg (eds.), *Antimicrobial Resistance: Issues and Options. Workshop Report, Forum on Emerging Infections, Division of Health Sciences Policy* (Washington, DC: National Academies Press, 1998).

52. World Medical Association, Statement on Resistance to Antimicrobial Drugs, Adopted by the 48th General Assembly, Somerset West, Republic of South Africa, October 1996.

53. Lord Soulsby, 16 November 1998, *Parliamentary Debates* (Lords), 5th ser. 594 (1997–8), col. 1044.

54. Lord McNair, *Parliamentary Debates* (Lords), 5th ser. 594 (1997–8), col. 1068 proposed the potential of hydrogen peroxide; for the contribution of Baroness Masham see cols. 1077–81.

55. Schnayerson and Plotkin, *The Killers Within*.

56. The General Report on the Activities of the European Union for 1997, Veterinary and Plant Health Legislation, Para. 606; published on the web at: **http://europa.eu.int/abc/doc/off/rg/en/1997/enx52197.htm**, accessed 1 December 2004.

57. These Food and Agriculture Organization figures were provided by Nancy Morgan, 'Repercussions of BSE on International Meat Trade. Global Market Analysis', **www.fao.org/ag/AGA/AGAP/FRG/Feedsafety/pub/Morgan%20bse.doc**, accessed 22 November 2004.

58. Schnayerson and Plotkin, *The Killers Within*, 142–3.

59. European Union Conference on 'The Microbial Threat', 9–10 September 1998, Copenhagen, Denmark, **www.ua.ac.be/main.asp?c=*ESAC&n=511&ct=ESACCONF01&e=t777**, accessed 22 November 2004. I am grateful Anna Lönnroth for clarifying this history for me and for highlighting the link between BSE and antimicrobial resistance concerns.

60. M. Ferech, M. Elseviers, R. Vander Stichele, and H. Goossens, 'Consumption of Antbiotics in Europe' accessible through **www.ua.ac.be/ESAC.**

61. Anita G. Carrie and George G. Zhanel, 'Antibacterial Use in Community Practice', *Drugs*, 57 (1999), 871–81 (p. 874).

62. Thus, shortly after the House of Lords report, a British government advisory panel issued a paper for doctors. Standing Medical Advisory Committee, Sub-Group on Antimicrobial Resistance, *The Path of Least Resistance* (London: Central Health Services Council, 1998).

63. 'Plan national pour préserver l'efficacité des antibiotiques', **www.sante.gouv.-fr/htm/actu/antibio/sommaire.htm**, accessed 1 December 2004. On the US position on streptococci see Ralph Gonzales, 'Principles of Appropriate Antibiotic Use for Treatment of Acute Respiratory Tract Infections in Adults: Background, Specific Aims, and Methods', *Annals of Internal Medicine*, 134 (2001), 479–86; Alan L. Bisno, 'Diagnosing Strep Throat in the Adult Patient: Do Clinical Criteria Really Suffice?', *Annals of Internal Medicine*, 139 (2003), 150–1; Robert J. Manasse, 'Evaluation of the Pacific Biotech CARDS STREP A Test for Detecting Group A Streptococci from Cases of Pharyngitis', *Journal of Clinical Microbiology*, 27 (1989), 1657–8.

64. *SuperBugs & SuperDrugs: A Strategic Guide to the Global Antimicrobials Industry, Innovation and Therapies* (North Adams, Mass.: SMI Publishing, October

2000), Product Code: R215-044. Abstract on the web **www.mindbranch.com/ listing/product/R215-044.html**, accessed 1 December 2004.

65. J. Coast, R. D. Smith, and M. R. Millar, 'An Economic Perspective on Policy to Reduce Antimicrobial Resistance', *Social Science and Medicine*, 46 (1998), 29–38.

66. Inge Kaul, Isabelle Grunberg, and Marc A. Stern, *Global Public Goods: International Cooperation in the 21st Century* (Oxford: Oxford University Press, 1999).

67. R. D. Smith and J. Coast, 'Antimicrobial Drug Resistance', in R. D. Smith, R. Beaglehole, D. Woodward, and N. Drager (eds.), *Global Public Goods for Health* (Oxford: Oxford University Press, 2003), 73–93.

68. The Harvard professor Thomas Francis O'Brien had been campaigning for years for a standard computerized approach to reporting resistance in hospital infections. He had begun such work as early as 1969. In 1980 he won the support of a Soviet colleague, and a committee was established under the auspices of WHO. Gradually the team at Brigham Women's Hospital in Boston developed a system they called WHONET. T. F. O'Brien, R. L. Kent, and A. A. Medeiros, 'Computer-Generated Plots of Results of Antimicrobial-Susceptibility Tests', *Journal of the American Medical Association*, 210 (1969), 84–92. T. F. O'Brien and J. M. Stelling, 'WHONET: An Information System for Monitoring Antimicrobial Resistance', *Emerging Infectious Diseases*, 1 (1995), 66.

69. 'Emerging and Other Communicable Diseases: Antimicrobial Resistance', WHA51.17, 21.2, World Health Assembly, 16 May 1988. I am grateful to the Library of WHO for supplying me with this.

70. WHO, *Global Strategy for Containment of Antibiotic Resistance* (Geneva: WHO, 2001).

71. *From Compliance to Concordance: Achieving Shared Goals in Medicine Taking* (London: Royal Pharmaceutical Society; Hoddesdon: Merck Sharp & Dohme, 1997). On the background to concordance see Jeremy A. Greene, 'Therapeutic Infidelities: "Noncompliance" Enters the Medical Literature', *Social History of Medicine*, 17 (2004), 327–43.

72. See P. Little, I. Williamson, G. Warner, C. Gould, M. Gantley, and A. L. Kinmonth, 'An Open Randomised Trial of Prescribing Strategies for Sore Throat', *British Medical Journal*, 314 (1997), 722–7. R. Mangione-Smith et al., 'Parent Expectations for Antibiotics, Physician–Parent Communication, and Satisfaction', *Archives of Pediatrics and Adolescent Medicine*, 155 (2001), 800–6. I am grateful to Brian Hurwitz for pointing me towards the work of Paul Little.

73. Susan Cant and Ursula Sharma, *A New Medical Pluralism? Alternative Medicines, Doctors, Patients and the State* (London: UCL Press, 1999).

74. **www.aware.md/media/documents/AWAREMediaKit2004.pdf**, accessed 1 December 2004. Alliance Working for Antibiotic Resistance Education, 'What is Aware', 1. AWARE is a project of the California Medical Association Foundation.

75. Department of Health Press Release,'Got A Cold? Don't Expect Antibiotics!', 29 October 1999, reference number: 1999/0644.

76. IPSOS UK Research, COI CASE STUDY—ANTIBIOTICS. I am grateful to Ogilvy and Mather for permission to use this document and to the Central Office of Information for permission to quote these results.
77. Stuart B. Levy, *The Antibiotic Paradox* (2nd edn. Cambridge, Mass.: Perseus Books), pp. vii–xii.
78. Stuart B. Levy, 'Antibiotic Resistance 1992–2002: A Decade's Journey', in Stacey L. Knobler, Stanley M. Lemon, Marjan Najafi, and Tom Burroughs (eds.), *The Resistance Phenomenon in Microbes and Infectious Disease Vectors: Implications for Human Health and Strategies for Containment* (Washington, DC: National Academies Press, 2003), 32–43.
79. IDSA, 'As Antibiotic Discovery Stagnates, a Public Health Crisis Brews: Bad Bugs, No Drugs' (Alexandria, Va.: Infectious Diseases Society of America, 2004).
80. M. Ashworth, R. Latinovic, J. Charlton, K. Cox, G. Rowlands, and M. Gulliford, 'Why Has Antibiotic Prescribing for Respiratory Illness Declined in Primary Care? A Longitudinal Study Using the General Practice Research Database', *Journal of Public Health*, 26 (2004), 268–74; J. A. Finkelstein, S. S. Huang, J. Daniel, S. I. Rifas-Shiman, K. Kleinman, D. Goldman, S. I. Pelton, A. DeMaria, R. Platt, 'Reduction in Antibiotic Use among US Children, 1996–2000', *Pediatrics*, 112 (2003), 620–7; L. F. McCaig and J. M. Hughes, 'Trends in Antimicrobial Drug Prescribing among Office-Based Physicians in the United States', *Journal of the American Medical Association*, 273 (1995), 214–19; Tom Wrigley, Alessandra Tinto, and Azeem Majeed, 'Age- and Sex-Specific Antibiotic Prescribing Patterns in General Practice in England and Wales, 1994 to 1998', *Health Statistics Quarterly*, 14 (2002), 14–20; for a note of scepticism see Michael E. Pichichero, 'Dynamics of Antibiotic Prescribing for Children', *Journal of the American Medical Association*, 287 (2002), 3133–5.
81. J. Stephenson, 'Icelandic Prescribers are Showing the Way to Bring Down the Rates of Antibiotic-Resistant Bacteria', *Journal of the American Medical Association*, 275 (1996), 175. See David Livermore, 'Can Better Prescribing Turn the Tide of Resistance?', *Nature Microbiology*, 2 (2004), 73–8. In 2001 a European Union survey found that, compared to ten years earlier, more of the public now knew that antibiotics did not affect viruses (up to 39.7% from 27.1% over the previous decade). See European Commission, Research Directorate-General, *Europeans, Science and Technology*, Eurobarometer 55.2 (Brussels: European Commission, 2001), 6.

Conclusion

1. There is now an increasingly rich literature on post-war consumer culture. See for instance Lizabeth Cohen, *A Consumers Republic: The Politics of Mass Consumption in Postwar America* (New York: Knopf, 2003).
2. Gunnar Biörck, 'The Next Ten Years in Medicine: Attempt at an Analysis of Factors Determining Medical and Social Development', *British Medical Journal*, 2 (3 July 1965), 7–11

3. See Aristotle, *Poetics*, paragraphs X and XI. In addition to the very numerous published editions such as Stephen Halliwell, *The Poetics of Aristotle: Translation and Commentary* (London: Duckworth, 1987), a translation of Aristotle's poetics is available on the world wide web, see **http://classics.mit.edu/-Aristotle/poetics.1.1.html#390**, accessed 5 November 2004.

Bibliography

Archives

Australia

UNIVERSITY OF NEW SOUTH WALES
Oral History Archive.

Czech Republic

ACADEMY OF SCIENCES OF THE CZECH REPUBLIC
Málek Memoirs.

France

PALAIS DE LA DÉCOUVERTE
Penicillin exhibition December 1945.

Italy

ISTITUTO SUPERIORE DI SANITA
UNRRA-funded penicillin laboratory.

Switzerland

WORLD HEALTH ORGANIZATION
Archives of WHO.

Bibliography

United Kingdom

BODLEIAN LIBRARY OXFORD

Dorothy Hodgkin papers.

BOOTS ARCHIVE

Coulthard Notes; papers relating to the early production of penicillin.

BRITISH LIBRARY

Alexander Fleming papers; British Library Sound Archive.

EDINBURGH UNIVERSITY

Michael Swann papers.

GLAXO SMITHKLINE

Glaxo papers relating to the early production of penicillin.

HOUSE OF LORDS RECORDS OFFICE

Beaverbrook papers.

ICI PLC

Company archives relating to penicillin and wartime promotion.

NATIONAL ARCHIVES

Wartime penicillin papers, Swann Committee, Sainsbury Committee, Penicillin Bill, Pharmacy and Medicines Bill.
Medical Research Council papers.
Ministry of Health papers.
Ministry of Supply papers.

NATIONAL CATALOGUING UNIT FOR THE ARCHIVES OF SCIENTISTS

Edward Abraham papers.

PFIZER LTD.

Kemball Bishop papers.

ROYAL SOCIETY
Florey papers.

ST MARY'S HOSPITAL
Medical School papers.

SCIENCE MUSEUM
Notebooks relating to the development of semisynthetic penicillins.

UNIVERSITY OF SUSSEX
Mass Observation Archive.

WELLCOME LIBRARY FOR THE HISTORY AND UNDERSTANDING OF MEDICINE
BMA archive; Patients' Association archive; Royal Army Medical Corps archive; Chain and Heatley papers.

United States

AMERICAN INSTITUTE FOR THE HISTORY OF PHARMACY, MADISON, WISCONSIN
Andrew Moyer papers.

AMERICAN PHILOSOPHICAL SOCIETY
Demerec papers.

AMERICAN SOCIETY OF MICROBIOLOGY, UNIVERSITY OF MARYLAND LIBRARY
David Perlman papers.

COLUMBIA UNIVERSITY
Medical Aid to China; René Dubos papers.

DUKE UNIVERSITY, JOHN W. HARTMAN CENTER
Medicine and Madison Avenue archives.

LIBRARY OF CONGRESS
Vannevar Bush papers.

MURRAY RESEARCH CENTER, HARVARD UNIVERSITY
Dataset relating to 'Health and Personal Styles Project'.

NATIONAL ARCHIVES
Wartime penicillin development; anti-trust activities in the 1950s; John Blair
papers.

PFIZER INC.
Penicillin Development papers.

ROCKEFELLER ARCHIVES
Funding of Florey laboratory.

UNITED NATIONS
UNRRA papers.

UNIVERSITY OF AUSTIN, TEXAS, TARLTON LAW LIBRARY
Walton Hamilton Papers.

UNIVERSITY OF PENNSYLVANIA
Alfred Newton Richards papers.

UNIVERSITY OF WISCONSIN IN MADISON
University archives, oral histories.

Printed Sources

Abraham, Edward. 'Chain, Ernst Boris 19 June 1906-12 August 1979'. *Biographical Memoirs of the Royal Society*, 29 (1983), 43–92.
___ 'Some Aspects of the History of the Penicillins and Cephalosporins'. Invitational ONR Lecture. *Journal of Industrial Microbiology and Biotechnology*, 22 (1999), 275–87.
___ Chain, E., Florey, H. W., Florey, M. E., Heatley, N. G., Jennings, M. A., and Sanders, A. G. 'Historical Introduction'. In H. W. Florey, E. Chain, N. G. Heatley, M. A. Jennings, A. G. Sanders, E. P. Abraham, and M. E. Florey (eds.), *Antibiotics*. Oxford: Oxford University Press, 1949, ii. 631–71.
Abraham, Edward, and Loder, P. B. 'History of Cephalosporin C'. In E. H. Flynn (ed.), *Cephalosporins and Penicillins; Chemistry and Biology*. New York: Academic Press, 1972, 3–11.

'Action Sought on Antibiotics after Babies' Deaths'. *The Times*, 14 April 1969.

'Acute Respiratory Infections: The Forgotten Pandemic. Communiqué from the International Conference on Acute Respiratory Infections, Held in Canberra, Australia, 7–10 July 1997'. *International Journal of Tuberculosis and Lung Diseases*, 2 (1998), 2–4.

Adams, David P. *The Greatest Good to the Greatest Number: Penicillin Rationing on the American Home Front, 1940–1945*. New York: Peter Lang, 1991.

'A Drug-Taking Culture'. *The Guardian*, 14 November 1967.

Anderson, E. S. 'Origin of Transferable Drug-Resistance Factors in the Enterobacteriaceae'. *British Medical Journal*, 2 (27 November 1965), 1289–91.

_____ 'Possible Importance of Transfer Factors in Bacterial Evolution'. *Nature*, 209 (5 February 1966), 637–8.

_____ 'Influence of the Delta Transfer Factor on the Phage Sensitivity of Salmonellae', *Nature*, 212 (19 November 1966), 795–9.

_____ 'The Ecology of Transferable Drug Resistance in the Enterobacteria', *Annual Review of Microbiology*, 22 (1968), 131–80.

_____ 'Drug Resistance in *Salmonella typhimurium* and its Implications'. *British Medical Journal*, 2 (10 August 1968), 333–9.

_____ and Lewis, M. J. 'Drug Resistance and its Transfer in *Salmonella typhimurium*', *Nature*, 206 (8 May 1965), 579–83.

Andrews, G. W. S., and Miller, J. *Penicillin and Other Antibiotics*. London: Todd, 1949.

Andrews, J. M., and Langmuir, A. D. 'The Philosophy of Disease Eradication'. *American Journal of Public Health*, 53 (1963), 1–6.

'A New Penicillin'. *British Medical Journal*, 2 (7 November 1959), 940.

'Antibiotics: Dangers of Misuse'. *Washington Post*, 8 August 1981.

'Antibiotics in the Barnyard'. *Fortune* (March 1952), 118–40.

'Antibiotic Resistance Survey: Report of Findings'. Conducted for the Royal Pharmaceutical Society by Business Diagnostics, September/October 1999.

Armstrong, David. 'The Patient's View'. *Social Science and Medicine*, 18 (1984), 737–44.

_____ 'Decline of the Hospital: Reconstructing Institutional Dangers'. *Sociology of Health and Illness*, 20 (1998), 445–57.

_____ 'The Myth of Concordance: Response to Stevenson and Scambler'. *Health*, 9 (2005), 23–7.

Armstrong, Donald B. 'Magic Bullets'. *Hygeia* (October 1938), 892.

Armstrong, G. L., Conn, L. A., and Pinner, R. W. 'Trends in Infectious Disease Mortality in the United States During the 20th Century'. *Journal of the American Medical Association*, 281 (1999), 61–6.

Arrow, Kenneth J. 'Uncertainty and the Welfare Economics of Medical Care'. *American Economic Review*, 53 (1963), 941–73.

Ashworth, M., Latinovic, R., Charlton, J., Cox, K., Rowlands, G., and Gulliford, M. 'Why Has Antibiotic Prescribing for Respiratory Illness Declined in Primary Care?

A Longitudinal Study Using the General Practice Research Database'. *Journal of Public Health*, 26 (2004), 268–74.

Auinger, P., Lamphear, B., Kalkwarf, H. J., and Mansour, M. E. 'Trends in Otitis Media among Children in the United States'. *Pediatrics*, 112 (2003), 514–20.

Austrian, Robert. 'Confronting Drug-Resistant Pneumococci'. *Annals of Internal Medicine*, 121 (1994), 807–9.

Avorn, Jerry, and Solomon, Daniel H. 'Cultural and Economic Factors That (Mis)Shape Antibiotic Use: The Nonpharmacologic Basis of Therapeutics'. *Annals of Internal Medicine*, 133 (2000), 128–35.

Ayliffe, Graham and English, Mary. *Hospital Infection: From Miasmas to MRSA*. Cambridge: Cambridge University Press, 2003.

Bacharach, A. L., and Hern, B. A. 'Chemistry and Manufacture of Penicillin'. In Alexander Fleming (ed.), *Penicillin*. London: Butterworth, 1946, 24–45.

Backus, M. P., and Stauffer, J. F. 'The Production and Selection of a Family of Strains in *Penicillium chrysogenum*', *Mycologia*, 47 (1955), 429–63.

———— and Johnson, M. J. 'Penicillin Yields from New Mold Strains'. *Journal of the American Chemical Society*, 68 (1946), 152–3.

Ballio, A., Chain, E. B., Dentice, D. I., Accadia, F., Rolinson, G. N., and Batchelor, F. R. 'Penicillin Derivatives of p-aminobenzylpenicillin'. *Nature*, 183 (17 January 1959), 180–1.

Balogh, Brian. 'Reorganising the Organisational Synthesis: Federal–Professional Relations in Modern America'. *Studies in American Political Development*, 5 (1991), 119–70.

Bankoff, George. *The Conquest of Disease*. London: Macdonald, 1946.

Baquero, Fernando. 'Pneumococcal Resistance to ß-lactam Antibiotics: A Global Geographic Overview'. *Microbial Drug Resistance*, 1 (1995), 115–20.

—— Baquero-Artigao, Gregorio, Canton, Rafael, and Garcia-Rey, Cesar. 'Antibiotic Consumption and Resistance Selection in *Streptococcus pneumoniae*'. *Journal of Antimicrobial Chemotherapy*, 50 (2002), Suppl. S2: 27–37.

Barber, Mary. 'Staphylococcal Infection Due to Antibiotic-Resistant Strains'. *British Medical Journal*, 2 (1947), 863–5.

—— 'The Incidence of Penicillin Sensitive Variant Colonies in Penicillinase Producing Strains of *Staphylococcus aureus*'. *Journal of General Microbiology*, 3 (1949), 274.

—— ' "Celbenin"-Resistant Staphylococci'. *British Medical Journal*, 2 (24 September 1960), 939.

—— 'Drug-Resistant Staphylococcal Infection'. *Journal of Obstetrics and Gynaecology in the British Empire*, 67 (1960), 727–32.

Barrett, F. F., McGehee, R. F., and Finland, M. 'Methicillin-Resistant *Staphylococcus aureus* at Boston City Hospital'. *New England Journal of Medicine*, 279 (1968), 441–8.

Bartrip, Peter. *Themselves Writ Large: The British Medical Association 1832–1966*. London: BMJ Publishing Group, 1996.

'Beecham's will have Million-a-Year Press Appropriation'. *World's Press News*, 14 July 1938.

Begley, Sharon. 'The End of Antibiotics'. *Newsweek* (28 March 1994), 47–52.

Bell, Robert. *Impure Science: Fraud, Compromise and Political Influence in Scientific Research*. New York: Wiley, 1992.

Benini, Aldo A., and Bradford-Benini, Janet. 'Ebola Virus: From Medical Emergency to Complex Disaster'. *Journal of Contingencies and Crisis Management*, 4 (1996), 10–19.

Benzenhöfer, Udo. 'Zum Paracelsusbild im Dritten Reich: Unter besonderer Berücksichtigung der Paracelsusfeier in Tübingen/Stuttgart im Jahre 1941'. In Ulrich Fellmeth and Andreas Kotheder (eds.), *Paracelsus - Theophrast von Hohenheim: Naturforscher, Arzt, Theologe*. Stuttgart: Wissenschaftliche Verlagsgesellschaft, 1993, 63–70.

Berlin, Isaiah. *The Hedgehog and the Fox: An Essay on Tolstoy's View of History*. New York: Bantam, 1957. First published 1953.

Berman, Stephen. 'Otitis Media in Developing Countries'. *Pediatrics*, 96 (1995), 126–31.

Bernal, John Desmond. 'Britain's Part in the New Scientific Industrial Revolution'. Newcastle-upon-Tyne: University of Newcastle-upon-Tyne, 1965.

Bernhauer, Konrad. *Gärungschemisches Praktikum*. Berlin: Julius Springer, 1936.

Bickel, Lennard. *Rise up to Life: A Biography of Howard Walter Florey who Gave Penicillin to the World*. London: Angus and Robertson, 1972.

Biörck, Gunnar. 'The Next Ten Years in Medicine: Attempt at an Analysis of Factors Determining Medical and Social Development'. *British Medical Journal*, 2 (3 July 1965), 7–11.

Bisno, Alan L. 'Diagnosing Strep Throat in the Adult Patient: Do Clinical Criteria Really Suffice?' *Annals of Internal Medicine*, 139 (2003), 150–1.

Blaxter, Mildred. *Mothers and Daughters: A Three Generation Study of Health Attitudes and Behaviour*. London: Heinemann, 1982.

——'Why do Victims Blame Themselves'. In Alan Radley (ed.), *Worlds of Illness: Biographical and Cultural Perspectives on the Worlds of Illness*. London: Routledge, 1993, 124–42.

——'Whose Fault is It? People's Own Conceptions of the Reasons for Health Inequalities'. *Social Science and Medicine*, 10 (1997), 747–56.

Bledsoe, Caroline H., and Goubaud, Monica F. 'The Reinterpretation and Distribution of Western Pharmaceuticals: An Example from the Mende of Sierra Leone'. In Sjaak Van Der Geest and Susan Reynolds Whyte (eds.), *The Context of Medicines in Developing Countries*. Dordrecht: Kluwer, 1988, 253–76.

Bloom, Samuel W. *The Word as Scalpel: A History of Medical Sociology*. Oxford: Oxford University Press, 2002.

Blum, Richard, and Blum, Eva. *Health and Healing in Rural Greece*. San Jose, Calif: Stanford University Press, 1965.

Bibliography

Blume, Stuart. *Insight and Industry: The Dynamics of Technological Change in Medicine.* Cambridge, Mass.: MIT Press, 1992.

Bogdan, H. A. 'Felix Marti Ibanez—Iberian Daedalus: The Man behind the Essays'. *Journal of the Royal Society of Medicine*, 86 (1993), 593–6.

Bornscheuer, U., and Buchholz, K. 'Highlights in Biocatalysis: Historical Landmarks and Current Trends'. *Engineering in Life Sciences*, 5 (2005), 309–23.

Bott, Elizabeth. *Family and Social Network.* 2nd edn. London: Tavistock, 1971.

Böttcher, Helmüth. *Wunderdrogen: Die abenteurliche Geschichte der Heilpilze.* Cologne: Kiepenheuer & Witsch, 1959.

Bovet, Daniel. *Une chimie qui guérit: histoire de la découverte dessulfamides.* Paris: Payot, 1988.

Brandt, Allan M. *No Magic Bullet: A Social History of Venereal Disease in the United States since 1880.* Oxford: Oxford University Press, 1985.

Branthwaite, A., and Pechère, J. C. 'Pan-European Survey of Patients' Attitudes to Antibiotic and Antibiotic Use'. *Journal of International Medical Research*, 24 (1996), 229–38.

Brewer, Gleb A., and Johnson, Marvin J. 'Activity and Properties of Para-aminobenzyl Penicillin'. *Applied Microbiology*, 1 (1953), 163–6.

Bridging a Gap: The Story of Boots Achievement in the Wartime Production of Penicillin. Nottingham: Boots, 1946.

Britten, Nicky. 'Patients' Demands for Prescriptions in Primary Care: Patients Cannot Take All the Blame for Overprescribing'. *British Medical Journal*, 310 (29 April 1995), 1084–5.

——— 'Lay Views of Medicines and their Influence on Prescribing: A Study in General Practice'. Doctoral thesis, London University, 1996.

Brock, Thomas. *The Emergence of Bacterial Genetics.* Cold Spring Harbor, NY: Cold Spring Harbor Laboratory Press, 1990.

Brown, Kevin. *Penicillin Man: Alexander Fleming and the Antibiotic Revolution.* Stroud: Sutton, 2004.

Brunner, R. 'In Memoriam: Konrad Bernhauer'. *Mitteilungen der Versuchsstation für das Gärungsgewerbe in Wien*, 2 (1976), 22.

Bud, Robert. 'Strategy in American Cancer Research after World War 2: A Case Study'. *Social Studies of Science*, 8 (1978), 425–59.

——— *The Uses of Life: A History of Biotechnology.* Cambridge: Cambridge University Press, 1994.

——— 'Penicillin and the New Elizabethans'. *British Journal for the History of Science*, 31 (1998), 305–33.

——— 'Antibiotics, Big Business and Consumers'. *Technology and Culture*, 46 (2005), 329–49.

——— Niziol, Simon, Boon, Tim, and Nahum, Andrew. *Inventing the Modern World.* London: Dorling Kindersley, 2000.

Burghart, R. 'Penicillin: An Ancient Ayurvedic Medicine'. In Sjaak Van Der Geest and Susan Reynolds Whyte (eds.), *The Context of Medicines in Developing Countries.*

Dordrecht: Kluwer, 1988, 289–98.

Burnet, Macfarlane. *The Natural History of Infectious Disease*. 2nd edn. Cambridge: Cambridge University Press, 1953.

Burns, Melanie, Bennett, J. W., and van Dijck, Piet W. M. 'Code Name Bacinol'. *ASM News*, 69 (2003), 25–31.

____ and van Dijck, Piet W. M. 'The Development of the Penicillin Production Process in Delft, the Netherlands, during World War II under Nazi Occupation'. *Advances in Applied Microbiology*, 51 (2002), 185–200.

Bush, Vannevar. 'The Case for Biological Engineering'. In Karl Compton (ed.), *Scientists Face the World of 1942*. New Brunswick, NJ: Rutgers University Press, 1942, 33–45.

____ *Science: The Endless Frontier*. Washington, DC: United States Government Printing Office, 1945.

Butler, Christopher C., Rollnick, Stephen, Pill, Roisin, Maggs-Rapport, Frances, and Stott, Nigel. 'Understanding the Culture of Prescribing: Qualitative Study of General Practitioners' and Patients' Perceptions of Antibiotics for Sore Throats'. *British Medical Journal*, 317 (5 September 1998), 637–42.

Cahal, M. F. 'What the Public Thinks of the Family Doctor: Folklore and Facts'. *GP* 25 (1962), 146–57.

Calder, Ritchie. *Medicine and Man: The History of the Art and Science of Healing*. London: George Allen and Unwin, 1958.

Calva, J., and Bojalil, R. 'Antibiotic Use in a Periurban Community in Mexico: A Household and Drugstore Survey'. *Social Science and Medicine*, 42 (1996), 1121–8.

Cannon, Geoffrey. *Superbug: Nature's Revenge: Why Antibiotics Can Breed Disease*. London: Virgin, 1995.

Cant, Susan, and Sharma, Ursula. *A New Medical Pluralism? Alternative Medicines, Doctors, Patients and the State*. London: UCL Press, 1999.

Carr, Harold. 'The Patients Association'. *Hospital and Health Management*, 4 (1963), 287–8.

Carrie, Anita G., and Zhanel, George G. 'Antibacterial Use in Community Practice: Assessing Quantity, Indications and Appropriateness, and Relationship to the Development of Antibacterial Resistance'. *Drugs*, 57 (1999), 871–81.

Cars, Otto, and Mölstad, Sigvard. 'Variation in Antibiotic Use in the European Union'. *The Lancet*, 357 (9 June 2001), 1851–3.

Casal, J., Fenol, A., Vicioso, M. D., and Munoz, R. 'Increase in Resistance to Penicillin in Pneumococci in Spain'. *The Lancet*, 1 (1 April 1989), 735.

Catron, Damon. 'Recent Development in Swine Nutrition'. *Veterinary Medicine*, 44 (May 1949), 215–20.

Central Health Services Council, Standing Medical Advisory Committee. *Staphylococcal Infections in Hospitals*. Report of the Subcommittee. London: HMSO, 1959.

Chain, E. B. 'Penicillinase Resistant Penicillins and the Problerm of the Penicillin Resistant Staphylococci'. In A. V. S. De Reuck and Margaret P. Cameron (eds.), *Resistance of Bacteria to the Penicillins: In Honour of Sir Charles Harington*. Ciba

Foundation Study Group 13. London: J. & A. Churchill, 1962, 3–18.

Chain, E. B. Paladino, S., Ugolini, F., Callow, D. S., and van der Sluis, J. 'A Laboratory Fermenter for Vortex and Sparger Aeration'. *Rendiconti Istitututo Superiore di Sanita* (English edition), 17 (1954), 61–86.

Chandler, Alfred. *Shaping the Industrial Century: The Remarkable Story of the Evolution of the Modern Chemical and Pharmaceutical Industries*. Cambridge, Mass.: Harvard University Press, 2005.

Chandler, D., and Dugdale, A. E. 'What do Patients Know about Antibiotics?' *The Lancet*, 2 (21 August 1976), 422.

'The Chemotherapy of Streptococcal Infections'. *The Lancet*, 230 (6 June 1936), 1303–4.

Chetley, Andrew. *A Healthy Business: World Health and the Pharmaceutical Industry*. London: Zed Books, 1990.

Chou, Y. J., Yip, W. C., Huang, N., Sun, Y. P., and Chang, H. J. 'Impact of Separating Drug Prescribing and Dispensing on Provider Behaviour: Taiwan's Experience'. *Health Policy and Planning*, A. 18 (2003), 316–29.

Čižman, Milan. 'The Use and Resistance to Antibiotics in the Community'. *International Journal of Antimicrobial Agents*, 21 (2003), 297–307.

Clark, A. J. *Patent Medicines*. London: FACT, 1938.

Clark, Ronald W. *The Life of Ernst Chain: Penicillin and Beyond*. London: Weidenfeld and Nicolson, 1985.

Clement & Johnson Ltd. *The Yadil Book: The Careful Study of this Book and the Use of Yadil Everywhere for Every Disorder will Save Hundreds of Thousands of Lives Every Year*. London: Clement & Johnson, 1922.

——*Tuberculosis: The Problem Solved: Yadil Antiseptic Cures & Prevents the White Scourge*. London: Clement & Johnson, 1923.

Coast, J., Smith, R. D., and Millar, M. R. 'An Economic Perspective on Policy to Reduce Antimicrobial Resistance'. *Social Science and Medicine*, 46 (1998), 29–38.

Cockburn, T. A. *The Evolution and Eradication of Infectious Diseases*. Baltimore: Johns Hopkins University Press, 1963.

Coghill, R. D., and Koch, R. S. 'Penicillin: A Wartime Accomplishment'. *Chemical and Engineering News*, 23 (1945), 2310.

——Stodola, F. H., and Wachtel, J. L. 'Chemical Modifications of Natural Penicillins'. In Hans T. Clarke, John R. Johnson, and Sir Robert Robinson (eds.), *The Chemistry of Penicillin*. Princeton: Princeton University Press, 1949, 680–7.

Cohen, I. Bernard. *Science, Servant of Man*. Boston: Little Brown, 1948.

Cohen, Lizabeth. *A Consumers Republic: The Politics of Mass Consumption in Postwar America*. New York: Knopf, 2003.

Col, N. F., and O'Connor, R. W. 'Estimating Worldwide Current Antibiotic Usage: Report of Task Force 1'. *Reviews of Infectious Diseases*, 9 (1987), Suppl. 3: S232–43.

Coleman, J. S., Katz, E., and Menzel, H. *Medical Innovation: A Diffusion Study*. Indianapolis: Bobbs-Merrill, 1966.

Collings, J. 'General Practice in England Today'. *The Lancet*, 1 (25 March 1950), 555–85.

Comanor, William S. 'The Political Economy of the Pharmaceutical Industry'. *Journal of Economic Literature*, 24 (1986), 1178–217.

Committee on the Costs of Medical Care. *Medical Care for the American People: The Final Report, Adopted October 31, 1932*. Chicago: University of Chicago Press, 1932.

Connell, Louise Fox. 'What We Now Know about Young Ears'. *Parents Magazine*, 29 (March 1954), 40–1.

'Conquering Streptococcus'. *New York Times*, 18 December 1936.

Cooper, Jill E. 'Of Microbes and Men: A Scientific Biography of René Jules Dubos'. Ph.D. dissertation, Rutgers University, 1998.

Cooper, Michael. *Prices and Profits in the Pharmaceutical Industry*. Oxford: Pergamon, 1966.

Cornwell, Jocelyn. *Hard-Earned Lives: Accounts of Health and Illness from East London*. London: Tavistock, 1984.

Costello, Peter. 'The Tetracycline Conspiracy: Structure, Conduct and Performance in the Drug Industry'. *Antitrust Law and Economics Review*, 1 (1968), 13–44.

Coulthard, C. E., Michaelis, R., Short, W. F., Sykes, G., Skrimshire, G. E. H., Standfast, A. F. B., Birkinshaw, J. H., and Raistrick, H. 'Notatin and Anti-bacterial Glucose-aerohydrogenase from Penicillium notatum Westling and Penicillium resticulosum sp. Nov.' *Biochemical Journal*, 39 (1945), 24–36.

Coy, Harold. *The Americans: A Story about People Democracy, Free Schools, Ice Cream, Airplanes, Social Security, Penicillin, Atomic Energy and All the Things that Make our Nation Great*. Boston: Little Brown, 1958.

Crawford, L. M. 'Comment on A. Linton, "The Swann Report and its Impact"'. In Charles H. Stuart-Harris and David M. Harris (eds.), *The Control of Antibiotic-Resistant Bacteria*. New York: Academic Press, 1982, 196.

Crellin, J. K. *A Social History of Medicines in the Twentieth Century: To be Taken Three Times a Day*. New York: Pharmaceutical Products Press, 2004.

Curtice, John and Jowell, Roger. 'Trust in the Political System'. In Roger Jowell, John Curtice, Alison Park, Lindsay Brook, Katarina Thomson, and Caroline Bryson (eds.), *British Social Attitudes: The 14th Report*. Aldershot: Ashgate, 1997, 89–109.

Cutler, Elliott C. 'The Chief Consultant in Surgery'. In B. Noland Carter (ed.), *Activities of Surgical Consultants*. Washington, DC: Office of the Surgeon General, Dept. of the Army, 1962–4, 19–238.

Damoiseaux, R. A., deMelker, R. A., Ausems, M. J., and van Belen, F. A. 'Reasons for Non-Guideline-Based Antibiotic Prescriptions for Acute Otitis Media in the Netherlands'. *Family Practice*, 16 (1999), 50–3.

'The Dangers of Misusing Antibiotics'. *The Guardian*, 3 February 1968.

Daston, Lorraine. 'The Moral Economy of Science'. *Osiris*, 2nd ser. 10 (1995), 1–26.

Datta, Naomi. 'Transmissible Drug Resistance in an Epidemic Strain of *Salmonella typhimurium*'. *Journal of Hygiene*, 60 (1962), 301–10.

Dauer, C. C. 'A Demographic Analysis of Recent Changes in Mortality, Morbidity, and Age Group Distribution in our Population'. In Iago Galdston (ed.), *The Impact of the Antibiotics on Medicine and Society*. Monograph 2, Institute of Social and Historical Medicine, New York Academy of Medicine. New York: International Universities Press, 1958, 98–120.

Dauer, C. C., and Serfling, R. E. 'Mortality from Influenza 1957–1958 and 1959–1960'. *American Review of Respiratory Diseases*, 83 (1961), 15–28.

Dauer, Holger. *Ludwig Fulda, Erfolgsschriftsteller: Eine mentalitätsgeschichtlich orientierte Interpretation populardramatischer Texte*. Tübingen: M. Niemeyer, 1998.

Davenport-Hines, R. P. T. *Sex, Death and Punishment: Attitudes to Sex and Sexuality in Britain since the Renaissance*. London: Collins, 1990.

＿＿and Slinn, Judy. *Glaxo: A History to 1962*. Cambridge: Cambridge University Press, 1992.

Davey, P. G., Bax, R. P., Newey, J., Reeves, D., Rutherford, D., Slack, R., Warren, R. E., Watt, B., and Wilson, J. 'Growth in the Use of Antibiotics in the Community in England and Scotland in 1980–93'. *British Medical Journal*, 312 (9 March 1996), 613.

Davidson, C. S. 'The Cocoanut Grove Disaster: Maxwell Finland'. *Journal of Infectious Diseases*, 125 (March 1972), Suppl.: 58–73.

Dawson, Marc H. 'The Social History of Africa in the Future'. *African Studies Review*, 30 (1987), 83–91.

Daykin, P. W. 'Antibiotic Usage in Veterinary Practice before Swann'. In Donald V. Jolly, David J. S. Miller, David B. Ross, and Peter D. Simm (eds.), *Ten Years on from Swann*. London: The Association of Veterinarians in Industries, 1981, 27–36.

'Deaths from Asian Influenza, 1957: A Report by the Public Health Laboratory Service Based on Records from Hospital and Public Health Laboratories'. *British Medical Journal*, 1 (19 April 1958), 915–18.

deForest Lamb, Ruth. *American Chamber of Horrors*. New York: Little and Ives, 1936.

Defries, Robert D. *The First Forty Years 1914–1955: Connaught Medical Research Laboratories*. Toronto: University of Toronto Press, 1968.

De Kruif, Paul. *The Sweeping Wind*. New York: Harcourt, 1962.

Dennis, Michael Aaron. 'Accounting for Research: New Histories of Corporate Laboratories and the Social History of American Science'. *Social Studies of Science*, 17(1987), 479–518.

＿＿'A Change of State: The Political Cultures of Technical Practice at the MIT Instrumentation Laboratory and the Johns Hopkins University Applied Physics Laboratory, 1930–1945'. Doctrol dissertation, Johns Hopkins University, 1991.

Deschepper, Reginald, Vander Stichele, Robert H., and Haaijer-Ruskamp, Flora M. 'Cross-Cultural Differences in Lay Attitudes and Utilisation of Antibiotics in a Belgian and a Dutch City'. *Patient Education and Counseling*, 48 (2002), 161–9.

'The Diary of a Tragedy'. *Evening Gazette* (Middlesbrough), 7 March 1968.

Dichter, Ernest. *Getting Motivated by Ernest Dichter: The Secret behind Individual Motivations by the Man Who was not Afraid to Ask 'Why?'*. New York: Pergamon Press, 1979.

'Disease Fights Back'. *The Economist*, 335 (20 May 1995), 15.

Divine, Robert. *Blowing on the Wind: The Nuclear Test Ban Debate*. New York: Oxford University Press, 1978.

Dixon, Bernard. 'Antibiotics on the Farm: Major Threat to Human Health'. *New Scientist* (5 October 1967), 33–5.

____ *What is Science For?* London: Collins, 1973.

____ 'Killer Bug Ate my Face'. *Current Biology*, 6 (1996), 493.

____ 'Don't Blame the Messenger'. *Current Biology*, 7 (1997), R2.

'Doctors Get the "Superbug" Drug'. *Daily Mail*, 17 September 1981.

'Doctors See a Split Personality'. *Business Week*, (22 February 1958), 160–70.

Dowell, Scott F., Kupronis, Benjamin A., Zell, Elizabeth R., and Shay, David K. 'Mortality from Pneumonia in Children in the United States, 1939 through 1996'. *New England Journal of Medicine*, 342 (2000), 1399–407.

Doyle, F. P. 'Some Contributions to Chemotherapy'. *Särtryck ur Farmaceutisk Revy*, 62 (1963), 443–63.

'Drug Resistance in Salmonellas'. *The Lancet*, 1 (19 June 1982), 1391–2.

Dubos, René. 'The Philosopher's Search for Health'. *Transactions of the Association of American Physicians*, 66 (1953), 31–41.

____ *Mirage of Health: Utopias, Progress, and Biological Change*. New York: Harper & Row, 1959.

____ and Dubos, Jean. *The White Plague: Tuberculosis, Man and Society*. Boston: Little Brown, 1952.

Eagleton, Terry. *Sweet Violence: The Idea of the Tragic*. Oxford: Blackwell, 2003.

Earl, Ernest. *Queen Mary's Hospital for Children*. Knebworth: Able, 1996.

'Edward Mellanby Celebrates New Hospitals Centre at Birmingham'. *Birmingham Post*, 4 July 1938.

Edwards, S. J. 'Antibiotics in the Treatment of Mastitis'. In Malcolm Woodbine (ed.), *Antibiotics in Agriculture: Proceedings of the University of Nottingham Ninth Easter School in Agricultural Science, 1962*. London: Butterworths, 1962, 43–57.

Elder, Albert. 'The Role of Government in the Penicillin Program'. In Albert Elder (ed.), *The History of Penicillin Production*. Chemical Engineering Progress Symposium Series No. 100. *Chemical Engineering Progress*, 66 (1970), 3–11.

Elek, S. D., and Fleming, P. C. 'A New Technique for the Control of Hospital Cross-Infection: Experience with BRL. 1241 in a Maternity Unit'. *The Lancet*, 2 (10 September 1960), 569–72.

Enright, M. C., Robinson, D. A., Randle, G., Feil, E. J., Grundmann, H., and Spratt, B. G. 'The Evolutionary History of Methicillin-Resistant *Staphylococcus aureus* (MRSA)'. *Proceedings of the National Academy of Science*, 99 (2002), 7687–92.

Eriksen, K. Riewerts, and Eriksen, Ingrid. 'Resistance to Newer Penicillins'. *British Medical Journal*, 1 (16 March 1963), 746.

Bibliography

European Commission, Research Directorate-General. *Europeans Science and Technology*, Eurobarometer 55.2. Brussels: European Commission, 2001.

Fabricant, Stephen J., and Hirschhorn, Norbert. 'Deranged Distribution, Perverse Prescription, Unprotected Use: The Irrationality of Pharmaceuticals in the Developing World'. *Health Policy and Planning*, 2 (1987), 204–13.

Falini, R. 'Biochemical Engineering in the Production of Fungal Metabolites'. In D. A. Hems (ed.), *Biologically Active Substances: Exploration and Exploitation*. Chichester: John Wiley, 1977, 33–48.

Falkow, S. *Infectious Multiple Drug Resistance*. London: Pion, 1975.

'F and M at the Min of Ag'. *Daily Mirror*, 29 April 1968.

Farrington, R. M. 'Fighting Death with"693": Medical Men are Tirelessly Testing a Miracle Drug Bordering on Witch Cures of the Middle Ages, That Promises to Wipe out Pneumonia'. *Star Weekly* (Toronto), 14 January 1939.

Fee, Elizabeth. 'Sin vs Science: Venereal Disease in Baltimore in the Twentieth Century'. *Journal of the History of Medicine and Allied Sciences*, 43 (1988), 141–64.

Feldman, Jack. 'What Americans Think about their Medical Care'. In American Statistical Association, *Proceedings of the Social Statistics Section 1958*. Washington, DC: American Statistical Association, 1959, 102–5.

Felmingham, D., and Washington, J. 'Trends in the Antimicrobial Susceptibility of Bacterial Respiratory Tract Pathogens: Findings of the Alexander Project 1992–1996'. *Journal of Chemotherapy*, 11 (1999), Suppl. 1: 5–21.

Ferguson, Anne. 'Commercial Pharmaceutical Medicine and Medicalization: A Case Study from El Salvador'. In Sjaak Van der Geest and Susan Reynolds Whyte (eds.), *The Context of Medicine in Developing Countries: Studies in Pharmaceutical Anthropology*. Dordrecht: Kluwer Academic Publishers, 1988, 19–46.

Ferry, Georgina. *Dorothy Hodgkin: A Life*. London: Granta, 1998.

Finerman, Ruthbeth, and Bennett, Linda A. 'Guilt, Blame and Shame: Responsibility in Health and Sickness'. *Social Science and Medicine*, 40 (1995), 1–3.

Finkelstein, J. A., Huang, S. S., Daniel, J., Rifas-Shiman, S. I., et al. 'Reduction in Antibiotic Use among US Children, 1996–2000'. *Pediatrics*, 112 (2003), 620–7.

Finland, M., Jones, W. J., Jr., and Barnes, M. W. 'Occurrence of Serious Bacterial Infections since Introduction of Antibacterial Agents'. *Journal of the American Medical Association*, 170 (1959), 2188–97.

Finlay, Mark R. 'Hogs, Antibiotics, and the Industrial Environment of Postwar Agriculture'. In Susan R. Schrepfer and Philip Scranton, (eds.), *Industrializing Organisms: Introducing Evolutionary History*. London: Routledge, 2004, 237–60.

'First A-Bomb Use Called the Century's No. 1 News Story'. *Christian Science Monitor*, 24 December 1999.

Fischetti, Vincent A. 'The Streptococcus and the Host: Present and Future Challenges'. *Advances in Experimental Medicine and Biology*, 418 (1997), 15–20.

'£5 million to Stop Foreigners Filching our Ideas', *Daily Herald*, 14 April 1948.

Fleisch, A, 'Antibiotika in Nahrungsmitteln'. *Schweize Ärtezeitung*, 49 (1959), 722.

Fleming, Alexander. 'On the Antibacterial Action of Cultures of a Penicillium, with Special Reference to their Use in the Isolation of *B. influenzae*'. *British Journal of Experimental Pathology*, 10 (1929), 226–36.

Forth, Wortgang, Gericke, Dietmar, and Klimmek, Reinhard. *Men & Fungi: Penicillin Research and Production in World War II Germany*. Munich: W. Zuckschwerdt, 2000. Translation of *Von Menschen und Pilzen* (1997).

Foster, J. W. 'Preface'. *Journal of Antibiotics*, 1 (1947), 1.

——'Three Days Symposium on Penicillin Production'. Separate issue of *Journal of Penicillin*, 1 (March 1947).

——'A View of Microbiological Science in Japan'. *Applied Microbiology*, 9 (1961), 434–51.

Fox, Daniel M. *Health Policies, Health Politics: The British and American Experience 1911–1965*. Princeton: Princeton University Press, 1986.

Franzen, Giep, and Brouwman, Margot. *The Mental World of Brands: Mind, Memory and Brand Success*. Henley-on-Thames: World Advertising Research Centre, 2001.

Fraser, Sir Ian. 'Penicillin: Early Trials in War Casualties'. *British Medical Journal*, 289 (22 December 1984), 1723–5.

——*Blood, Sweat and Cheers*. London: BMJ, 1989.

Freeman, Howard E., and Reeder, Leo G. 'Medical Sociology: A Review of the Literature'. *American Sociological Review*, 22 (1957), 73–81.

Freidson, Eliot. 'The Development of Design by Accident', in R. H. Elling and M. Sokoloska (eds.), *Medical Sociologists at Work*. New Brunswick, NJ: Transaction Books, 1978, 115–32.

Freund, Michaela. 'Women, Venereal Disease and the Control of Female Sexuality in Post-War Hamburg'. In Roger Davidson and Lesley A. Hall (eds.), *Sex, Sin and Suffering: Venereal Disease and European Society since 1870*. London: Routledge, 2001, 205–19.

From Compliance to Concordance: Achieving Shared Goals in Medicine Taking. London: Royal Pharmaceutical Society; Hoddesdon: Merck Sharp & Dohme, 1997.

Fügnerová, M. K. 'Health Services and the Two Year Plan'. *Czechoslovakia* (January 1947), 455–8.

Fujii, R. 'Changes in Antibiotic Consumption in Japan during the Past 40 Years'. *Japanese Journal of Antibiotics*, 37 (1984), 2261–70.

Fulda, Ludwig. *Das Wundermittel: Komödie in drei Aufzügen*. Stuttgart: J. G. Cotta'sche Buchhandlung Nachfolger, 1920.

'Future of Methicillin'. *British Medical Journal*, 1 (2 February 1963), 280–2.

Galdston, Iago. *Behind the Sulfa Drugs: A Short History of Chemotherapy*. New York: Appleton-Century, 1943.

——(ed.). *The Impact of the Antibiotics on Medicine and Society*. Monograph 2, Institute of Social and Historical Medicine, New York Academy of Medicine. New York: International Universities Press, 1958.

Gallup Poll Ltd., Social Surveys. 'Report on the National Health Service Medical Service: Report Prepared on Behalf of the "The Daily Telegraph"'. In *A Review of the Medical Services in Great Britain* (Porritt Report). London: Social Assay, on behalf of the Medical Services Review Committee, 1963.

Garfield, Simon. *Our Hidden Lives. The Remarkable Diaries of Post-War Britain.* London: Ebury, 2005.

Garrett, Laurie. *The Coming Plague: Newly Emerging Diseases in a World out of Balance.* Harmondsworth: Penguin, 1995.

Garrity, Joseph. 'Soldiers without Weapons'. *Eighth Army News*, 8 June 1945.

Garrod, L. P. 'The Waning Power of Penicillin'. *British Medical Journal*, 2 (1947), 874.

——'Mary Barber 3 April 1911–11 September 1965'. *Journal of Pathology and Bacteriology*, 92 (1996), 603–10.

Gaudillière, Jean-Paul. *Inventer la biomédecine: la France, l'Amérique et la production des savoirs du vivant (1995–1965).* Paris: La Découverte, 2002.

——and Gausemeier, B. 'Molding National Research Systems: The Introduction of Penicillin to Germany and France'. *Osiris*, 20 (2005), 180–202.

George, Peter. *Dr Strangelove, or, How I Learned to Stop Worrying and Love the Bomb.* London: Transworld, 1963.

Gilks, Charles F. 'HIV and Pneumococcal Infection in Africa: Clinical, Epidemiological and Preventative Aspects'. *Transactions of the Royal Society of Tropical Medicine and Hygiene*, 91 (1997), 627–31.

Gilson, Lucy. 'Trust and the Development of Health Care as a Social Institution'. *Social Science and Medicine*, 56 (2003), 1453–68.

Girstenbrey, Wilhelm. 'Der Aufstieg der Gruenenthal gmbh mit dem "Wundermittel" Penicillin'. *die Waage*, 22 (1983), 126–32.

Godber, Sir George. 'Opening Address'. In *Prevention of Hospital Infection: The Personal Factor. Report of a Conference Held in London on 19 June 1963.* London: Royal Society of Health, 1963, 1–3.

Goldsmith, Margaret. *The Road to Penicillin: A History of Chemotherapy.* London: Lindsay Drumond, 1946.

Gonzales, Ralph. 'Principles of Appropriate Antibiotic Use for Treatment of Acute Respiratory Tract Infections in Adults: Background, Specific Aims, and Methods'. *Annals of Internal Medicine*, 134 (2001), 479–86.

Good, Mary-Jo Delvecchio, and Good, Byron J. 'Clinical Narratives and the Study of Contemporary Doctor–Patient Relationships'. In Gary L. Albrecht, Ray Fitzpatrick, and Susan C. Scrimshaw (eds.), *Handbook of Social Studies in Health and Medicine.* London: Sage, 2000, 243–58.

Goossens, Herman, Ferech, Matus, Vander Stichele, Robert, Elseviers, Monique, and the ESAC Project Group. 'Outpatient Antibiotic Use in Europe and Association with Resistance'. *The Lancet*, 365 (12 February 2005), 579–87.

Green, F. H. K., and Covell, Gordon. *Medical Research: Medical History of the Second World War.* London: HMSO, 1953.

Greenberg, Selig. 'The Decline of the Healing Art'. In Marion Sanders (ed.), *The Crisis in American Medicine*. New York: Harpers, 1960, 20–9.

Greene, Alan J., and Schmitz, Andrew J. 'Meeting the Objective'. In Albert Elder (ed.), *The History of Penicillin Production*. Chemical Engineering Progress Symposium Series No. 100. *Chemical Engineering Progress*, 66 (1970), 80–97.

Greene, Jeremy A. 'Therapeutic Infidelities: "Noncompliance" Enters the Medical Literature'. *Social History of Medicine*, 17 (2004), 327–43.

Greenwood, D. 'Resistance to Antimicrobial Agents: A Personal View'. *Journal of Medical Microbiology*, 47 (1998), 751–5.

Gualandi, Giuseppe. 'Il Centro Internazionale di Chimica Microbiológica ed il suo capo E. B. Chain'. In *Domenico Marotta nel 25° anniversario della morte: rendiconti Accademia Nazionale delle Scienze detta dei XL 23* (1999), 211–13.

Guthe, T., and de Vries, J. L. 'Surveillance Reports: Epidemiological/Serological Evaluation of Tropical Yaws Following Mass Penicillin Campaigns'. World Health Organization Report GES/SR/662 WHO/VDT/66.336.

Habermas, Jürgen. *The Theory of Communicative Action*, i: *Reason and Rationalization of Society*, trans. Thomas McCarthy. London: Heinemann, 1984.

Hackett, C. J. 'Yaws'. In E. Sabben-Clare, D. J. Bradley, and K. Kirkwood (eds.), *Health in Tropical Africa during the Colonial Period: Based on the Proceedings of a Symposium Held at New College Oxford 21–23 March 1977*. Oxford: Oxford University Press, 1980, 62–92.

Hafferty, F., and McKinlay, J. (eds.). *The Changing Character of the Medical Profession: An International Comparison*. New York: Oxford University Press, 1993.

Halliwell, Stephen. *The Poetics of Aristotle: Translation and Commentary*. London: Duckworth, 1987.

Hancher, L. *Regulating for Competition: Law and the Pharmaceutical Industry in the United Kingdom and France*. Oxford: Oxford University Press, 1990.

Hansman, D. 'Type Distribution and Antibiotic Sensitivity of Pneumococci from Carriers in Kiriwina, Trobriand Islands (New Gornea)'. *Medical Journal of Australia*, 14 (1972), 771–3.

—— and Bullen, M. M. 'A Resistant Pneumococcus'. *The Lancet*, 2 (29 July 1967), 264–5.

Hanson, Elizabeth. *The Rockefeller University Achievement: A Century of Science for the Benefit of Mankind, 1901–2001*. New York: Rockefeller University Press, 2001.

Harbarth, Stephan, Albrich, Werner, and Brun-Buisson, Christian. 'Outpatient Antibiotic Use and Prevalence of Antibiotic-Resistant Pneumococci in France and Germany: A Sociocultural Perspective'. *Emerging Infectious Diseases*, 8 (2002), 1460–7.

Hardin, Garrett. 'The Tragedy of the Commons'. *Science*, 162 (13 December 1968), 1243–8.

Harington, Sir Charles. 'Opening Remarks'. In *Ciba* G. E. W. Wolstenholme and Cecilia M. O'Connor (eds.), *Foundation Symposium on Drug Resistance in Microorganisms: Mechanisms of Development*. London: J. & A. Churchill, 1957, 3.

Harpole, James. 'A Surgeon's Case-Book'. *Sunday Graphic*, 2 October 1938.

Harris, Richard. *The Real Voice*. New York: Macmillan, 1964.

Harris, Seymour E. *The Economics of American Medicine*. New York: Macmillan, 1964.

Harrison, Mark. *Medicine & Victory: British Military Medicine in the Second World War*. Oxford: Oxford University Press, 2004.

Harrison, Polly F., and Lederberg, Joshua (eds.). *Antimicrobial Resistance: Issues and Options. Workshop Report, Forum on Emerging Infections, Division of Health Sciences Policy*. Washington, DC: National Academies Press, 1998.

Harrison, Ruth. *Animal Machines: The New Factory Farming Industry*. London: Vincent Stuart, 1964.

Hastings, A. Baird, and Shimkin, Michael B. 'Medical Research Mission to the Soviet Union: Part II'. *Science*, 103 (24 May 1946), 637–44.

Heagney, Brenda. *Half a Century of Penicillin: An Australian Perspective*. Canberra: The Royal Australasian College of Physicians, 1991.

'Health Propaganda'. *The Lancet*, 220 (14 February 1931), 357.

Heaman, E. A. *St Mary's: The History of a London Teaching Hospital*. Montreal: McGill University Press, 2003.

Heinecke, Horst (ed.). *Dokumente zu den Anfängen der Penicillin-Forschung in Deutschland*. Erfurt: Akademie Gemeinnütziger Wissenschaften zu Erfurt, 2001.

Helm, Toby. 'Tragic Allergy to Light Drives Kohl Wife to Suicide'. *Daily Telegraph*, 6 July 2001.

Helman, C. G. ' "Feed a Cold, Starve a Fever": Folk Models of Infection in an English Suburban Community, and their Relation to Medical Treatment'. *Culture, Medicine and Psychiatry*, 2 (1978), 107–37.

Herring Jr., George C. *Aid to Russia 1941–1946: Strategy, Diplomacy and the Origins of the Cold War*. New York: Columbia University Press, 1973.

Herzlich, Claudine, and Pierret, Janine. *Illness and Self in Society*, trans. Elborg Forster. Baltimore: Johns Hopkins University Press, 1987.

Hewitt, W. L. 'Penicillin: Historical Impact on Infection Control'. *Annals of the New York Academy of Sciences*, 145 (1967), 212–15.

Hobby, Gladys L. *Penicillin: Meeting the Challenge*. New Haven: Yale University Press, 1985.

Hodgson, Helen. 'A Patients' Group'. *Sunday Times*, 25 November 1962.

Hoge, James F. 'An Appraisal of the New Drug and Cosmetic Legislation from the Viewpoint of the Industries'. *Law and Contemporary Problems*, 6 (1939), 111–28.

Hohn, Maria. *GIs and Frauleins: The German American Encounter in 1950s West Germany*. Chapel Hill: University of North Carolina Press, 2002.

Holmberg, S. D., Osterholm, M. T., Senger, K. A., and Cohen, M. L. 'Drug Resistant Salmonella from Animals Fed Anti-microbials'. *New England Journal of Medicine*, 311 (1984), 617–22.

Homburg, Ernst. 'De "Tweede Industriële Revolutie": een problematisch historisch concept'. *Theoretische Geschiedenis*, 13 (1986), 367–85.

Hoogerheide, J. C. 'Address by the Symposium Co-sponsor'. *Biotechnology and Bioengineering Symposium*, 4i (1973), p. vii.

Horby, P., Rushdy, A., Graham, C., and O'Mahoney, M., on Behalf of the PHLS. 'PHLS Overview of Communicable Diseases 1999'. *Communicable Diseases and Public Health*, 4 (2001), 8–17.

Hounshell, David, and Smith, John K. *Science and Corporate Strategy: Du Pont R & D, 1902–1980*. Cambridge: Cambridge University Press, 1988.

Howie, James. 'Gonorrhoea: A Question of Tactics'. *British Medical Journal*, 2 (22 December 1979), 1631–2.

—— 'The Situation Then and Now'. In Donald V. Jolly, David J. S. Miller, David B. Ross, and Peter D. Simm (eds.), *Ten Years on from Swann*. London: The Association of Veterinarians in Industry, 1981, 3–26.

Hoy, Sue Ellen. *Chasing Dirt: The American Pursuit of Cleanliness*. New York: Oxford University Press, 1995.

Hughes, D. 'Exploiting Genomics, Genetics and Chemistry to Combat Antibiotic Resistance'. *Nature Reviews Genetics*, 4 (2003), 432–41.

Hughes, W. Howard. 'Methods of Administration', in Alexander Fleming (ed.), *Penicillin: Its Practical Application*. London: Butterworth, 1946, 93–104.

Ibsen, Henrik. *Ghosts*. In *Ghosts and Other Plays*, trans. Peter Watts. London: Penguin, 1964.

IDSA. 'As Antibiotic Discovery Stagnates, a Public Health Crisis Brews: Bad Bugs, No Drugs'. Alexandria, Va.: Infectious Diseases Society of America, 2004.

Idsøe, O., and Guthe, T. 'Penicillin Side Reactions and Fatalities'. Presented at the 5th International Congress of Chemotherapy, Vienna, 26 June to 1 July 1967. WHO paper WHO/VDT/67.340.

Illiffe, John. *East African Doctors: A History of the Modern Profession*. Cambridge: Cambridge University Press, 1978.

Immergut, Ellen M. *Health Politics: Interests and Institutions in Western Europe*. Cambridge: Cambridge University Press, 1992.

'Influenzal Pneumonia'. *British Medical Journal*, 2 (29 November 1958), 1342–3.

Institute for Motivational Analysis. *A Psychological Study of the Doctor–Patient Relationship*. Submitted to California Medical Association. Sacramento: California Medical Association, 1950.

—— *A Research Study on Pharmaceutical Advertising*. New York: Pharmaceutical Advertising Club, 1955.

Interim Commission to the First World Health Assembly. Report 'Venereal Diseases'. *Official Records of the World Health Organization*, 9 (1948).

Irving, David I. (ed.). *The Secret Diaries of Hitler's Doctor*, rev. and abridged by Susanna Scott-Gall. London: Grafton, 1990.

Jackson, Charles O. *Food and Drug Legislation in the New Deal*. Princeton: Princeton University Press, 1970.

Jacobs, J., Livsey, T. J., and Stephens, B. J. 'Methicillin Spray and Staphylococcal Carriage in a Neonatal Unit'. *Journal of Obstetrics and Gynaecology in the British Commonwealth*, 71 (1964), 543–55.

Jeaves, Arnold. 'Disease You Need No Longer Dread', *Everybody's*, 25 July 1938.

Jefferys, Margot, Brotherton, J. H., and Cartwright, Ann. 'Consumption of Medicines on a Working-Class Housing Estate'. *British Journal of Preventive and Social Medicine*, 14 (1960), 64–76.

Jevons, Patricia. ' "Celbenin"-Resistant Staphylococci'. *British Medical Journal*, 1 (14 January 1961), 124–5.

Johnson, Judith A. *Infectious Diseases: Emerging and Reemerging Threats to Public Health in the United States*. Washington, DC: Congressional Research Service, 1995.

Jolly, Donald V., Miller, David J. S., Ross, David B., and Simm, Peter D. *Ten Years on from Swann*. London: The Association of Veterinarians in Industries, 1981.

Jones, Edgar. *The Business of Medicine: The Extraordinary History of Glaxo, a Baby Food Producer, Which Became One of the World's Most Successful Pharmaceutical Companies*. London: Profile, 2001.

Jones, S. G., and Howard, J. 'Stories about "Doomsday Killer Bugs": The Aftermath'. *British Medical Journal*, 312 (17 February 1996), 441.

Jukes, Thomas H. 'Antibiotics in Feeds'. *Science*, 204 (6 April 1978), 8.

—— 'Antibiotics, Resistance and Animal Growth: Another View'. *The Sciences* (April 1980), 24–6.

Kaempffert, Waldemar. 'On Great Discoveries and What Precedes Them'. *New York Times*, 22 August 1948.

Kahn Jr., E. J. *All in a Century: The First Hundred Years of Eli Lilly and Company*. Indianapolis: Eli Lilly, 1976.

Kallet, Arthur, and Schlink, Frederik. *100,000,000 Guinea Pigs: Dangers in Everyday Foods, Drugs and Cosmetics*. New York: Vanguard Press, 1933.

Kamp, G. A. G., La Riviere, J. W. M., and Verhoeven, W. (eds.). *'Albert Jan Kluyver: His Life and Work, Biographical Memoranda, Selected Papers, Bibliography and Addenda*. Amsterdam: North-Holland Publishing Company, 1959.

Karpf, Anne. *Doctoring the Media: The Reporting of Health and Medicine* (London: Routledge, 1988).

Kato, K. 'Occurrence of Penicillin-Nucleus in Culture Broths'. *Journal of Antibiotics*, 6 (1953), 130–6.

—— 'Further Notes on Penicillin-Nucleus'. *Journal of Antibiotics*, 6 (1953), 184–5.

Kaul, Inge, Grunberg, Isabelle, and Stern, Marc A. *Global Public Goods: International Cooperation in the 21st Century*. Oxford: Oxford University Press, 1999.

Kay, Lily E. 'Selling Pure Science in Wartime: The Biochemical Genetics of G. W. Beadle'. *Journal of the History of Biology*, 22 (1989), 73–101.

—— *The Molecular Vision of Life: Caltech, the Rockefeller Foundation, and the Rise of the New Biology*. Oxford: Oxford University:Press, 1993.

Keilin, D., and Hartree, E. F. 'Properties of Glucose Oxidase (Notatin)'. *Biochemical Journal*, 42 (1948), 221–9.

Kingston, William. 'Streptomycin, Schatz v. Waksman, and the Balance of Credit for Discovery'. *Journal of the History of Medicine and Allied Sciences*, 59 (2004), 441–62.

Kirk, Beate. *Der Contergan-Fall: Eine unvermeidbare Arzneimittelkatastrophe*. Stuttgart: Wissenschafts-Verlag, 1999.

Kislak, J. W., Razavi, L. M. B., Daly, A. K., and Finland, M. 'Susceptibility of Pneumococci to Nine Antibiotics'. *American Journal of Medical Science*, 250 (1965), 261–8.

Kleinmann, Arthur. *Patients and Healers in the Context of Culture*. Berkeley and Los Angeles: University of California Press, 1980.

Klugman, Keith. 'Pneumococcal Resistance to Antibiotics'. *Clinical Microbiology Reviews*, 3 (1990), 171–96.

Knowles, J. (ed.). *Doing Better and Feeling Worse*. New York: W. W. Norton, 1977.

Koenig, Joseph. *Die Penicillin-V Story. Eine Erfindung aus Tirol als Segen für die Welt*. Innsbruck: Haymon Verlag, 1984.

Koestler, Arthur. *The Sleepwalkers: A History of Man's Changing Vision of the Universe*. London: Hutchinson, 1959.

Kogan, Herman. *The Long White Line*. New York: Random House, 1963.

Kohler, Robert E. *Partners in Science: Foundations and Natural Scientists, 1900–1945*. Chicago: University of Chicago Press, 1991.

_____ *Lords of the Fly: Drosophila Genetics and the Experimental Life*. Chicago: Chicago University Press, 1994.

Koornhof, Hendrik J., Wasas, Avril, and Klugman, Keith. 'Antimicrobial Resistance in Streptococcus pneumoniae: A South African Perspective'. *Clinical Infectious Diseases*, 15 (1992), 84–94.

Koos, E. L. *The Health of Regionsville*. New York: Columbia University Press, 1954.

Koprowski H. 'Future of Infectious and Malignant Diseases'. In Gordon Wolstenholme (ed.), *Man and his Future*. London: Ciba Foundation, 1963, 196–216.

Koštio, Josef. 'O "Českem" Penicilinu'. *Chemické Listy*, 84 (1990), 827–42.

Krause, Richard M. 'Introduction to Emerging Infectious Diseases: Stemming the Tide'. In Richard M. Krause (ed.), *Emerging Infections: Biomedical Research Reports*. New York: Academic Press, 1998, 1–22.

Krécmâery, V., Rosival, L., and Watanabe, T. *Bacterial Plasmids and Antibiotic Resistance: International Symposium on Infectious Antibiotic Resistance 1971*. Prague: Avicenum, 1972.

Lamberton Harper, John. *America and the Reconstruction of Italy, 1945–1948*. Cambridge: Cambridge University Press, 1986.

Lappé, Marc. *Germs That Won't Die*. Garden City, NY: Anchor Press, 1982.

Lasagna, Louis. *The Doctor's Dilemmas*. New York: Harper, 1962.

Laurence, William L. 'Drug for Staph: Widespread Germ Succumbs to New Synthetic Penicillin'. *New York Times* (12 March 1961), section 4.

Lavin, B., Haug, M., and Balgrave, L. L., and Breslau, N. 'Change in Student Physicians' Views on Authority Relations with Patients'. *Journal of Health and Social Behavior*, 28 (1987), 258–72.

Lawless, Peter. 'Along the Broad Highway to Health: Bringing back Physical Well-Being to the Youth of Britain'. *Morning Post*, 14 February 1933.

Bibliography

Lawrence, Ghislaine, (ed.). *Technologies of Modern Medicine: Proceedings of a Seminar Held at the Science Museum, London, March 1993*. London: Science Museum, 1994.

Lax, Eric. *The Mould in Dr Florey's Coat*. New York: Henry Holt, 2004.

Lazell, H. G. *From Pills to Penicillin*. London: Heinemann, 1975.

Lechevalier, Hubert. 'The Search for Antibiotics at Rutgers University'. In John Parascandola (ed.), *The History of Antibiotics: A Symposium*. 113–24. Madison: American Institute for the History of Pharmacy, 1980, 113–24.

Lederberg, Joshua. 'Medical Science, Infectious Disease and the Unity of Humankind'. *Journal of the American Medical Association*, 260 (1988), 684–5.

———'Pandemic as a Natural Evolutionary Phenomenon'. In Arien Mack (ed.), *In Time of Plague: The History and Social Consequences of Lethal Epidemic Disease*. New York: New York University Press, 1991, 21–38.

———'Viruses and Humankind: Intracellular Symbiosis and Evolutionary Competition'. In Stephen Morse (ed.), *Emerging Viruses*. New York: Oxford University Press, 1993, 3–9.

———'*Escherichia coli*', in Robert Bud and Deborah Jean Warner (eds.), *Instruments of Science: An Historical Encyclopedia*. New York: Garland, 1998, 230–2.

———Shope, R. E., and Oaks, S. C. (eds.), *Emerging Infections: Microbial Threats to Health in the United States*. Washington, DC: National Academy Press, 1992.

Lederer, Susan, and Parascandola, John. 'Screening Syphilis: Dr Ehrlich's Magic Bullet Meets the Public Health Service'. *Journal of the History of Medicine and Allied Sciences*, 53 (1998), 345–70.

Le Fanu, James. *The Rise and Fall of Modern Medicine*. London: Little, Brown, 1999.

Levy, Stuart B. 'Survey of a Conference: Turista or not Turista'. In Stuart B. Levy, Royston B. Clowes, and Ellen L. Koenig (eds.), *International Plasmid Conference on Molecular Biology, Pathogenicity and Ecology of Bacterial Plasmids*. New York: Plenum Press, 1981, 676–7.

———*The Antibiotic Paradox: How Miracle Drugs are Destroying the Miracle*. New York: Plenum Press, 1992; 2nd edn. 2002.

———'Antibiotic Resistance 1992–2002: A Decade's Journey'. In Stacey L. Knobler, Stanley M. Lemon, Marjan Najafi, and Tom Burroughs (eds.), *The Resistance Phenomenon in Microbes and Infectious Disease Vectors. Implications for Human Health and Strategies for Containment*. Washington, DC: National Academies Press, 2003, 32–43.

Liebenau, Jonathan. 'The British Success with Penicillin'. *Social Studies of Science*, 17 (1987), 69–86.

Lief, Stella. 'Chairman's Address'. Annual Meeting of the National Antivaccination League. *Vaccination Observer* (July–September 1963), 26–7.

Lindee, M. Susan. *American Science and the Survivors at Hiroshima*. Chicago: University of Chicago Press, 1999.

Lines, Mary. 'From Wonder Drug to Potential Killer. Penicillin Allergies, 1941 to 1960'. M.Sc. thesis, London Centre for the History of Science, Technology and Medicine, University of London, 1999.

Linton, A. H. 'Antibiotic Resistance: The Present Situation Reviewed'. *Veterinary Record*, 100 (1977), 354–60.

——— 'The Role of Meat in the Spread to Man of Pathogenic and Antibiotic-Resistant Bacteria'. *Meat Hygienist*, 25 (February/March 1980), 22–7.

——— 'Has Swann Failed?' *Veterinary Record*, 108 (1981), 328–31.

Lipset, Seymour Martin, and Schneider, William. *The Confidence Gap: Business, Labor and Government in the Public Mind*. New York: Free Press, 1982.

Lipsky, Eleazar. *The Scientists*. London: Longman Green, 1959.

Liss, R. H., and Batchelor, F. R. 'Economic Evaluations of Antibiotic Use and Resistance: A Perspective Report of Task Force 6'. *Reviews of Infectious Diseases*, 9 (1987), S297–S312.

Litsios, Socrates. 'René J. Dubos and Fred L. Soper: Their Contrasting Views on Vector and Disease Eradication'. *Perspectives in Biology and Medicine*, 41 (1997), 138–49.

Little, P. S., Williamson, I., Warner, G., Gould, C., Gantley, M., and Kinmonth, A. L. 'An Open Randomised Trial of Prescribing Strategies for Sore Throat'. *British Medical Journal*, 314 (1997), 722–7.

Little, R. B., Dubos, René, Hotchkiss, R. D., Bean, C. W., and Miller, W. T. 'The Use of Gramicidin and Other Agents for the Elimination of the Chronic Form of Bovine Mastitis'. *American Journal of Veterinary Research*, 11 (1941), 305–12.

Livermore, David. 'Can Better Prescribing Turn the Tide of Resistance?' *Nature Microbiology*, 2 (2004), 73–8.

Loefler, J. P. 'Microbes, Chemotherapy, Evolution, and Folly'. *The Lancet*, 348 (21 December 1996), 1703–4.

Logan, W. P. D. *General Practitioners' Records: An Analysis of the Clinical Records of Eight Practices during the Period April 1951 to March 1952*. GRO Studies on Medical and Population Subjects 7. London: HMSO, 1953.

——— and Brook, E. *The Survey of Sickness 1943–1952*. Studies of Medical and Population Subjects 12. London: HMSO, 1957.

Loomis, Charles P., and Beegle, J. Allan. *Rural Social Systems: A Textbook in Rural Sociology and Anthropology*. New York: Prentice Hall, 1950.

Löwy, Ilana. 'Immunology and Literature in the Early Twentieth Century: *Arrowsmith* and *The Doctor's Dilemma*'. *Medical History*, 32 (1988), 314–32.

Lundbeck. H., Plazsikowski, U., and Silverstolpe, L. 'The Swedish Salmonella Outbreak of 1953'. *Journal of Applied Bacteriology*, 18 (1955), 535–48.

Lupton, Deborah. 'Consumerism, Reflexivity and the Medical Encounter'. *Social Science and Medicine*, 45 (1997), 373–81.

Lutts, Ralph H. 'Chemical Fallout: Rachel Carson's Silent Spring, Radioactive Fallout and the Environmental Movement'. *Environmental Review*, 9 (1985), 214–25.

Lutz, E. H. G. *Penicillin: Die Geschichte eines Heilmittels und seines Entdeckers Alexander Fleming*. Bad Worishofen: Kindler, 1954

Lyons, Champ. 'Penicillin Therapy of Surgical Infections in the US Army'. *Journal of the American Medical Association*, 123 (1943), 1007–18.

Bibliography

McCaig, L. F., Besser, Richard E., and Hughes, James M. 'Antimicrobial Drug Prescription in Ambulatory Care Settings, United States, 1992–2000', *Emerging Infectious Diseases*, 9 (2003), 432–7.

——and Hughes, J. M. 'Trends in Antimicrobial Drug Prescribing among Office-Based Physicians in the United States'. *Journal of the American Medical Association*, 273 (1995), 214–19.

McCray, W. Patrick. 'Large Telescopes and the Moral Economy of Recent Science'. *Social Studies of Science*, 30 (2000), 685–711.

McDermott, Walsh. 'The Problem of Staphylococcal Infection'. *British Medical Journal*, 2 (3 October 1956), 837–40.

MacFadyen, Richard E. 'Thalidomide in America: A Brush with Tragedy'. *Clio Medica*, 11 (1976), 79–93.

——'The FDA's Regulation and Control of Antibiotics in the 1950s: The Henry Welch Scandal, Felix Marti-Ibanez. and Charles Pfizer & Co.' *History of Medicine*, 53 (1979), 159–69.

Macfarlane, Gwyn. *Howard Florey: The Making of a Great Scientist.* Oxford: Oxford University Press, 1979.

——*Alexander Fleming: The Man and the Myth.* London: Chatto and Windus, 1984.

McGraw, Donald I. 'The Golden Staph: Medicine's Response to the Challenge of the Resistant Staphylococci in the Mid-Twentieth Century'. *Dynamis*, 4 (1984), 219–37.

McKeown, T. *The Role of Medicine: Dream. Mirage or Nemesis?* London: Nuffield Provincial Hospitals Trust, 1976.

McKie, Gerry. 'Patterns of Social Trust in Western Europe and their Genesis'. In Karen Cook (ed.), *Trust in Society*. New York: Russell Sage, 2001, 245–82.

McKinlay, John B., and McKinlay, Sonja M. 'The Questionable Contribution of Medical Measures to the Decline of Mortality in the United States in the Twentieth Century'. *Health and Society*, 55 (1977), 405–28.

——and Marceau, L. D. 'The End of the Golden Age of Doctoring'. *International Journal of Health Services*, 32 (2002), 379–416.

Mackintosh, J. *Trends of Opinion about the Public Health 1901–51*. Oxford: Oxford University Press, 1953.

Maddox, John. 'Obituary: Thomas Hughes Jukes (1906–99)'. *Nature*, 402 (2 December 1999), 478.

Maeder, Thomas. *Adverse Reactions.* New York: William Morrow, 1994.

'Major Trends in U.S. Food Supply, 1909–99'. *Food Review*, 23 (2000), 9–15.

Malek, Walter Ullmann. *The United States in Prague, 1945–1948*. Boulder, Colo.: East European Quarterly: distributed by Columbia University Press, 1978.

Management Sciences for Health. *Interventions and Strategies to Improve the Use of Antimicrobials in Developing Countries*. Geneva: WHO, 2001.

Manasse, Robert J. 'Evaluation of the Pacific Biotech CARDS STREP A Test for Detecting Group A Streptococci from Cases of Pharyngitis'. *Journal of Clinical Microbiology*, 27 (1989), 1657–8.

Mangione-Smith, R., McGlynn, E. A., Elliott, M. N., McDonald, L., Franz, C. E., and Kravitz, R. L. 'Parent Expectations for Antibiotics, Physician–Parent Communication and Satisfaction'. *Archives of Pediatrics and Adolescent Medicine*, 155 (2001), 800–6.

Marchand, Roland. *Advertising the American Dream: Making Way for Modernity, 1920–1940*. Berkeley and Los Angeles: University of Califomia Press, 1985.

Marcus, Alan. *Cancer from Beef: DES, Federal Food Regulation and Consumer Confidence*. Baltimore: Johns Hopkins University Press, 1994.

Marinker, Marshall. 'The Doctor and his Patient: An Inaugural Lecture'. Leicester: Leicester University Press, 1975.

Martell, Louise K. 'Maternity Care during the Post-World War II Baby Boom'. *Western Journal of Nursing Research*, 21 (1999), 387–404.

Massell, Benedict F. *Rheumatic Fever and Streptococcal Infection: Unravelling the Mysteries of a Dread Disease*. Cambridge, Mass.: Harvard University Press, 1997.

Masters, David. *Miracle Drug: The Inner History of Penicillin*. London: Eyre and Spottiswoode, 1946.

Mastro, Julius J. 'The Pharmaceutical Manufacturers' Association. The Ethical Drug Industry and the 1962 Drug Amendments: A Case Study of Congressional Action and Interest Group Reaction'. Ph.D. thesis, New York University, 1993.

Maurois, André. *The Life of Sir Alexander Fleming: Discoverer of Penicillin*. London: Jonathan Cape, 1959.

Mayne, H. G. 'The Army Medical Services'. In Franklin Mellor (ed.), *Casualties and Medical Statistics: History of the Second World War United Kingdom Medical Services*. London: HMSO, 1972, 91–454.

Mazzaglia, G., Caputi, A. P., Rossi, A., Bettoncelli, G., Stefanini, G., Ventriglia, G., Nardi, R., Brignoli, O., and Cricelli, C. 'Pharmacoepidemiology and Prescription: Exploring Patient- and Doctor-Related Variables Associated with Antibiotic Prescribing for Respiratory Infections in Primary Care'. *European Journal of Clinical Pharmacology*, 59 (2003), 651–7.

Mechanic, David. 'Changing Medical Organization and the Erosion of Trust'. *Milbank Quarterly*, 74 (1996), 171–89.

Meehan, Patricia. *A Strange Enemy People: Germans under the British 1945–50*. London: Peter Owen, 2001.

Melrose, Dianna. *Bitter Pills: Medicine and the Third World Poor*. Oxford: Oxfam, Public Affairs Unit, 1983.

'The Men who Fought It'. *Evening Gazette* (Middlesbrough), 7 March 1968.

Mines, Samuel. *Pfizer: An Informal History*: New York: Pfizer, 1978.

Ministry of Health (England and Wales). *The Influenza Epidemic in England and Wales 1957–1958*. Reports on Public Health and Medical Subjects No. 100. London: HMSO, 1960.

'"Miracle" Drug saves Life of W'ton Girl'. *Express and Star* (Wolverhampton), 9 September 1938.

Miškova, Alena, and Svobodny, Petr. 'Hermann Hubert Knaus, 1892–1970'. In Monika Gettler and Alena Miškova (eds.), *Prager Professoren 1938–1948*. Essen: Klartext, 2001, 429–41.

Misztal, B. *Trust in Modern Societies*. Cambridge: Polity Press, 1996.

Mizoguchi, Hazime. 'Penicillin Production and the Reconstruction of the Pharmaceutical Industry'. In Shigeru Nakayama (ed.), *A Social History of Science and Technology in Contemporary Japan*, 2 vols. Melbourne: Transpacific Press, 2005. ii. 541–51.

Moberg, C. L. 'Rene Dubos: A Harbinger of Microbial Resistance to Antibiotics'. *Microbial Drug Resistance*, 2 (1996), 287–97.

_____ and Cohn, Zanvil. 'René Jules Dubos'. *Scientific American* (May 1991), 58–65.

Mol, H. *Antibiotics and Milk*. Rotterdam: A. A. Balkema, 1975.

Mooij, Anne. *Out of Otherness: Characters and Narrators in the Dutch Venereal Disease Debates 1850–1990*. Translated from the Dutch by Beverley Jackson. Amsterdam: Rodopi, 1998.

Moore, Joseph Earle. 'Venereology in Transition'. *British Journal of Venereal Diseases*, 32 (1956), 217–25.

Morley, David. *Paediatric Priorities in the Developing World*. London: Butterworth, 1973.

Morrell, David. 'As I Recall'. *British Medical Journal*, 317 (1998), 40–5.

Morrell, Jack. *Science at Oxford 1914–1939: Transforming an Arts University*. Oxford: Clarendon Press, 1997.

Morse, Stephen (ed.). *Emerging Viruses*. New York: Oxford University Press, 1993.

Moser, R. H. *Diseases of Medical Progress*. Springfield, Ill.: Charles Thomas, 1959.

Moskowitz, Milton. 'Wonder Profits in Wonder Drugs'. *The Nation*, 184 (1957), 357.

Mudd, Stuart. 'Staphylococcic Infections in the Hospital and Community'. *Journal of the American Medical Association*, 166 (1956), 1177–8.

Muggeridge, Malcolm. 'London Diary'. *New Statesman* (3 August 1962), 139–40.

Munch-Petersen, C., and Boundy, E. 'Yearly Incidence of Penicillin-Resistant Staphylococci in Man since 1942'. *Bulletin of the World Health Organization*, 26 (1962), 241–52.

Murard, L., and Zylbermann, P. *L'Hygiène dans la République: la santé en France ou l'utopie contrariée*. Paris: Fayard, 1996.

Mygind, N., Meistrup-Larsen, K. L., Thomsen, J., Thomsen, V. F., Josefsson, K., and Sorenson, H. 'Penicillin in Acute Otitis Media: A Double-Blind Placebo-Controlled Trial'. *Clinical Otolaryngology*, 6 (1981), 5–13.

National Academy of Sciences. *The Effects on Human Health of Subtherapeutic Use of Antimicrobials in Animal Feeds*. Washington, DC: National Academy of Sciences, Office of Publications, 1980.

National Research Council. *The Use of Drugs in Food Animals*. Washington, DC: National Academy Press, 1999.

'Nationalized Doctors?' *Time* (21 June 1937), 26–30.

Nayler, J. H. 'Early Discoveries in the Penicillin Series'. *Trends in the Biochemical Sciences*, 16 (1991), 195–7.

Needham, Joseph. 'Science in South-West China'. *Nature*, 152 (3 July 1943), 9–10; (10 July 1943), 36–37.

Nelkin, Dorothy, and Gilman, Sander. 'Placing Blame for Devastating Disease'. *Social Research*, 55 (1988), 361–78.

Netherthorpe, Lord. *Report of the Joint Committee on Antibiotics in Animal Feeding to the Agricultural Research Council and the Medical Research Council*. London: HMSO, 1962.

Neushul, Peter. 'Science, Government and the Mass Production of Penicillin'. *Journal of the History of Medicine and Allied Sciences*, 48 (1993), 371–95.

——'Fighting Research: Army Participation in the Clinical Testing and Mass Production of Penicillin during the Second World War', in Roger Cooter, Mark Harrison, and Steve Sturdy (eds.), *War, Medicine and Modernity*. Stroud: Sutton, 1998, 203–24.

'New Drug Arrests Roosevelt Jr's Sinus Trouble'. *Newsweek* (26 December 1936), 8.

'New Warning on Risk from Antibiotic in Animal Feed'. *Nature*, 280 (5 July 1979), 4.

Nguyen-Van-Tam, Jonathan S., and Hampson, Alan W. 'The Epidemiology and Clinical Impact of Pandemic Influenza'. *Vaccine*, 21 (2003), 1762–8.

Nicholls, Alice. 'Lord Nuffield's Gift of an Iron Lung to any Hospital or Institution in the Empire, November 1938: An Appropriate Gift for the Colonies?'. MA dissertation, Birkbeck College, University of London, 2000.

Nicol, C. S. 'Venereal Diseases: Moral Standards and Public Opinion', *British Journal of Venereal Diseases*, 39 (1963), 169–70.

Niu Yahua. ['The Manufacture of Penicillin in China in 1940s']. *Zhonghua yi shi za zhi*, 31 (2001), 184–8.

North, E. A., and Christie, R. 'Observations on the Sensitivity of Staphylococci to Penicillin'. *Medical Journal of Australia*, 2 (1945), 44–6.

Novick, Richard. 'Use of BRL 1241'. *The Lancet*, 2 (29 October 1960), 978.

——'Analysis by Transduction of Mutations Affecting Penicillinase Formation in *Staphylococcus aureus*'. *Journal of General Microbiology*, 33 (1963), 121–36.

——'Antibiotics: Use in Animal Feed'. *Science*, 204 (1 June 1978), 908.

——'The Situation is Completely Out of Hand'. *New York Times*, 3 July 1978.

——'Antibiotics: Wonder Drugs or Chicken Feed'. *The Sciences* (July–August 1979), 14–17.

Obaseiki-Ebor, E. E., Akerele, J. O., and Ebea, P. O. 'A Survey of Antibiotic Outpatient Self-Medication'. *Journal of Antimicrobial Chemotherapy* (1987), 759–63.

O'Brien, T. F., Kent, R. L., and Medeiros, A. A. 'Computer-Generated Plots of Results of Antimicrobial-Susceptibility Tests'. *Journal of the American Medical Association*, 210 (1969), 84–92.

——and Stelling, J. M. 'WHONET: An Information System for Monitoring Antimicrobial Resistance'. *Emerging Infectious Diseases*, 1 (1995), 66.

Office of Technology Assessment. *Drugs in Livestock Feed*. Washington, DC: US Office of Technology Assessment, 1979.

——*Impacts of Antibiotic-Resistant Bacteria: 'Thanks to Penicillin, He will Come Home!'* Publication OTA-H-6297. Washington, DC: Office of Technology Assessment, 1995.

Olins, Wally. *On B®and*. London: Thames and Hudson, 2003.

O'Neill, Onora. *A Question of Trust*. Cambridge: Cambridge University Press, 2002.

Onuma, Hiroyuki. 'The Development of the Physical Training and Recreation Policy in Britain 1937–1939: Mainly Concerned in the Measures of National Fitness Council'. *Japanese Journal of Sports History*, 7 (1994), 1–17.

Orero, A., Gonzalez, J., and Prieto, J. 'Antibiotics in Spanish Households: Medical and Socioeconomic Implications'. *Medicina Clinica*, 109 (1997), 782–5.

Osler, William. *The Principles and Practice of Medicine*. 4th edn. New York: Appleton, 1901.

Oswald, N. C., Shooter, R. A., and Curwen, M. P. 'Pneumonia Complicating Asian Influenza'. *British Medical Journal*, 2 (29 November 1958), 1305–11.

Oswin, Maureen. *The Empty Hours: A Study of the Week-End Life of Handicapped Children in Institutions*. Harmondsworth: Penguin, 1973.

Owen, S. P. 'Industrial Fermentations'. *Annual Review of Microbiology*, 14 (1960), 99–120.

Packard, Vance. *The Hidden Persuaders*. Harmondsworth: Penguin, 1960. First published 1957.

Pappworth, M. H. 'Human Guinea Pigs: A Warning.' *Twentieth Century* (Autumn 1962), 66–75.

——*Human Guinea Pigs*. London: Routledge, 1967.

Parascandola, John (ed.). *The History of Antibiotics: A Symposium*. Madison: American Institute for the History of Pharmacy, 1980.

——'The Introduction of Antibiotics into Therapeutics'. In Yosio Kawakita, Shizu Sakai, and Yasuo Otsuka (eds.), *History of Therapy: Proceeding of the 10th Internation Symposium on the Comparative History of Medicine—East and West, September 8–September 15, 1985*. Ishiyaku: Euroamerica, 1990, 261–81.

——'John Mahoney and the Introduction of Penicillin to Treat Syphilis'. *Pharmacy in History*, 43 (2001), 1–56.

——and Ihde, Aaron J. 'Edward Mellanby and the Antirachitic Factor'. *Bulletin of the History of Medicine*, 51 (1977), 507–15.

Parsons, Talcott. *The Social System*. London: Routledge and Kegan Paul, 1951.

Pates, E. W. 'A Visit to Barnard Castle', *Glaxo Staff Bulletin*, 96, April 1946.

Pavin, Melinda, Nurgozhin, Tafgat, Hafner, Grace, Yusufy, Farruh, and Laing, Richard. 'Prescribing Practices of Rural Primary Health Care Physicians in Uzbekistan'. *Tropical Medicine and International Health*, 8 (2003), 182–90.

Pechère, Jean Claude. 'Patients' Interviews and Misuse of Antibiotics'. *Clinical Infectious Diseases*, 33 (2001), Suppl. 3: S170–3.

'Penicillin', *The Times*, 31 August 1942.

'Penicillin'. *Time*, 8 February 1943.

'Penicillin Administration in Wartime Surgery', in *Statistical Report on the Health of the Army 1943–45*. London: HMSO, 1948, 281–8.

'Penicillin and Modern Research', *The Lancet*, 1 (14 January 1950), 76–7.

Penicillin: Its Properties, Uses and Preparations. London: Pharmaceutical Press, 1946.

' "Penicillin Won't be Ready for Second Front"—M.P.', *Daily Mirror*, 14 February 1944.

'Penicillium'. *The Times*, 27 August 1942.

Perlman, D. 'How Penicillin Research Came to the University of Wisconsin'. *Mortar and Quill*, 15/1 (1978–9), 5–8.

Pescosolido, Bernice A., Tuch, Stephen A., and Martin, Jack A. 'The Profession of Medicine and the Public: Examining Americans' Changing Confidence in Physician Authority from the Beginning of the "Health Care Crisis" to the Era of Health Care Reform'. *Journal of Health and Social Behavior*, 42 (2001), 1–16.

Peterson, O. L., Andrews, L. P., Spain, R. S., and Greenberg, B. G. 'An Analytical Study of North Carolina General Practice'. *Journal of Medical Education*, 31 (1956), 1–165.

'Pharmaceutical Euphoria'. *The Guardian*, 21 October 1967.

Phillips, Simon. 'Jesse Boot and the Rise of Boots the Chemists'. *The Pharmaceutical Journal*, 264 (2002), 925–28.

Pichichero, Michael E. 'Dynamics of Antibiotic Prescribing for Children'. *Journal of the American Medical Association*, 287 (2002), 3133–5.

Pieroth, Ingrid. *Penicillin herstellung: von den Anfängen bis zur Gross production*. Stuffgart: Wissenchaftliche Verlagsgessellschaft, 1992.

Pieters, Toine. *Interferon: The Science and Selling of a Miracle Drug*. London: Routledge, 2004.

Pill, R., and Stott, N. C. H. 'Concepts of Illness Causation and Responsibility: Some Preliminary Data from a Sample of Working Class Mothers'. *Social Science and Medicine*, 16 (1982), 43–52.

——— 'Preventive Procedures and Practices among Working-Class Women: New Data and Fresh Insights'. *Social Science and Medicine*, 21 (1985), 975–93.

Pincher, Chapman. 'The Big Penicillin Robbery'. *Daily Express*, 6 November 1959.

Platt, Jennifer. *Social Research in Bethnal Green*. London: Macmillan, 1971.

'Pneumonia Yields to New Chemical'. *New York Times*, 9 September 1939.

'Pneumococcal Vaccines'. WHO Position Paper. *Weekly Epidemiological Record*, 74 (1999), 177–84.

Pope, Willliam J. ' "Yadil": An Exposure'. *Daily Mail*, 22 July 1924.

Porritt, A. E. and Mitchell, G. A. G. 'Penicillin and Sulphonamides in Prophylaxis'. In *Penicillin Therapy and Control in 21 Army Group*. London: Published under the Direction of the Director of Medical Services, 21 Army Group, May 1945.

Porter, D. (ed.). *Social Medicine and Medical Sociology in the Twentieth Century*. Amsterdam: Rodopi, 1997.

Preston, R.. *The Hot Zone*. New York: Random House, 1994.

Putnam, Robert D. *Bowling Alone: The Collapse and Revival of American Community*. New York: Simon and Schuster, 2000.

Quirke, Viviane. 'Experiments in Collaboration: The Changing Relationship between Scientists and Pharmaceutical Companies in Britain and in France, 1935–1965'. D.Phil thesis, Oxford University, 1999.

'Racket in Fake Drug Smashed in Germany'. *New York Times*, 21 April 1946.

Radford, Tim. 'Medicine and the Media: Influence and Power of the Media'. *The Lancet*, 347 (1996), 1533–5.

Radley, Alan. *Making Sense of Illness*. London: Sage, 1994.

Raper, Kenneth B. 'The Penicillin Saga Remembered'. *ASM News*, 44 (1978), 645–53.

_____ 'Research in the Development of Penicillin'. In E. C. Andrus et al. (eds.), *Science in World War II: Advances in Military Medicine*. Boston: Little, Brown, 1948, 723–45.

Rasmussen, Nicolas. 'The Moral Economy of the Drug Company–Medical Scientist Collaboration in Interwar America'. *Social Studies of Science*, 34 (April 2004), 161–85.

Ravenholt, R. T., and La Veck, G. D. 'Staphylococcal Disease: An Obstetric, Pediatric and Community Problem'. *American Journal of Public Health*, 46 (1956), 1287–96.

Reed, Stuart. '300 Years of Cod Liver Oil'. *Pharmaceutical Historian*, 18 (1988), 6–7.

Reeder, Leo G. 'The Patient-Client as a Consumer: Some Observations on the Changing Professional–Client Relationship'. *Journal of Health and Social Behavior*, 13 (1972), 406–12.

Reiser, Stanley Joel. *Medicine and the Reign of Technology*. Cambridge: Cambridge University Press, 1978.

Rentschler, E. 'Pabst Redesigned: Paracelsus'. *Germanic Review*, 66 (1991), 16–24.

Rettew, Raymond G. *A Quiet Man from Chester County*. West Chester, Pa.: Chester County Historical Society, 1975.

Richmond, Mark. 'Why has Swann Failed?'. *British Medical Journal*, 1 (28 June 1980), 1615.

Robinson, K. L. 'Use of Antibiotics in Feeds: The Value of Antibiotics for Growth of Pigs'. In Malcolm Woodbine (ed.), *Antibiotics in Agriculture: Proceedings of the University of Nottingham Ninth Easter School in Agricultural Science*. London: Butterworths, 1962, 285–302.

Roizin, Paul, and Brandt, Allan (eds.). *Morality and Health*. London: Routledge, 1997.

Rolinson, G. N. 'Evolution of β-Lactamase Inhibitors'. *Review of Infectious Diseases*, 13 (1991), Supp.: 727–32.

_____ 'Forty Years of β-lactam Research'. *Journal of Antimicrobial Chemotherapy*, 41 (1998), 589–603.

Rosebury, Theodor. *Microbes and Morals: The Strange History of Venereal Disease*. London: Secker and Warburg, 1971.

Rosenberg, Charles. E. *No Other Gods*. Baltimore: Johns Hopkins University Press, 1976.

Rosencrantz, Barbara. 'Coverage of Antibiotic Resistance in the Popular Literature 1950 to 1994'. Appendix to *Impacts of Antibiotic-Resistant Bacteria: 'Thanks to Penicillin He will Come Home!'*. Publication OTA-H–6297. Washington, DC: Office of Technology Assessment, 1995.

Rothman, David. 'Suing the Stranger'. *Transactions of the College of Physicians of Philadelphia*, ser. 5/13 (1991), 263–72.

——*Beginnings Count: The Technological Imperative in American Health Care*. Oxford: Oxford University Press, 1997.

Rountree, Phyllis M. 'History of Staphylococcal Infection in Australia'. *Medical Journal of Australia*, 2 (1978), 543–6.

Ryan, Frank. *Virus X. Understanding the Real Threat of the New Pandemic Plagues*. London: HarperCollins, 1996.

Sá-Leão, Raquel, Vilhelmsson, Sigurdur E., de Lencastre, Hermínia, Kristinsson, Karl G., and Alexander Tomasz. 'Diversity of Penicillin-Nonsusceptible Streptococcus pneumoniae Circulating in Iceland after the Introduction of Penicillin-Resistant Clone Spain 6B–2'. *Journal of Infectious Diseases*, 186 (2002), 966–75.

Savage, Mildred. *In Vivo*. London: Longmans 1965. First published 1964.

Sawao, Kinichiro, and Murao, Sakaguchi. 'A Preliminary Report on a New Enzyme. "Penicillin-amidase"'. *Journal of Agricultural Chemical Society* (Japan), 23 (1950), 411.

Scambler, Graham (ed.). *Habermas, Critical Theory and Health*. London: Routledge, 2001.

Schell, Orville. *Modern Meat: Antibiotics, Hormones and the Pharmaceutical Farm*. New York: Random House, 1984.

Schlesinger, Mark. 'A Loss of Faith: The Sources of Reduced Political Legitimacy for the American Medical Profession'. *Milbank Quarterly*, 80 (2002), 185–235.

Schnayerson, Michael, and Plotkin, Mark. *The Killers Within: The Deadly Rise of Drug-Resistant Bacteria*. London: Time Warner, 2003.

Schneider, W. G., and Valenta, Z. 'Karel František Wiesner'. *Biographical Memoirs of the Royal Society*, 37 (1991), 463–90.

Schneierson, Stanley. 'Hazards of Antibiotics'. *Consumer Reports* (April 1953), 162–4.

'Scientists Quit Panel in Dispute over Livestock'. *New York Times*, 23 January 1979.

Scott, J. G., Cohen, D., DiCicco-Bloom, B., Orzano, A. J., Jaen, C. R., and Crabtree, B. F. 'Antibiotic Use in Acute Respiratory Infections and the Ways Patients Pressure Physicians for a Prescription'. *Family Practice*, 50 (2001), 853–8.

Selwyn, Sydney. *The Beta-lactam Antibiotics: Penicillins and Cephalosporins in Perspective*. London: Hodder and Stoughton, 1980.

Semba, Richard D. 'Vitamin A as "Anti-Infective" Therapy, 1920–1940'. *Journal of Nutrition*, 129 (1999), 783–91.

Seven Seas Health Care. *A History of British Cod Liver Oils: The First Fifty Years with Seven Seas*. Cambridge: Martin Books, 1984.

Shama, Gilbert, and Reinarz, Jonathan. 'Allied Intelligence Reports on Wartime German Penicillin Research and Production'. *Historical Studies in the Physical and Biological Sciences*, 32 (2002), 347–67.

Shapin, Steve.'Who is the Industrial Scientist? Commentary from Academic Sociology and from the Shop-Floor in the United States, ca. 1900–ca. 1970'. In Karl Grandin, Nina Wormbs, Anders Lundgren, and Sven Widmalm (eds.), *The Science–Industry Nexus: History, Policy, Implications*. Nobel Symposium 123. New York: Science History Publications, 2005, 337–63.

Sheehan, John C. *The Enchanted Ring: The Untold Story of Penicillin*. Cambridge, Mass.: MIT Press, 1982.

Shimkin, Michael. 'Roads to OZ. I.: A Personal Account of Some USSR Medical Exchanges and Contacts 1942–1962'. *Perspectives in Biology and Medicine*, 22 (1979), 565–8 .

Shlaes, David M. 'The Abandonment of Antibacterials: Why and Wherefore?'. *Current Opinion in Pharmacology*, 3 (2003), 470–3.

——Levy, D., and Archer, G. 'Antimicrobial Resistance: New Directions'. *ASM News*, 57 (1991), 455–8.

Simmons, H. E., and Stolley, Paul D. 'This is Medical Progress? Trends and Consequences of Antibiotic Use in the United States'. *Journal of the American Medical Association*, 227 (1974), 1023–8.

Simmons, Ozzie G. 'Popular and Modern Medicine in Mestizo Communities of Coastal Peru and Chile'. *Journal of American Folklore*, 68 (1955), 57–71.

Slater, Patrick. *Survey of Sickness. October 1943 to December 1945: A Report on a Series of Surveys on the State of Health of the Civilian Population between these Dates, Made for the Ministry of Health*. London: GRO, 1946.

Smith, David F., and Diack, H. Lesley, with Pennington, T. Hugh, and Russell, Elizabeth M. *Food Poisoning, Policy, and Politics: Corned Beef and Typhoid in Britain in the 1960s*. Woodbridge: Boydell Press, 2005.

Smith, E. Lester. 'British Penicillin Production'. *Transactions of the Society of Chemical Industry*, 65 (1946), 308–13.

Smith, H. Williams, and Halls, Sheila. 'Observations on Infective Drug Resistance in Britain'. *British Medical Journal*, 1 (29 January 1966), 266–9.

Smith, Richard D., and Coast, J. 'Antimicrobial Drug Resistance'. In R. D. Smith, R. Beaglehole, D. Woodward, and N. Drager (eds.), *Global Public Goods for Health*. Oxford: Oxford University Press, 2003, 73–93.

Sokoloff, Boris. *Penicillin: A Dramatic Story*. London: George Allen and Unwin, 1946.

Somers, Herman Miles, and Somers, Anne Ramsay. *Doctors, Patients, and Health Insurance: The Organization and Financing of Medical Care*. Washington, DC: Brookings Institution, 1961.

Sommer, Karel. *UNRRA a Československo*. Opava: Slezský ústav AV ČR, 1993.

Somogyi, J. C. 'Antibiotics in Agriculture and Human Health'. In *Antibiotics in Agriculture: Proceedings of the 5th Symposium of the Group of European Nutritionists in Jouy-en-Josas April 25–27 1966*. Basel: Karger, 1968, 204–6.

Sontag, Susan. *AIDS and its Metaphors*. New York: Farrar Straus Giroux, 1989.

Soper, F. L. 'Rehabilitation of the Eradication Concept in Prevention of Communicable Diseases'. *Public Health Reports*, 80 (1965), 855–69.

Soulsby, Lord (chair). *Resistance to Antibiotics and Other Antitmicrobiial Agents.* Seventh Report of the Select Committee on Science and Technology, House of Lords. 17 March 1998. House of Lords paper 81-I.

Spellberg, B., Powers, J. H., Brass, E. P., Miller, L. G., and.Edwards, J. E., Jr. 'Trends in Antimicrobial Drug Development: Implications for the Future'. *Clinical Infectious Diseases*, 38 (2004), 1279–86.

Spink, Wesley W. *Infectious Diseases: Prevention and Treatment in the Nineteenth and Twentieth Centuries*. London: W. M. Dawson, 1978.

Standing Medical Advisory Committee, Sub-Group on Antimicrobial Resistance. *The Path of Least Resistance*. London: Central Health Services Council, 1998.

Stanton, Jennifer (ed.). *Innovations in Health and Medicine: Diffusion and Resistance in the Twentieth Century*. London: Routledge, 2002.

Starr, Paul. *The Social Transformation of American Medicine*. New York: Basic Books, 1982.

Steffen, Craig H. 'Penicillins and Staphylococci: A Historical Interaction'. *Perspectives in Biology and Medicine*, 35 (1991–2), 596–608.

Steiger, Victor, and Hansen, A. Victor. 'A Definition of Comprehensive Medicine'. *Journal of Health and Human Behavior*, 2 (1961), 82–6.

Stephenson, J. 'Icelandic Prescribers are Showing the Way to Bring Down the Rates of Antibiotic-Resistant Bacteria'. *Journal of the American Medical Association*, 275 (1996), 175.

Stevenson, Fiona, and Scambler, Graham. 'The Relationship between Medicine and the Public: The Challenge of Concordance'. *Health*, 9 (2005), 5–21.

Stewart, G. T. ' "Celbenin"-Resistant Staphylococci'. *British Medical Journal*, 2 (8 October 1960), 1085.

——— 'Toxicity of the Penicillins'. *Postgraduate Medical Journal*, 40 (3 July 1964), Suppl.: 160–9.

——— *The Pencillin Group of Drugs*. Amsterdam: Elsevier, 1965.

——— Butcher, Brian T., and McGovern, John P. 'Penicillin Allergy: The Nature of the Problem'. In Gordon T. Stewart and John P. McGovern (eds.), *Penicillin Allergy: Clinical and Immunologic Aspects.* Springfield, Ill.: Charles C. Thomas, 1970, 176–91.

——— and Rolt, R. J. 'Evolution of Natural Resistance to the Newer Penicillins'. *British Medical Journal*, 1 (2 February 1963), 308–11.

Stivers, T. 'Participating in Decisions about Treatment: Overt Parent Pressure for Antibiotic Medication in Pediatric Encounters'. *Social Science and Medicine*, 54 (2002), 1111–30.

Stratchounski, L. S., Andreeva, I. V., Ratchina, S. A., Galkin, D. V., Petrotchenkova, N. A., Demion, A. A., Kuzin, V. B., Kusnetsova, S. T., Likhatcheva, R. Y., Nedogoda, S. V., Ortenberg, E. A., Belikov, A. S., and Toropova, J. A. 'The Inventory of Antibiotics in Russian Home Medicine Cabinets'. *Clinical Infectious Diseases*, 15 (2003), 498–505.

Strausbaugh, Larry J. 'Emerging Infectious Diseases: No End in Sight'. *American Journal of Infection Control*, 26 (1998), 3–4.

Sturchio, Jeffrey (ed.). *Values and Visions: A Merck Century*. Rahway, NJ.: Merck, 1991.

Sturdy, Steve (ed.). *Medicine, Health and the Public Sphere in Britain, 1600–2000*. London: Routledge, 2002.

Sturgess, Ray. 'The Magic Bottle'. *Pharmaceutical Journal*, 263 (1999), 1015–17.

Stursberg, Peter. *Lester Pearson and the American Dilemma*. Toronto: Doubleday Canada, 1980.

SuperBugs & SuperDrugs: A Strategic Guide to the Global Antimicrobials Industry, Innovation and Therapies. North Adams, Mass.: SMI Publishing, October 2000.

Swackhamer, Gladys V. *Choice and Change of Doctors. A Study of the Consumer of Medical Services*. New York: Committee on Research on Medical Economics, 1939.

Swann, John P. 'The Search for Synthetic Penicillin during World War 2'. *British Journal for the History of Science*, 16 (1983): 154–88.

—— *Academic Scientists and the Pharmaceutical Industry*. Baltimore, MD: Johns Hopkins University Press, 1988.

Swann, M. M. *Report of the Joint Committee on the Use of Antibiotics in Animal Husbandry and Veterinary Medicine*. London: HMSO, 1969.

Tansey, E. M., and Reynolds, L. M. (eds.). *Post-Penicillin Antibiotics: From Acceptance to Resistance?* Wellcome Witnesses to Twentieth Century Medicine 6. London: Wellcome Institute for the History of Medicine, 2000.

Taylor, A. J. P. *Beaverbrook*. London: Hamish Hamilton, 1992.

Taylor C. E, 'The Doctor's Role in Rural Health Care'. *International Journal of Health Services*, 6 (1976), 219–30.

Taylor-Goody, Peter. 'Attachment to the Welfare State'. In Roger Jowell, Lindsay Brook, Bridget Taylor and Gillian Prior (eds.), *British Social Attitudes: The 8th Report*. Aldershot; Dartmouth Publishing, 1991, 23–42.

Tejada de Rivero, David A. 'Alma-Ata Revisited'. *Perspectives in Health Magazine*, 8/2 (2003).

Temin, Peter. *Taking your Medicine: Drug Regulation in the United States*. Cambridge, Mass.: Harvard University Press, 1980.

Temkin, Elizabeth. 'Rooming-in: Redesigning Hospitals and Motherhood in Cold War America'. *Bulletin of the History of Medicine*, 76 (2002), 271–98.

Thackray, Arnold, Sturchio, Jeffrey L., Carroll, P. Thomas, and Bud, Robert. *Chemistry in America, 1876–1976: Historical Indicators*. Dordrecht: Reidel, 1984.

Threlfall, E. J., Ward, L. R., Frost, J. A., and Willshaw, G. A. 'Spread of Resistance from Food Animals to Man: The UK Experience'. *Acta Veterinaria Scandinavica*, 93 (2000), Suppl.: 63–8; discussion 68–74.

____Ward, L. R., Ashley, A. S., and Rowe, B. 'Plasmid-Encoded Trimethoprim Resistance in Multiresistant Epidemic *Salmonella typhimurium* Phage Types 204 and 193 in Britain'. *British Medical Journal*, 280 (17 May 1980), 1210–1.

Tomes, Nancy. *The Gospel of Germs: Men, Women, and the Microbe in American Life*. Cambridge, Mass.: Harvard University Press, 1998.

____ 'Merchants of Health: Medicine and Consumer Culture in the United States, 1900–1940'. *Journal of American History*, 88 (2001), 519–47.

Tousijn, W. 'Medical Professionalisation in Italy: A Comparative Perspective'. In I. Hellberg, M. Saks, and C. Benoit (eds.), *Professional Identities in Transition: Cross-Cultural Dimensions*. Sodertalje: Almqvist & Wiksell, 1999, 107–19.

____ 'Medical Dominance in Italy: A Partial Decline'. *Social Science and Medicine*, 55 (2002), 733–41.

Trends in the Supply and Demand of Medical Care. Study Paper no. 5. US Congress Joint Economic Committee, 10 November 1959. Washington, DC: US Government Printing Office, 1959.

Trostle, James. 'Inappropriate Distribution of Medicines by Professionals in Developing Countries'. *Social Science and Medicine*, 42 (1996), 1117–20.

Trueta, Joseph. *Trueta: Surgeon on War and Peace: The Memoirs of Joseph Trueta*, trans. Meli and Michael Strubell. London: Gollancz, 1980.

Truman, Harold. *Year of Decisions 1945*. London: Hodder and Stoughton, 1955.

Tucker, Anthony. 'Anti-antibiotics'. *The Guardian*, 30 January 1967.

____ 'Issues Raised by the Inquiry into the Farm Use of Antibiotics'. *The Guardian*, 13 July 1968.

Turner, Thomas B. 'Japan and Korea'. In *Civil Affairs/Military Government Public Health Activities*. Vol. viii of Ebbe Curtiss Hoff (ed.), *Preventive Medicine in World War II*. Washington, DC: Office of the Surgeon General, Dept. of the Army, 1976, 659–707.

Turnidge, John, and Christiansen, Keryn. 'Antibiotic Use and Resistance: Proving the Obvious'. *The Lancet*, 365 (12 February 2005), 548–9.

'20th Century Seer'. *Time* (15 May 1944), 61–8.

Tyabjim, N. 'Gaining Technical Know-how in an Unequal World: Penicillin Manufacture in Nehru's India'. *Technology and Culture*, 45 (2004), 331–49.

US Congress, Senate. *Administered Prices in the Drug Industry*, Hearings before the Subcommittee on Antitrust and Monopoly of the Committee on the Judiciary, 86th Congress, 1st and 2nd sessions, 1960–1.

____ Subcommittee on Antitrust and Monopoly. *Report of the Study on Administered Prices in the Drug Industry*, 87th Congress, 1st session, 1961.

US Federal Trade Commission. *Economic Report on Antibiotics Manufacture*. Washington, DC: US Government Printing Office, 1958.

van Buchem, F. L., Dunk, J. H., and van't Hof, M. A. 'Therapy of Acute Otitis Media: Myringotomy. Antibiotics or Neither'. *The Lancet*, 2 (24 October 1981), 883–7.

Van Nistelrooij, H. J. M., Krijgsman, J., de Vroom, E., and Oldendof, C. 'Penicillin Update—Industrial'. In Richard I. Mateles (ed.), *Penicillin: A Paradigm for Biotechnology*. Chicago: Candida, 1998, 85–91.

Vansittart, Peter. *In the Fifties*. London: John Murray, 1995.

Vickers, H. R., Bagratuni, L., and Alexander, S. 'Dermatitis Caused by Penicillin in Milk'. *The Lancet*, 1 (15 February 1958), 351–2.

von Borstel, R. C., and Steinberg, Charles M. 'Alexander Hollaender: Myth and Mensch'. *Genetics*, 143 (1996), 1051–6.

Wainwright, Milton. 'Hitler's Penicillin'. *Perspectives in Biology and Medicine*, 47 (2004), 189–98.

Waksman, Selman. 'What is an Antibiotic or Antibiotic Substance?' *Mycologia*, 39 (1947), 565–9.

Waldbott, George L. 'Anaphylactic Death from Penicillin'. *Journal of the American Medical Association*, 139 (1949), 526–7.

Walter, Carl. 'The Personal Factor in Hospital Hygiene'. In *Prevention of Hospital Infection*. London: Royal Society of Health, 1963, 37–46.

Watanabe, T. 'Infectious Drug Resistance'. *Scientific American*, 217 (1967), 19–28.

Wax, Murray. 'On Public Dissatisfaction with the Medical Profession: Personal Observations'. *Journal of Health and Human Behavior*, 3 (1962), 152–6.

Webster, Charles. *The Problems of Health Care: The National Health Service before 1957*, vol. i of *The National Health Services since the War*. London: HMSO, 1988.

——*Government and Health Care: The National Health Service 1958–1979*, vol. ii of *The Health Services since the War*. London: The Stationery Office, 1996.

Wehrbein, H. L. 'Therapy in Gonorrhea: An Historical Review'. *Annals of Medical History*, 7 (1935), 492–7.

Weindling, Paul. *Epidemics and Genocide in Eastern Europe 1890–1945*. Oxford: Oxford University Press, 1999.

Welch, Henry. 'Antibiotics 1943–1955: Their Development and Role in Present-Day Society'. In Iago Galdston (ed.), *The Impact of the Antibiotics on Medicine and Society*. Monograph 2, Institute of Social and Historical Medicine, New York Academy of Medicine. New York: International Universities Press, 1958, 70–87.

Wellings, Kaye, and Wadsworth, Jane. 'Aids and the Moral Climate'. In Roger Jowell, Sharon Witherspoon, and Lindsay Brook (eds.), *British Social Attitudes: The 7th Report*. London: Gower, 1990, 10–26.

Wells, Percy. 'Some Aspects of the Early History of Penicillin in the United States'. *Journal of the Washington Academy of Sciences*, 65 (1975), 96–101.

——Lynch, D. F. J., Herrick, H. T., and May, O. E. 'Translating Mold Fermentation Research to Pilot Plant Operation'. *Chemical and Metallurgical Engineering*, 44 (April 1937), 188–90.

Wells, Wyatt C. *Antitrust and the Making of the Postwar World*. New York: Columbia University Press, 2002.

White, Hayden. *The Historical Imagination in Nineteenth-Century Europe*. Baltimore: Johns Hopkins University Press, 1973.

Whitney, Cynthia G., and Klugman, Keith P. 'Vaccines as Tools against Resistance: The Example of Pneumococcal Conjugate Vaccine'. *Seminars in Pediatric Infectious Diseases*, 15 (2004), 86–93.

Whorton, James C. '"Antibiotic Abandon": The Resurgence of Therapeutic Rationalism'. In John Parascandola (ed.), *The History of Antibiotics: A Symposium*. Madison: American Institute for the History of Pharmacy, 1980, 125–36.

Whyte, S. R. 'Penicillin, Battery Acid and Sacrifice: Cures and Causes in Nyole Medicine'. *Social Science and Medicine*, 16 (1982), 2055–64.

Widmann, Georg Rudolf. *Das ärgerliche Leben und schreckliche Ende des vielberüchtigten Ertzschwartzkünstlers D. Johannis Fausti...und einem Anhange von den Lapponischen Wahrsager-Pauken, etc.* Nuremberg, 1681.

Williams, Bryan. 'Discussion'. *Journal of Obstetrics and Gynaecology in the British Empire*, 67 (1960), 738.

Williams, Glen. 'WHO: The Days of the Mass Campaigns'. *World Health Forum*, 9 (1988), 7–23.

Williams, Mark. 'Elsie the Cow Changed Industry's Image: Ad Age Ranks Icon among Century's Best'. *Cincinnati Enquirer*, 23 October 1999.

Williams, R. *A Protestant Legacy: Attitudes to Death and Illness among Older Aberdonians*. Oxford: Clarendon Press, 1990.

Williams, R. E. O. 'Investigations of Hospital-Acquired Staphylococcal Disease and its Control in Great Britain'. *Proceedings of the National Conference on Hospital-Acquired Staphylococcal Disease, Sponsored by US PHS and NAS Atlanta Georgia*. Washington, DC: US DHEW, CDC, 1958, 11–29.

—— 'Hospital Infection'. In Philips S. Brachman and Theodore C. Eickhoff (eds.), *Proceedings of the International Conference on Nosocomial Infections, Center for Diseases Control, August 3–6 1970*. Chicago: American Hospital Association, 1971, 1–10.

—— *Microbiology for the Public Service: Evolution of the Public Health Laboratory Service 1939–1980*. London: Public Health Laboratory Service, 1985.

Williams, Simon J., and Calnan, Michael. 'The "Limits" of Medicalization? Modern Medicine and the Lay Populace in "Late" Modernity'. *Social Science and Medicine*, 42 (1996), 1609–20.

Williams, Trevor. *Howard Florey: Penicillin and After*. Oxford: Oxford University Press, 1984.

Willoughby, John. 'The Sexual Behavior of American GIs during the Early Years of the Occupation of Germany'. *Journal of Military History*, 62 (1998), 155–74.

Winstanley, Michael. 'Cow Punch: Antibiotics in Milk through Treatment of Cows'. *The Guardian*, 25 June 1963.

Wise, Richard. 'β-Lactamase Inhibitors'. *Journal of Antimicrobial Chemotherapy*, 9 (1982), Supp. B. 31–40.

——, Ossman, Elizabeth A., and Littlefield, Dwight R. 'Personal Reflections on Nosocomial Infections and the Development of Hospital Surveillance'. *Reviews of Infectious Diseases*, 11 (1989), 1005–19.

317

Witkop, Bernhard. 'Paul Ehrlich and his Magic Bullets—Revisited'. *Proceedings of the American Philosophical Society*, 143 (1999), 540–57.

Wolstenholme, G. E. W., and O'Connor, Cecilia M. (eds.). *The CIBA Foundation Symposium on Drug Resistance in Micro-organisms: Mechanisms of Development.* London: J. & A. Churchill, 1957.

Wondrák, E. 'Die Pharmaindustrie von Hitlers Leibarzt Dr. T. Morell während des Zweiten Weltkrieges in Olmutz: Gab es ein Olmutzer Penicillin?' *Acta Universitatis Palackianae Olumuciencis Chemica*, 32 (1993), 127–37.

Wood, M. 'The Politicization of Antimicrobial Resistance'. *Current Opinion in Infectious Diseases*, 11 (1998), 649–51.

Woods, Abigail. *A Manufactured Plague: The History of Foot and Mouth Disease in Britain.* London: Earthscan, 2004.

Woodward, Kevin. *Antibiotics: The Resistance Issue.* London: PJB Publications, 1999.

World Health Organization. *Global Strategy for Containment of Antibiotic Resistance.* Geneva: WHO, 2001.

——Expert Committee on the Public Health Aspect of the Use of Antibiotics in Food and Feedstuffs, *The Public Health Aspects of the Use of Antibiotics in Food and Feedstuffs: Report of an Expert Committee*, meeting held in Geneva 11–17 December 1962. Geneva: World Health Organization, 1963.

'Worldwide Abuse of Antibiotics Poses Threat: 150 Experts Say'. *Washington Post*, 5 August 1981.

Wrigley, Tom, Tinto, Alessandra, and Majeed, Azeem. 'Age- and Sex-Specific Antibiotic Prescribing Patterns in General Practice in England and Wales, 1994 to 1998'. *Health Statistics Quarterly*, 14 (2002), 14–20.

Yagisawa, Yukimasa. 'Early History of Antibiotics in Japan'. In John Parascandola (ed.), *The History of Antibiotics: A Symposium.* Madison: American Institute for the History of Pharmacy, 1980, 69–90.

Yermolieva, Z., Kaplun, T., and Levitov, M. 'Penicillin Crustosin'. *American Review of Soviet Medicine*, 2 (February 1945), 247–50.

Yoshioka, Alan, 'Streptomycin in Postwar Britain: A Cultural History of a Miracle Drug'. In M. Gijswijt-Hofstra, G. M. Van Heteren, and E. M. Tansey (eds.), *Biographies of Remedies: Drugs, Medicines and Contraceptives in Dutch and Anglo-American Healing Cultures.* Amsterdam: Rodopi, 2002, 203–27.

Young, J. T. 'Illness Behaviour: A Selective Review and Synthesis'. *Sociology of Health and Illness*, 26 (2004), 1–31.

Zola, I. K. 'Medicine as an Institution of Social Control'. *Sociological Review*, 10 (1972), 487–504.

Penicillin Index